Molecular Diagnosis of Genetic Diseases

METHODS IN MOLECULAR MEDICINE™

John M. Walker, SERIES EDITOR

METHODS IN MOLECULAR MEDICINE™

Molecular Diagnosis of Genetic Diseases

Edited by
Rob Elles
*Regional Molecular Genetics Laboratory, St. Mary's Hospital,
Manchester, UK*

Humana Press ❄ Totowa, New Jersey

© 1996 Humana Press Inc.
999 Riverview Drive, Suite 208
Totowa, New Jersey 07512

This publication is printed on acid-free paper. ∞
ANSI Z39.48-1984 (American Standards Institute) Permanence of Paper for Printed Library Materials.

Cover illustration: Fig. 3 from Chapter 8, "Risk Analysis," by Andrew P. Read.

Printed in the United States of America. 10 9 8 7 6 5 4 3 2 1

Library of Congress Cataloging in Publication Data

Main entry under title:

Methods in molecular medicine™.

Molecular diagnosis of genetic diseases / edited by Rob Elles.
    p. cm. — (Methods in molecular medicine™)
    Includes index.
    ISBN 0-89603-346-5 (alk. paper)
    1. Genetic disorders—Molecular diagnosis—Laboratory manuals. I. Elles, Rob. II. Series.
        [DNLM: 1. Hereditary Diseases—diagnosis. 2. Genetic Screening. 3. Genetic Techniques.
QZ 50 M71835 1996]
    RB155.6.M65 1996
    616'.042—dc20
    DNLM/DLC   96-3091
    for Library of Congress   CIP

Preface

Many previous volumes concerned with methodology in human genetics have been written by research scientists and naturally reflect that culture. *Molecular Diagnosis of Genetic Diseases* aims to diverge from previous titles by presenting contributions that cover a key method in detail, but are set in the context of a diagnostic area or genetic disease. In this format, the book attempts to cover nearly all of the most common genetic disease diagnostics that are offered as services by clinical molecular genetics laboratories, thus contributing a reasonably comprehensive handbook for this type of center. Most of the authors are active scientists working in clinical diagnostics. The methods reflect their working experience in attempting to assure robust, reliable results, and to include essential controls, quality standards, and interpretive guides.

Molecular Diagnosis of Genetic Diseases is primarily aimed at scientists, clinicians, and technologists working in clinical molecular genetics, especially those working in, or with, diagnostic laboratories. Others who will find the book useful include students and scientific workers at the interface of research genetics and diagnostics, forensic scientists, and biotechnologists. Those concerned with the commercial development of the diagnostic field and with regulation or improvement in standards in molecular genetics, both in professional bodies or government agencies, will also be interested in this book. In addition, scientists planning to develop novel molecular genetic diagnostics in countries with little or no experience in this field will find the book a useful starting point.

The chapters form a practical guide to the introduction of new diagnostic areas into the laboratory and provide a bench book for day-to-day use and the development of laboratory-specific standard operating procedures. Finally, chapters have been included with the notion of stimulating fresh thinking about molecular genetic diagnostics in the context of risk analysis and genetic counseling and to consider the internal and external quality standards that will have to apply for the public and patients to have confidence in genetic testing.

Rob Elles

Contents

vii

Contributors

MANJEET BOLLA • *Division of Cardiovascular Genetics, Department of Medicine, University College London Medical School, London, UK*

DAVID J. COCKBURN • *DNA Laboratory, Oxford Medical Genetics Laboratories, Churchill Hospital, Oxford, UK*

JOHN A. CROLLA • *Wessex Regional Genetics Laboratory, Salisbury District Hospital, Wiltshire, UK*

IAN N. M. DAY • *Division of Cardiovascular Genetics, Department of Medicine, University College London Medical School, London, UK*

JOY D. A. DELHANTY • *Galton Laboratory, Department of Genetics and Biometry, University College, London*

ROB ELLES • *Regional Molecular Genetics Laboratory, St. Mary's Hospital, Manchester, UK*

LUCY A. ELLIS • *DNA Laboratory, Clinical Genetics Unit, St. James's University Hospital, Leeds, UK*

IAN M. FRAYLING • *Colorectal Cancer Unit, Imperial Cancer Research Fund, St. Mark's Hospital, Middlesex, UK*

COLIN A. GRAHAM • *Regional Genetics Centre, Belfast City Hospital, Belfast, Northern Ireland*

VILMUNDUR GUDNASON • *Division of Cardiovascular Genetics, Department of Medicine, University College London Medical School, London, UK*

LEMA HADDAD • *Division of Cardiovascular Genetics, Department of Medicine, University College London Medical School, London, UK*

ALAN H. HANDYSIDE • *Human Embryology Laboratory, Institute of Obstetrics and Gynecology, Royal Postgraduate Medical School, Hammersmith Hospital, London, UK*

JOYCE C. HARPER • *Galton Laboratory, Department of Genetics and Biometry, University College, London and Institute of Obstetrics and Gynecology, London, UK*

JOHN F. HARVEY • *Wessex Regional Genetics Laboratory, Salisbury District Hospital, Wiltshire, UK*

ALISON J. M. HILL • *Regional Genetics Centre, Belfast City Hospital, Belfast, Northern Ireland*

STEVE E. HUMPHRIES • *Division of Cardiovascular Genetics, Department of Medicine, University College London Medical School, London, UK*

LAUREN KERZIN-STORRAR • *Department of Medical Genetics, St. Mary's Hospital, Manchester, UK*

KIM J. LEACH • *DNA Laboratory, Clinical Genetics Unit, St. James's University Hospital, Leeds, UK*

Y. M. DENNIS LO • *Nuffield Department of Clinical Biochemistry, John Radcliffe Hospital, Oxford, UK*

GERALDINE MALONE • *Pediatric Genetics Unit, Royal Manchester Children's Hospital Manchester, UK*

HELEN MIDDLETON-PRICE • *North East Thames Regional DNA Laboratory, Institute of Child Health, London, UK*

ROGER MOUNTFORD • *Regional Molecular Genetics Laboratory, Liverpool Women's Hospital, Liverpool, UK*

JAYNE S. NOBLE • *DNA Laboratory, Clinical Genetics Unit, St. James's University Hospital, Leeds, UK*

SANDRA O'DELL • *Division of Cardiovascular Genetics, Department of Medicine, University College London Medical School, London, UK*

JOHN M. OLD • *Institute of Molecular Medicine, John Radcliffe Hospital, Oxford, UK*

SIMON C. RAMSDEN • *Regional Molecular Genetics Laboratory, St. Mary's Hospital, Manchester, UK*

PIERRE F. RAY • *Human Embryology Laboratory, Institute of Obstetrics and Gynecology, Royal Postgraduate Medical School, Hammersmith Hospital, London, UK*

ANDREW P. READ • *Department of Medical Genetics, St. Mary's Hospital, Manchester, UK*

DAVID O. ROBINSON • *Wessex Regional Genetics Laboratory, Salisbury District Hospital, Wiltshire, UK*

ANDREW J. ROWAN • *Cancer Genetics Laboratory, Imperial Cancer Research Fund, London, UK*

MARTIN SCHWARZ • *Pediatric Genetics Unit, Royal Manchester Children's Hospital, Manchester, UK*

ANNEKE SELLER • *DNA Laboratory, Oxford Medical Genetics Laboratories, Churchill Hospital, Oxford, UK*

PAUL J. SINNOTT • *Regional Tissue Typing Laboratory, St. Mary's Hospital, Manchester, UK*

SUSAN A. R. STENHOUSE • *Northern Regional Genetics Service, Newcastle Upon Tyne, UK*

GRAHAM R. TAYLOR • *DNA Laboratory, Clinical Genetics Unit, St. James's University Hospital, Leeds, UK*

ANDREW J. WALLACE • *Regional Molecular Genetics Laboratory, St. Mary's Hospital, Manchester, UK*

ROS E. WHITTALL • *Division of Cardiovascular Genetics, Department of Medicine, University College London Medical School, London, UK*

1

An Overview of Clinical Molecular Genetics

Rob Elles

1. Introduction

Clinical molecular genetics has only recently become recognizable as a diagnostic discipline in its own right—gradually becoming distinct from its academic- and research-based origins. This chapter seeks to give some shape and context to the contributions that follow and add to previously published ideas of how diagnostic laboratories are structured and evolving *(1,2)*. The chapter largely draws on the UK experience of the field and does not claim to be authoritative on developments in North America, Europe, Australasia, or other parts of the world.

2. Clinical Molecular Genetics and Other Diagnostic Disciplines

Diagnosis of genetic disease usually involves a consideration of the inherited nature of the condition and therefore often involves a family study. This imposes unique disciplines and requirements on the molecular diagnostic laboratory which distinguishes it from other categories of clinical laboratory. The family is the unit of study in contrast to the individual. This will remain true even when mutation screening takes over from linkage analysis.

Furthermore, inheritance across generations and horizontally in the extended kindred gives the information generated by the genetic laboratory a lasting relevance. It places on the laboratory a responsibility for long-term and careful storage and retrieval of clinical information. For instance this requirement may be met by a report format suitable for long-term access deposited in the individual or the family file held by the genetic counseling service.

Similarly, key samples must be reliably stored and readily retrievable. Such long-term sample storage provides a challenge in terms of space, safety, and reliability, and data storage and retrieval (*see* Section 7.4.).

From: *Methods in Molecular Medicine: Molecular Diagnosis of Genetic Diseases*
Edited by: R. Elles Humana Press Inc., Totowa, NJ

As well as this long-term cycle of storage and testing, a molecular genetics laboratory also requires the flexibility to respond to urgent clinical needs. These include prenatal diagnosis (PND) and carrier detection tests during pregnancy. In the neonatal period, cystic fibrosis (CF) mutation screening is an example of a test which may be urgently required in order to influence management of the child's condition. In addition some presymptomatic programs (e.g., Huntington's disease [HD]), which are set in a rigorous counseling protocol, require a rapid results service (*see* Section 3.5.).

Both of these disciplines of urgent and long-term testing require clear lines of communication with clinicians and the clinical genetics infrastructure. For PND, one key individual who can coordinate the patient and the family doctor, obstetric, genetic counseling, and laboratory services is important for their smooth provision. A second example is the existence of a reliable mechanism for the clinical service and the laboratory to coordinate and prioritize testing within a family and ensure the availability of key samples required in a linkage or carrier detection study. This may be achieved by a regular meeting between individual counselors/clinicians and the laboratory scientist responsible for a particular diagnostic area.

The establishment of voluntary family registers in the United Kingdom has provided a structure which lends itself to the long-term continuity of contact required for effective counseling and carrier and presymptomatic testing within the extended family (*see* Chapter 11). A geographical area-based structure for genetic services serving populations of 1–4 million prevents duplicated provision of services and gives an effective catchment size for genetic diseases all of which are relatively rare.

However, diagnostic testing at a distance is quite possible as long as the requirements and limitations of testing are appreciated. The referring clinicians must understand that there may be a requirement for a correct diagnosis in an index case, for key specimens, the need to establish informativeness, the error rates inherent in the test, and the lag time in some procedures (mutation screening for example). The laboratory must be aware of the degree of urgency in a particular case and be realistic about quoting turnaround times for the test.

The widespread implications of genetic testing also impose a requirement for a reference point to the social and ethical considerations connected with the generation of this type of data. Practically this means a close working relationship between the laboratory and the clinic—usually clinical geneticists and nonclinical counselors.

3. Categories of Test

Clinical molecular genetics testing falls into five main categories. The mix of cases within these categories will to some extent define the resources required in the laboratory and the characteristics of the laboratory.

3.1. Differential Diagnostic Testing

This category includes differential diagnosis for the X-linked muscular dystrophies and for some of the neurological disorders where neurological symptoms exist for example to differentiate HD from other rare conditions, to confirm or exclude Fragile X (FraX) disease as a cause of mental retardation, and to clarify a diagnosis or suspicion of CF or Angelman/Prader Willi syndrome. A feature of these molecular tests is that they are often highly specific but not highly sensitive. For example failure to detect a deletion in Duchenne or Becker muscular dystrophy (DMD/BMD) does not exclude the diagnosis because a high proportion of these remaining cases may be the result of a point mutation.

3.2. Carrier Detection Within Families

These tests are relevant for instance where an index case exists for congenital adrenal hyperplasia owing to 21-hydroxylase deficiency and carrier detection is required for a sibling or close blood relative. Molecular genetic testing is a powerful tool for this kind of diagnosis and may be the only method suitable for deriving carrier information. Linkage-based carrier testing in DMD may involve introducing risks derived from biochemical and pedigree data and the complex calculations require skills in using and interpreting the computer-based statistical packages available for this type of analysis (*see* Chapter 8).

3.3. Carrier Detection Within Populations

Molecular testing for autosomal recessive diseases may not be the most efficient way of carrier testing in populations—for hemoglobinopathies for instance. However in some cases like CF, it is the only method available and may be sufficiently efficient to be effective (*see* Chapter 5 for methods). Molecular genetics laboratories set up to handle this type of program must be capable of handling relatively large numbers of cases and have the sample processing, testing, and reporting systems appropriate for the task. The limitations on this kind of program are based on social acceptability, the existence of an adequate counseling service, and cost effectiveness in detecting heterozygotes couples.

3.4. PND

A demand for PND from parents is usually apparent for severe childhood onset diseases where there is a poor prognosis and no effective treatment. The demand on the molecular genetics laboratory is to cope with an urgent test in pregnancy in a situation where the test may be complex. The answer is to have a close collaboration with the clinicians ideally to gather the required specimens from the index case and from family members prior to the requirement for PND. The laboratory then has the opportunity to ascertain in advance the tests required (i.e., to make the family informative for a linkage-based test or to define the genetic mutations involved). The prenatal test can then proceed in a more controlled fashion with a faster and more predictable turnaround time.

3.5. Presymptomatic Diagnosis

Presymptomatic diagnosis for adult onset disorders also requires a close liaison between the laboratory and the referring clinicians. Counseling protocols may place the test in the urgent category once a decision to proceed has been taken by the patient. An example of this is HD. It is felt to be of paramount importance to minimize the period of anxiety prior to receiving the result. The laboratory must be in a position to meet these demands *(3)*. Other tests may require extensive effort before a test can be offered to the family, for instance in familial adenomatous polyposis coli or familial breast–ovarian cancer, the work involved in finding the mutation is a considerable undertaking.

4. Introducing New Genetic Tests

The human genome project is generating a huge amount of data and characterizing genes capable of producing human disease at an impressive rate. This presents an enormous challenge to the molecular diagnostic laboratory in terms of the possible choice of diagnostic areas to resource and develop. However a number of constraints and considerations impose themselves in these choices.

4.1. Disease Frequency and Patient Demand for Testing

The first diagnostic tests to be developed naturally tended toward those diseases that are most frequent, for instance the hemoglobinopathies—DMD and CF. There is, however, a relationship between the demand for testing and the perceived individual burden of a disease. This may depend on whether it is treatable or not, causes mental or physical handicap, its age of onset, average impairment of function, and loss of life years and life quality. Hemophilia A, although as prevalent as DMD, does not present a large demand for molecular carrier detection or prenatal diagnosis at least to UK laboratories. Families may consider that the problem of HIV contamination of factor VIII has been controlled and the disease is treatable and does not warrant PND.

4.2. Resource/Benefit Trade Off

Given current technologies, the choice of a diagnostic area may be dictated by the available resources in the laboratory. For instance, hydrocephalus is perceived to be a serious condition with a considerable patient demand for carrier testing and PND. However, the offer of a service is tempered by the low detection rate of mutations in the L1CAM gene owing to possible genetic het-

Table 1
Comparison of Mutation Detection Services for CF and Hydrocephalus

Gene screened	Number of exonic fragments to screen	Mutations detected by SSCP/ heteroduplex analysis (%)	Estimated turnaround time (wk)	Estimated cost (US$)	Cost/ mutation found (US$)
CFTR	20	98[a]	32	1100	1122
LICAM	27	18[b]	32	1475	8194

[a]Screening of 20 exonic fragments detects approx 98% of mutations in UK populations.
[b]Detection rate in the cases referred (S. Ramsden, personal communication).

erogeneity, phenocopies, and the laborious nature of screens given current strategies. These tests may involve a single-stranded conformational polymorphism (SSCP)/heteroduplex analysis or denaturing gradient gel electrophoresis (DGGE) prescreen followed by sequencing and development of a mutation-specific assay. Laboratories may attempt to alter the resource/benefit ratio by selecting the diagnostic criteria acceptable for a referral to be accepted. In the case of hydrocephalus, perhaps referrals by limiting to clear X-linked familial cases. In contrast, rare mutation screening for CF provides a high detection rate (>95%) and the demand for testing is high. Typical referrals are the result of equivocal diagnosis of CF or for carrier screening where only one mutation segregating in a family is recognized. The cost per mutation detected is much less for CF than for L1CAM (Table 1), although the cost of detection should be divided by the average number of persons who will take up and benefit from the test. Without doubt the resource/benefit equation will alter rapidly as new technologies to find unknown and uncommon mutations in genes come on-stream in the future.

4.3. Technical Difficulty

Other criteria which may be considered are the degree of technical difficulty involved in an analysis and the current level of sophistication of the laboratory. For example, strategies of analysis involving RNA as the analytical material may not be tenable. In the same way, linkage-based risk analysis using computer programs may not be an expertise available in the laboratory.

4.4. Clinical Limitations

Other problems may be exterior to the laboratory. For instance, it may be difficult to set up a linkage-based service for a familial cancer like neurofibromatosis type 2 (bilateral meningioma) where early death may mean that families are frequently fragmented and the key samples are simply unavailable. Similarly, if the clinical infrastructure to collect key specimens and clinical diagnostic and pedigree information is not available, then providing a service is difficult. Thus, the choice of a laboratory service may be closely tied to local clinical expertise, interests, and resources.

4.5. Rare Disorders Versus Population Screening

Clinical molecular genetics laboratories began by being mostly concerned with diagnosis of relatively rare disorders in an index case and in carrier testing within the immediate family—persons at high prior risk of carrying and perhaps expressing the disease gene in question. The possibility now exists for genetic diagnosis among the general population at relatively low prior risk of carrier status in relevant recessives and of genetic susceptibility to common diseases. Chapters 5, 16, and 19 discuss techniques relevant to population-based screens in CF and cardiovascular disease. These programs have not yet taken hold on a large scale. However if they do, they will signal a profound shift in the scale and organization of the clinical molecular genetics laboratories that undertake them and indeed of the services required to counsel those screened. Laboratory and clinical genetic services are faced with the choice of entering these areas which will greatly change the nature and emphasis of their work.

5. Services for Rarer Disorders

Limited demand because of the rarity of a disorder limits efficiency by slowing the development of expertise and by not allowing batch efficiencies in a reasonable turnaround time. One answer to this problem is to widen the catchment population for a service speciality. In the United Kingdom, most laboratories serving a National Health Service (NHS) Region of 1–4 million people provide core services for CF, DMD, FraX, and HD, but only one or two laboratories specialize in rarer disorders such as mitochondrial myopathies or α-1 antitrypsin deficiency. These more specialized services may develop in the public sector by the adoption of formal or informal arrangements between centers to promote sample flows.

6. Relationship Between Research and Diagnostic Service

Molecular diagnostics has a short transfer time from the research laboratory to the service laboratory (largely because new diagnoses are usually new applications of a generic DNA-based technology). This transfer time may involve a validation period of only a few weeks from the publication of a characterized gene to the new diagnostic test—the trinucleotide repeat expansion mutation in HD is a case in point. It is not surprising that there is often a close relationship between university academic research teams and diagnostic facilities. In many examples research groups take on the initial cohort of diagnostic cases.

These studies form an integral part of the search for or characterization of a gene, the spectrum of pathological mutations within it, and the range of expressed phenotypes. However, for a variety of reasons, such as the ending of research potential, increasing demand, changing interests, or medico–legal considerations, research laboratories invariably and quite properly wish to pass on diagnostic work to diagnostic facilities. Physical and organizational links between the research and diagnostic laboratories are then of enormous benefit in facilitating this transfer of technology and application. Similarly, the diagnostic service may be of benefit to the research effort in providing infrastructure facilities, a continuity of expertise in the technology, a resource for laboratory quality, and access to a DNA sample bank and its associated clinical information.

The initial application of a new diagnosis is usually itself of research interest and it is in this level of development that the diagnostic laboratory is most active. In the public sector the controllers or purchasers of health care may be quite rigorous in their approach to this kind of research. They may require or commission it as an evaluation to determine whether outcomes in terms of the costs and benefits to the persons tested are sufficiently great to allow additional resources for a new service development *(4–6)*.

7. Space Requirements
for the Clinical Molecular Genetics Laboratory

The technological base of clinical molecular genetics has yet to stabilize making it difficult to make statements on specialized facilities that will be required in the future. However, the current situation can be outlined together with an idea on whether the requirements will diminish or grow.

7.1. Specialized Facilities for Specimen Handling

Handling facilities are required to receive and process specimens (mostly blood, but also prenatal samples, solid tissues, and mouthwashes). The space must take account of the biohazard associated with these specimens. This hazard is generally a population frequency risk of HIV and hepatitis B, unless certain high-risk groups are being routinely dealt with.

Specimen preparation requires centrifugation facilities and may involve handling hazardous chemicals (phenol and chloroform) depending on the chemistry chosen. Parts of the process may be dealt with by automated equipment.

The clinical and data processing involved in sample handling must not be overlooked and access is required to the laboratory database via a computer terminal, and sufficient space must be provided for a clean and dry area within the sample preparation room separated from the actual sample handling facility for efficient clerical procedures to be carried out.

A laboratory serving a population of 4 million people may expect to receive 60–70 samples/wk, but this obviously will depend heavily on the clinical infrastructure available, the mix of disease categories offered as a laboratory service, and whether a population screening program is being offered. The ideal is for a separate room to be provided for sample handling to give a physical separation of the biological and chemical hazards involved from other laboratory activities, to provide a clear barrier to contamination by polymerase chain reaction (PCR) products, and to provide an efficient environment for the clerical procedures required.

7.2. General Operations

Adequate space is required for general operations including PCR, polyacrylamide and agarose gel electrophoresis, restriction enzyme digestion, centrifugation, Southern blotting, silver staining, and chemiluminescent imaging techniques. Specialized areas required for these activities include containment for chemical hazards and a clean area for setting up PCRs.

7.3. Radioisotopes

Although the trend has been away from radioisotope techniques in recent years, the use of ^{32}P and ^{33}P and ^{35}S is still required for Southern blotting, certain fragment sizing techniques, and the Protein Truncation Test. These techniques are still standard for instance in sizing FraX and myotonic dystrophy alleles and in sequencing. The ideal is a separate room for radioisotope handling requiring fume extract, sealed floors, nonabsorbent working surfaces, and so on to meet national and local isotope handling regulations.

7.4. Storage

The accumulation of an archived bank of DNA specimens is an inevitable consequence of setting up a clinical molecular genetics service and thought needs to be given to suitable storage facilities. DNA is inherently stable and very low temperatures are not required. However, a storage temperature of –20°C or below is recommended. A DNA bank of 25,000 specimens stored in 2-mL cryotubes racked in vertical towers in a chest freezer occupies approx 0.5 m^3 of freezer space. This space should be doubled if a policy of splitting samples for safety from fire, security, or other incident is adopted. The duplicate bank should be in a separate part of the building for extra protection against the possibility of serious mishap (7). A bank serving 4 million people can be expected to grow at a rate of up to 2500–3500 samples/yr (5000–7000 including duplicates). Account must be taken of the heat generated from freezers in planning storage space.

7.5. Imaging

Radioisotope imaging requires specialized instrumentation or standard autoradiography. Autoradiography requires access to a $-70°C$ freezer and facilities for developing standard X-ray films. In addition, ethidium bromide stained gels must be visualized and recorded under UV illumination. These operations require constant access to a darkroom which is standard to a molecular genetics laboratory.

7.6. Instrumentation

Recently, more automated instrumentation has become important in molecular genetics. Fluorescent labeling techniques coupled with automated detection allow analysis of sequencing gels and fragment analysis for microsatellites, SSCP, and similar techniques. Space needs to be allowed for this type of instrumentation and associated computer and printing equipment.

7.7. Microbiology

PCR has largely taken over from the use of recombinant DNA probes in clinical molecular genetics. However, facilities to propagate plasmid or cosmid DNA in bacteria are required for some techniques including analysis of FraX disease, myotonic dystrophy, and Angelmann/Prader Willi syndromes and for fluorescent *in situ* hybridization studies. The alternative may be to purchase these materials commercially. These facilities may be available in association with academic research programs involved in cloning and screening for DNA sequences from libraries. Otherwise these facilities will have to be provided. The space will need to account for national and local regulations covering the handling of genetically manipulated organisms. Generally these operations require precautions appropriate to the lowest level of containment consistent with good microbiological practice and will not require negative pressure rooms, extraordinary equipment, or room fixtures. Nevertheless the ideal situation is a separate laboratory devoted to microbiological work.

7.8. Other Space Requirements

The clinical molecular genetics laboratory also requires access to adequate office, information, and communication facilities and preparation, autoclave, and storage areas.

8. Equipment and Choices of Technology

The technology in molecular genetics is shifting, but a number of key technologies will be important in the next 5 yr and these may be borne in mind in the choices of capital equipment purchased and in setting up techniques. The technologies which are likely to become more important are:

1. Rapid fluorescent sequencing and fragment analysis;
2. Nonradioactive hybridization techniques—imaging systems;
3. Kit-based diagnostic systems;
4. Automated sample handling devices;
5. Information technologies—access to the Internet;
6. Laboratory databases and reporting systems.

9. Staffing of the Clinical Molecular Genetics Laboratory

The staffing of molecular diagnostic laboratories has reflected the research origins of the discipline. In many cases those first employed in diagnostics, at least in the United Kingdom, came from a research background and in the years following, graduate scientists have largely been employed. It is still true that the nature of the work is relatively nonroutine and automation and kit-based technologies have yet to make a major impact on molecular genetic testing. Because of this, a number of characteristics are required of the core staff in a laboratory: an ability to innovate and troubleshoot, a deep understanding of the technology, result interpretation, data and risk analysis, and the relationship between the laboratory and clinical genetics. These criteria dictate that the time of relatively skilled and motivated graduates is available to the laboratory either directly running the diagnostic service or overseeing its activities. Academic scientists may be able to give this input at least at the beginning of the service.

9.1. Growth in Staffing in the United Kingdom

The last 8–10 yr have seen a steady growth in public sector (NHS) laboratories in the United Kingdom. Table 2 indicates this growth and illustrates that most of this expansion has been by employing graduate scientists. The other grades of staff commonly found in this kind of laboratory are technical support workers and short-term funded workers on academic research assistant scales or the same type of NHS scientific scale as the graduate scientists.

9.2. Training

In the United Kingdom since 1990, 2-yr postgraduate training programs accredited and controlled by the UK Clinical Molecular Genetics Society (CMGS), have become available. This training is workplace based and relies on the achievement of competences. It should give the trainee a wide experience of the main diagnostic areas and techniques but also includes a theoretical program and a research project. This is one route to the main career grade for diagnostic scientists. Specialist career grade training qualifications by examination are available to allow molecular geneticists to achieve Membership of the Royal College of Pathologists (MRCPath). Postqualification Continued Professional Development by attendance at accredited meetings or participa-

Table 2
Growth in UK Staffing from 1986–1994[a]

Category of staff	1986	1994	Change (%)
Qualified graduate scientists	15	107	+613
Trainee graduate scientists	—	14	—
Technical/support workers	5	27	+440
Academic-related staff/short-term funded graduate staff	18	38	+111

[a]Source UK Clinical Molecular Genetics Society (CMGS) survey.

tion in approved relevant activities has become a recent requirement for the laboratory scientist. In North America, the American Board of Medical Genetics and the Canadian College of Medical Genetics accredit training programs for clinical molecular geneticists *(8)*.

9.3. Individual Skills

One characteristic of molecular diagnostics in recent years has been a constant change within the technology (Southern blotting to PCR) and in the method of diagnosis (linkage to direct mutation analysis). This shifting ground has dictated that staff retain a contact with the research base and develop an individual expertise in a diagnostic area. For the diagnostic laboratory this may have the strength of allowing up-to-the minute research developments to be quickly brought into service and for building quality into tests. The weakness is that this expertise may be embodied in one person who may move on and damage the overall capability of what remain relatively small laboratories in most cases. This problem of overspecialization can be overcome by deliberately spreading responsibilities as laboratories expand. It also will diminish as techniques become more standardized, automated, and kit-based, and some work in the laboratory becomes relatively deskilled from graduate scientist to technician level.

10. Audit

As part of the evaluation of the effectiveness of molecular genetic diagnosis, it has become necessary to standardize the collection of workload and activity data. In the United Kingdom, audit data is collected by the CMGS. The three main categories of data are samples entering the laboratory for testing or archiving, tests indicated as genotypes, and output as reports. The definition of samples is self-explanatory but the working definition of genotypes and reports is more problematic and worth outlining.

A genotype is the sequence, variant, or mutation data generated by one PCR reaction or Southern blot track. In many cases the definition is straightforward, but in some cases is somewhat complicated. A multiplex of nine exons amplified from the dystrophin gene would count as one genotype. An Amplification Refractory Mutation System test may involve two PCR reactions but counts as one genotype for audit purposes as both reactions are required to produce a result.

A report is defined as the answer to one clinical question in one individual. A family-specific report for DMD may include the characterization of the dystrophin mutation in the index case and say two carrier tests on female relatives. This would count as three reports for audit. When a couple is tested for informativeness in advance of a pregnancy this counts as one report because in this context the results on one individual are meaningless without those of their partner. The value of standardized audit data is in allowing the laboratory to track trends in workload, provide accurate costs, and make internal and external comparisons (Tables 3 and 4).

10.1. UK Trends

Although the number of UK laboratories submitting audit returns had stabilized by 1990, the audit figures demonstrate an impressive increase in activity over the next 3-yr period. Samples processed doubled and reports issued rose by approaching 200%. The fact that genotypes only rose by a factor of 45% reflects the move away from linkage-based tests, the increased emphasis on PCR technology, a reduced failure rate, and an increase in low prior risk–population-based tests (CF and FraX). Over a similar period, the number of services available increased by 65%, but most of these comprise relatively rare disorders.

11. Quality Issues—External Quality Assessment

An emphasis in diagnostics is a systematic attempt to assess and control the quality of tests. To this end, a number of single disease external quality assessment (EQA) exercises have been undertaken *(9)*. In addition North America, Australasia, the United Kingdom, and parts of Europe are some way into setting up standing multidisease EQA systems involving testing reference specimens and some form of interpretation of the results or of theoretical results (*see* Chapter 20).

11.1. Internal Quality Assurance

Internal quality assurance includes all the controls and checks that a laboratory builds into its procedures to prevent sample mix-up and to ensure a consistent and adequate quality of testing. Some examples of these measures are given in Chapter 20.

Table 3
UK Activity Statistics from 1990–1994[a]

Activity indicator	1990	1993–1994	Change, %
Samples processed	19,446	42,505	+118
Genotypes	101,379	146,562	+45
Reports issued	8551	24,618	+188
Number of laboratories submitting audit returns	25	27	+8

[a]Source CMGS surveys.

Table 4
UK Service Categories Offered from 1988–1993[a]

	1988	1991	1993
Number of services offered	32	49	81

[a]Source CMGS surveys.

11.2. Laboratory Accreditation

In the United States, several individual states, most notably New York, have developed accreditation systems for diagnostic molecular genetics laboratories. The accreditation requires that the materials used (probes or PCR marker systems) meet certain standards (e.g., having well-established recombination frequencies between the marker and the disease in question). It also requires the staff to be qualified specialists.

In the United Kingdom, an independent company set up by the Royal College of Pathologists–College of Pathologists Accreditation trains inspectors and has the power to accredit facilities. Inspection includes examination of the effectiveness of the management structure, the equipment and facilities available in the laboratory, and safety and maintenance standards. Also the quality and consistency of documentation relating to the tracking of specimens through the laboratory, staff facilities, and training are examined. Although accreditation is only in the earliest stages of development in the United Kingdom, the pressure to become accredited will increase from the public sector health service purchasing organizations which fund genetic services.

12. Role of the Professional Bodies

In the United Kingdom, a number of professional bodies have had an interest in the development of clinical molecular genetics over the last 10 yr. Of note are the Clinical Genetics Society, the Association of Clinical Cytogeneticists, and the Royal College of Pathologists. The American College of Medical Genetics and the American College of Pathologists have broadly similar roles in the United States. The UK professional body with the most direct interest in the field is the CMGS. Since 1987, the CMGS has organized laboratory-based scientists mostly working in NHS diagnostic laboratories. The society promotes the discipline through training, audit, quality assessment schemes, best practice guidelines, and scientific meetings.

13. Conclusions

Clinical molecular genetics will continue to grow as the benefits of testing become apparent, as the number of possible tests increases, and as they become available to new populations. The technology will change and become more kit-based and automated. However, for some time the discipline will retain and enjoy its close links with the research community as the human genome project reaches its successive goals.

Whatever scientific and technical developments bring, scientists working in this field will continue to be anxious that the testing they carry out should be provided in an adequate counseling framework and after an informed debate on the social and ethical impact of the introduction of genetic testing. They also will be concerned to retain the confidence of the public in genetic testing by promoting an improving standard of quality in all the centers involved.

Acknowledgments

My thanks to Andrew Read, Simon Ramsden, and Andrew Wallace for discussion during the preparation of this chapter.

References

1. Harris, R., Elles, R., Craufurd, D., Dodge, A., Ivinson, A., Hodgkinson, K., et al. (1989) Molecular genetics in the National Health Service in Britain. *J. Med. Genet.* **26,** 219–225.
2. Rona, R. J., Swan, A. V., Beech, R., Wilson, O. M., Kavanagh, F. B., Brown, C., et al. (1992) DNA probe technology: implications for service planning in Britain. *Clin. Genet.* **42,** 186–195.
3. Tyler, A., Ball, D., and Craufurd, D., on behalf of the United Kingdom Huntington's Disease Prediction Consortium (1992) Presymptomatic testing for Huntington's disease in the United Kingdom. *Br. Med. J.* **304,** 1593–1596.
4. MacDonald, F., Morton, D. G., Rindl, P. M., Haydon, J., Cullen, R., Gibson, J., et al. (1992) Predictive diagnosis of familial adenomatous polyposis with linked DNA markers: population based study. *Br. Med. J.* **304,** 869–872.
5. Elles, R. G., Hodgkinson, K. A., Mallick, N. P., O'Donoghue, D. J., Read, A. P., Rimmer, S., Watters, E. A., and Harris, R. (1994) Diagnosis of adult polycystic kidney disease by genetic markers and ultrasonographic imaging in a voluntary family register. *J. Med. Genet.* **31,** 115–120.

6. Read, A. P., Kerzin-Storrar, L., Mountford, R. C., Elles, R. G., and Harris, R. (1986) A register based system for gene tracking in Duchenne muscular dystrophy. *J. Med. Genet.* **23,** 581–586.

7. Yates, J., Malcolm, S., and Read, A. P. (1989) Guidelines for DNA banking: report of a working party of the Clinical Genetics Society. *J. Med. Genet.* **26,** 245–250.

8. Andrews, L. B., Fullarton, J. E., Holtzman, N. A., and Motulsky, A. G. (eds.) (1994) *Assessing Genetics Risks—Implications for Health and Social Policy,* National Academy Press, Washington, DC, pp. 202–233.

9. Cuppens, H. and Cassimans, J. J. (1995) A Quality Control Study of CFTR Mutation Screening in 40 different European Laboratories. *Eur. J. Hum. Genet.,* **3,** 235–245.

2

PCR Techniques for Deletion, Linkage, and Mutation Analysis in Duchenne/Becker Muscular Dystrophy

Roger Mountford

1. Introduction

Duchenne muscular dystrophy (DMD) and Becker muscular dystrophy (BMD) are allelic disorders caused by mutations in the dystrophin gene. The molecular genetic analysis of these disorders is among the most difficult encountered in a routine diagnostic laboratory. The analysis is made difficult by the size and structure of the gene, which is 2.4 Mb in size, and comprises 79 exons encoding a 14-kb mRNA transcript *(1,2)*. The exons are all small (<200 bp), whereas the introns vary from 109 bp to >200 kb. The interpretation of results is hampered further by the incidence of new mutation (approximately one-third of DMD cases), the greater than normal level of recombination across the gene (approx 10% *[3,4]*), and finally the occurrence of a significant level of germline mosaicism *(5,6)*.

1.1. Strategy

It is difficult to define a set procedure for the analysis of all DMD/BMD cases, since the exact tests performed will depend on the pedigree structure and the availability of key samples. However, the following set of guidelines will cover most cases seen in a diagnostic laboratory.

1.1.1. Mutation Detection

Approximately two-thirds of boys with DMD and a similar proportion of affected males with BMD have a deletion of one or more exons of the dystrophin gene *(7,8)*. The deletions vary in size and location, but are clustered in two "hot spots," the major site encompassing exons 45–52, and a minor

From: *Methods in Molecular Medicine: Molecular Diagnosis of Genetic Diseases*
Edited by: R. Elles Humana Press Inc., Totowa, NJ

region including exons 3–19. Deletions are detected using a multiplex poly-merase chain reaction (PCR) method *(9)*, in which 18 exons are analyzed in two separate PCR reactions. These exons were chosen to include the two dele-tion "hot spots," and this system is estimated to identify approx 98% of all deletions. Further exons can be studied to increase the sensitivity of the test or to define the extent of deletions identified by the initial screen. However, full characterization of a deletion may require analysis with cDNA probes.

A further 5–10% *(7)* of affected males have a duplication of one or more exons, and the remainder are assumed to have point mutations. The duplica-tions have traditionally been detected using dosage estimation of cDNA-probed Southern blots. Autoradiograph signals from blots have proven very difficult to quantify, and many laboratories do not screen routinely for duplications. Alternatively, duplications can be detected using pulsed-field gel electrophore-sis (PFGE) *(see* Chapter 17) or by RNA analysis, but these methods are labor-intensive, technically demanding procedures that are used in very few routine laboratories. However, the advent of automated fluorescent dosage analysis will make duplication screening a reality for more laboratories in the future.

Point mutation screening is very difficult given the size of the gene. Muta-tions can be identified systematically in patients using reverse transcriptase-polymerase chain reaction (RT-PCR) analysis of illegitimate transcripts of the gene in peripheral lymphocytes followed by the use of the protein truncation test *(10,11)* *(see* Chapter 4). However, this system is only used in a research context, and has not been transferred to a routine diagnostic setting. Some point mutations may be identified by single-stranded conformational polymorphism (SSCP)/heteroduplex analysis on the 18 exons used for the multiplex deletion screening assay. This system requires no extra resources in the laboratory in terms of primers. However, there is no evidence for clustering of such mutations *(12,13)*, and therefore, this approach has a limited detection rate.

1.2. Direct Carrier Detection
1.2.1. Deletion Detection

If a deletion is detected in a family, then carrier detection can be performed using one of a number of direct tests. The simplest method is to analyze the family with one or more polymorphisms from within the deleted region *(14)*. If a woman is heterozygous for the appropriate marker, then she cannot be a car-rier (excluding germline mosaicism—*see* Section 1.2.3.). If a woman is a car-rier, this can manifest itself as a failure to inherit a maternal allele for the appropriate marker, although this is dependent on the right combination of alleles being present in the woman's parents. This approach is quick and effec-tive, but is limited because there are no markers available for all the deleted regions *(see* Table 1), and those that are used may not always be informative.

Table 1
Sequences of Primers for Multiplex Deletion Screen[a]

Exon	Product, bp	Forward primer, 5'–3'	Reverse primer, 5'–3'
5' Reaction			
1	535	GAA GAT CTA GAC AGT GGA TAC ATA ACA AAT GCA TG	TTC TCC GAA GGT AAT TGC CTC CCA GAT CTG AGT CC
19	459	TTC TAC CAC ATC CCA TTT TCT TCC A	GAT GGC AAA AGT GTT GAG AAA AAG TC
3	410	TCA TCC ATC ATC TTC GGC AGA TTA A	CAG GCG GTA GAG TAT GCC AAA TGA AAA TCA
8	360	GTC CTT TAC ACA CTT TAC CTG TTG AG	GGC CTC ATT CTC ATG TTC TAA TTA G
13	238	AAT AGG AGT ACC TGA GAT GTA GCA GAA AT	CTG ACC TTA AGT TGT TCT TCC AAA GCA G
6	202	CCA CAT GTA GGT CAA AAA TGT AAT GAA	GTC TCA GTA ATC TTC TTA CCT ATG ACT ATG G
4	196	TTG TCG GTC TCC TGC TGG TCA GTG	CAA AGC CCT CAC TCA AAC ATG AAG C
3' Reaction			
48	506	TTG AAT ACA TTG GTT AAA TCC CAA CAT G	CCT GAA TAA AGT CTT CCT TAC CAC AC
44	426	GTT GTG TGT ACA TCG TAG GTG TGT A	TCC ATC ACC CTT CAG AAC CTG ATC T
51	388	GAA ATT GGC TCT TTA GCT TGT GTT TC	GGA GAG TAA AGT GAT TGG TGG AAA ATC
43	357	GAA CAT GTC AAA GTC ACT GGA CTT CAT GG	ATA TAT GTG TTA CCT ACC CTT GTC GGT CC
45	307	CTT TCT TTG CCA GTA CAA CTG CAT GTG	CAT TCC TAT TAG ATC TGT CGC CCT AC
50	271	CAC CAA ATG GAT TAA GAT GTT CAT GAA T	TCT CTC TCA CCC AGT CAT CAC TTC ATA G
53	212	TTG AAA GAA TTC AGA ATC AGT GGG ATG	CTT GGT TTC TGT GAT TTT CTT TTG GAT TG
47	181	CGT TGT TGC ATT TGT CTG TTT CAG TTA C	GTC TAA CCT TTA TCC ACT GGA GAT TTG
42	155	CAC ACT GTC CGT GAA GAA ACG ATG ATG	TTA GCA CAG AGG TCA GGA GCA TTG AG
60	139	AGG AGA AAT TGC GCC TCT GAA AGA GAA CG	CTG CAG AAG CTT CCA TCT GGT GTT CAG G
52	113	AAT GCA GGA TTT GGA ACA GAG GCG TCC	TTC GAT CCG TAA TGA TTG TTC TAG CCT C

[a]Adapted from ref. 9.

An alternative direct carrier detection method is to use fluorescent *in situ* hybridization (FISH) of standard metaphase chromosome spreads with cosmid probes specific for given dystrophin exons *(15)*. If a carrier has a deletion that includes the relevant cosmid, then she will show a signal on only one of her X chromosomes, whereas a noncarrier will have a signal on both. A number of cells (minimum 10) are analyzed to rule out false-negative results owing to hybridization failure. This direct technique has advantages over the use of polymorphic markers in that a result is more certain. However, cosmids are not currently available for all the deleted exons, and the size of the deletion is critical. If the deletion does not encompass the whole of the region complementary to the cloned DNA in the cosmid, then the labeled cosmid will hybridize to the deleted chromosome and the test becomes invalid. Therefore, if the cosmid includes an exon at either end of the deletion, then an affected boy or an obligate carrier should be tested to validate the test in each specific family. This method will usually be performed in, or in conjunction with, a cytogenetics laboratory.

Other direct tests include the use of PFGE *(16)* or RT-PCR analysis of ectopic dystrophin transcripts *(10,11)*. PFGE is a very effective method of detecting deletion carriers and, in addition, has the ability to detect duplications. However it requires a positive commitment to the technology. This method is considered in more detail in Chapter 17. Analysis of ectopic dystrophin RNA transcripts from peripheral lymphocytes is a potentially useful method of carrier detection, but is technically difficult. The effect of X chromosome inactivation on such low levels of transcript is not understood, and therefore, it is not possible to say a woman is not a carrier with complete certainty.

A new method of deletion detection is the use of automated fluorescent DNA analysis to measure dosage on PCR products using the exons of the multiplex deletion screen *(17,18)*. This involves the use of modified fluorescent primers or the incorporation of a fluorescent-labeled nucleotide in the multiplex PCR assay. The number of cycles of amplification is kept below 24 to ensure the reaction is still in the logarithmic phase. The levels of fluorescence in each exon can then be analyzed and compared with each other either visually using peak heights or statistically using peak areas. The ratio of a deleted exon to nondeleted exons in a carrier would be approximately half that in a noncarrier. This method is new, but the technique has proven to be accurate and is being introduced into routine service laboratories.

1.2.2. Point Mutation Detection

If a point mutation has been detected in a family, then carrier detection should be carried out using an appropriately designed assay. If the mutation alters a restriction enzyme site, then a simple assay based on the enzyme should be used. If no restriction site is involved, a modified oligonucleotide primer can be designed to create a novel restriction site involving either the normal or mutant sequence, or alternatively, primers may be designed for an amplification refractory mutation system (ARMS)-based assay (*see* Chapter 5). If these methods are not possible, then an assay using allele-specific oligonucleotides (ASOs) specific for the normal or mutant sequence can be used, or finally direct sequencing of potential carriers can be performed.

1.2.3. Germline Mosaicism

Interpretation of all direct carrier tests is complicated by the presence of germline mosaicism. It has been demonstrated that where the mother of an affected male has been shown not to be a carrier by any one of the direct detection methods available using somatic material, she still has a 5% chance of having another affected child *(5,6)*. Therefore, the mother of an affected male can never be told she is definitely not a carrier.

If a woman is definitely a carrier and her affected son(s) has inherited the grand-paternal haplotype for some/all markers across the gene, then there is a chance that the grandfather could have been a germinal mosaic carrier. This has implications for any maternal aunts of affected males. Cases of grand-paternal mosaicism have been demonstrated, but there are no figures available for its frequency.

1.3. Indirect Carrier Detection

If no mutation is detectable in a family or a direct test is uninformative, then carrier detection and prenatal diagnosis can be carried out indirectly using linked markers. There are over 20 intragenic polymorphisms described in the dystrophin gene (Table 2). These range from restriction fragment length polymorphisms (RFLPs) with two alleles to highly polymorphic microsatellite markers. They can be used to track the disease through a family, but interpretation of the results is complicated by the high level of intragenic recombination and by the high frequency of new mutations. There are two recombination "hot spots" located in introns 3 and 44 of the dystrophin gene.

Ideally, when carrying out linkage analysis, markers from the 5' and 3' ends of the gene plus a marker between introns 3 and 44 should be used to reduce the possibility of double recombinants going undetected. However, not all families are informative with this combination of markers.

The results of linked marker analysis can be combined with details of the pedigree and information on serum creatinine kinase levels to produce relative carrier risks. Such risks are often calculated using the MLINK option of the LINKAGE computer program *(19)* (*see* Chapter 8).

Table 2
Sequences of Primers for Dystrophin-Specific Markers

Marker	Forward primer, 5'–3'	Reverse primer, 5'–3'
DYSI	ACT GTA AAT GAA ATT GTT TTC TAA GTG CC	GTT AAC AAA ATG TCC TTC AGT TCT ATC C
DYSII	TGA GTA CTT GCA CAC AAA GC	TAG TGT TTT CCT AAG GGG TT
pERT 84-1/*MaeIII*	CAG GGA TGC AAA GGA ACT GGG	CAG TTT GTT TAA CAG TCA CTC
NM7/73	ATC CCA TCC TGT TCT ATT TT	ACT GGC ATG CAT TAT TTT GT
pERT 87-1/*BstNI*	CTA TCA TGC CTT TGA CAT TCC AG	CTC AAT AAG AGT TGG ATT CAT TC
pERT87-15/*BamHI*	TCC AGT AAC GGA AAG TGC	ATA ATT CTG AAT AGT CAC AAA AAG
pERT87-8/*TaqI*	GTC AGT TGG TCA GTA AAA GCC	CCA ATT AAA ACC ACA GCA G
pERT87-15/*XmnI*	GAC TGG AGC AAG GGT CGC C	ACA ATT TCC CTT TCA TTC CAG
pERT87-15 *TaqI*	GAC TTT CGA TGT TGA GAT TAC TTT CCC	AAG CTT GAG ATG CTC TCA CCT TTT CC
Ca1a/*PstI*	GAA TGG CCT GCC CTT GGG GAT TCA G	AGT GTT AAG TTC TTT GAG TTC TGT CTC AAG
Cf23a/*TaqI*	ATT CAG CAG GGG GTG AAT CTG A	GTT GTA AGT TGT CTC CTC TTT GC
Exon 43 TA	GAA CAT GTC AAA GTC ACT GGA CTT CAT GG	ATA TAT GTG TTA CCT ACC CTT GTC GGT CC
STR44	TCC AAC ATT GGA AAT CAC ATT TCA A	TCA TCA CAA ATA GAT GTT TCA CAG
Exon 45-SSCP	CTT TCT TTG CCA GTA CAA CTG CAT GTG	CAT TCC TAT TAG ATC TGT CGC CCT AC
STR45	GAG GCT ATA ATT CTT TAA CTT TGG C	CTC TTT CCC TCT TTA TTC ATG TTA C
Exon 48/*MseI*	AAG CTT GAA GAC CTT GAA GAG C	CCT GAA TAA AGT CTT CCT TAC CAC AC
DXS997	TGG CTT TAT TTT AAG AGG AC	GTT TTC AGT TTC CTG GGT
STR49	CGT TTA CCA GCT CAA AAT CTC AAC	CAT ATG ATA CGA TTC GTG TTT TGC
STR50	AAG GGT TCC TCC AGT AAC AGA TTT GG	TAT GCT ACA TAG TAT GTC CTC AGA C
Exon 53-SSCP	TTG AAA GAA TTC AGA ATC AGT GGG ATG	CTT GGT TTC TGT GAT TTT CTT TTG GAT TG
DMD1	TGT CTG TCT TCA GTT ATA TG	ATA ACT TAC CCA AGT CAT GT
J66	GCA GCT ATA TGT TTC CCA AGA TTG A	GAG GTT CTT TGG AGG AAT AC
STR62/63	TTC TTC GTC GAT ACC CCC ATT CCA	CTC TTT GAG TTT GAA GTT ACC TGA
STRHI	ACG ACA AGA GTG AGA CTC TG	ATA TAT CAA ATA TAG TCA CTT AGG
MP1P	ATC AGA GTG AGT AAT CGG TTG G	ATC TAG CAG CAG GAA GCT GAA TG
3/DYS	GAA AGA TTG TAA ACT AAA GTG TGC	GGA TGC AAA ACA ATG CGC TGC CTC

2. Materials

Analytical-grade reagents should be used at all stages, unless otherwise indicated.

2.1. Multiplex Deletion Screening

1. 10X PCR buffer: 670 mM Tris-HCl, pH 8.3, 166 mM ammonium sulfate, 500 mM KCl, 37 mM magnesium chloride, and 0.85 mg/mL bovine serum albumin (BSA). Filter sterilize and store as 1-mL aliquots at –20°C.
2. Deoxynucleoside triphosphates (dNTPs): Dissolve 10 mg of individual nucleotides (Sigma, St. Louis, MO) in sterile dH$_2$O to a concentration of 20 mM, and mix together to form an equimolar mix of all four dNTPs. Store 400-µL aliquots at –20°C. Avoid excessive freezing and thawing.
3. Oligonucleotide primers: Primers may be synthesized "in-house," cleaved from their CpG column, and deprotected in ammonium hydroxide. These can be stored for several years at –70°C. Prepare a 10X working stock of all the primer pairs at a concentration of 2.5 µM.
4. *Taq* polymerase: The author uses BRL (Life Technologies, Gaithersburg, MD) enzyme for all laboratory uses, but can also recommend BCL (Boehringer Mannheim, Mannheim, Germany) and Perkin-Elmer (Foster City, CA).
5. Agarose: Use a mixture of ordinary electrophoresis-grade agarose (Boehringer Mannheim) and NuSieve low-gelling-temperature agarose (FMC, Rockland, ME).
6. TBE electrophoresis buffer: Make as a 10X stock solution, 0.89M Tris, 0.89M boric acid, and 0.02M EDTA (pH 8.0). Store at room temperature.
7. 5X TBE gel loading buffer: 5 mL 10X TBE, 4.9 mL glycerol, 0.1% SDS, 3 mg bromophenol blue, and 15 mg xylene cyanole. Store at room temperature.
8. Agarose electrophoresis equipment: Wide minisubcell system, 15 × 10 cm (Bio-Rad, Hercules, CA).

2.2. SSCP Analysis

1. PCR materials: Use the same PCR materials as multiplex analysis except:
   a. 10X PCR buffer: 670 mM Tris-HCl, pH 8.3, 166 mM ammonium sulfate, 37 mM magnesium chloride, 0.85 mg/mL BSA. Filter sterilize and store as 1-mL aliquots at –20°C.
   b. Oligonucleotides: Prepare a 10X working stock of all the primer pairs at a concentration of 5 µM.
2. Formamide loading buffer: 10 mL formamide, 200 mL 0.5M EDTA (pH 8.0), 3 mg bromophenol blue, and 15 mg xylene cyanole. Store at room temperature.
3. Acrylamide: Use 49:1 acrylamide/bis-acrylamide mix. The author uses a 40% ready-mixed solution (Sigma).
4. Ammonium persulfate: Prepare a 10% solution that can be stored at 4°C for up to 48 h.
5. Polyacrylamide electrophoresis equipment: Model SA system 32 × 20 cm (Life Technologies).
6. Silver-staining solution A: 10% ethanol (industrial-grade) and 0.5% acetic acid. Prepare on the day of use. Store at room temperature.

7. Silver-staining solution B: 0.1% $AgNO_3$. Prepare a 10X stock solution of 1% $AgNO_3$, and store at room temperature in a brown bottle. 1X solution should be stored in clear bottles at room temperature, but away from light. The 1X solution may be reused until efficiency of staining falls.

8. Silver-staining solution C: 1.5% NaOH, 0.15% formaldehyde. This solution is labile. Add the formaldehyde immediately (i.e., within 3 min) before use.

9. Silver-staining solution D: 0.75% Na_2CO_3. Prepare a 10X stock of 7.5% Na_2CO_3. Store at room temperature.

10. Cellophane sheets (Hoefer Scientific Instruments, San Francisco, CA).

11. Drying frame and platform (Hoefer).

2.3. Microsatellite Analysis

1. PCR materials: Use the same PCR materials as SSCP analysis.

2. Restriction enzymes supplied by Boehringer Mannheim, Life Technologies, and New England Biolabs (Beverley, MA). Restriction enzymes are supplied with their own reaction buffers. Store at –20°C.

3. Phenol/chloroform: Equilibrate phenol in 100 mM Tris, pH 8.0. Prepare a 50:50 solution of this phenol with chloroform. Store at 4°C.

4. Acrylamide: Use a 19:1 acrylamide/bis-acrylamide mix. The author uses a 40% ready-mixed solution (Acugel-National Diagnostics, Atlanta, GA).

5. Polyacrylamide electrophoresis equipment: ATTO AE6210 20 × 14 cm slab gel system (Genetic Research Instrumentation, Dunmow, Essex, UK).

6. Silver staining (*see* Section 2.2., items 6–9).

3. Methods

PCR is a very powerful technique where contamination of the reaction by very low levels of DNA from an external source can lead to erroneous results. Great care should be taken to avoid such contamination (*see* Note 1).

Oligonucleotide primers: Precipitate a 400-µL aliquot of primer in ammonium hyroxide solution by adding 13 µL of 3M sodium acetate and 1 mL of absolute ethanol. Cool to –70°C for 1 h, and spin in a bench-top centrifuge for 15 min. Resuspend the primer in 200 µL of sterile dH_2O, estimate the concentration by measuring the OD_{260nm}, and dilute to the appropriate concentration (2.5 µM for multiplex primers, and 5 µM for all other uses). All the multiplex primer pairs are diluted together to give a mixed 10X working stock.

3.1. Mutation Screening

3.1.1. Multiplex Deletion Screening

3.1.1.1. PCR CONDITIONS

The final concentrations of the reaction components are: 67 mM Tris, pH 8.3, 50 mM KCl, 16.6 mM NH_4SO_4, 3.7 mM $MgCl_2$, 85 µg/mL BSA, 0.25 µM each primer, 3 mM dNTPs, 20–50 ng of genomic DNA, 1 U of *Taq* polymerase in a total volume of 10 µL (*see* Note 2).

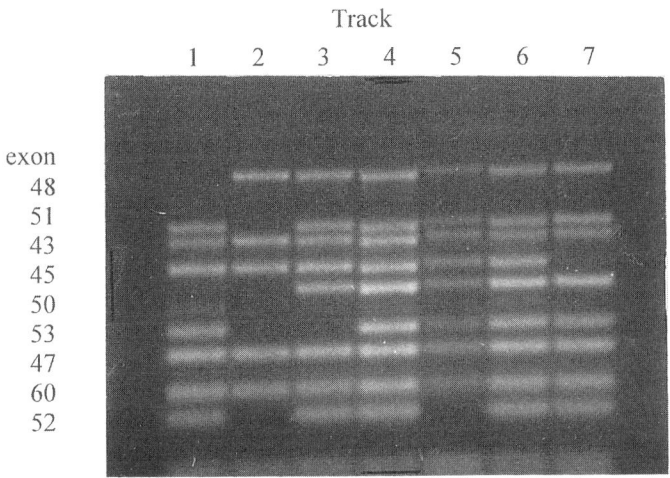

Fig. 1. Screening for dystrophin deletions using the multiplex PCR method. Track 1, deletion of exons 48–50; Track 2, deletion of exons 50–53; Track 3, deletion of exon 53; Tracks 4 and 6, no deletion; Track 5, deletion of exon 52; and Track 7, deletion of exon 45.

1. Prepare a master mix of all the components, except the DNA. Aliquot 8 μL into a thin-walled 0.5-mL Eppendorf tube.
2. Add 2 μL of DNA solution (10–25 ng/μL) (*see* Note 3).
3. Add one drop of light paraffin oil, and place on a PCR machine with a preheated block at 94°C (*see* Note 4).
4. PCR cycling conditions: Initial denaturation: 94°C for 3 min, followed by 30 cycles of 94°C for 1 min, 60°C for 1 min, and 72°C for 2, 3, or 4 min. (The synthesis time is extended by 1 min every 10 rounds.) Final synthesis: 72°C for 5 min.
5. Add 2.5 μL of 5X TBE loading buffer.
6. Load 6 μL of reaction on a 2% agarose gel (1% Nusieve/1% BCL agarose), and carry out electrophoresis at 100 mA for approx 1 h with ethidium bromide (0.5 mg/mL) in both the gel and the TBE running buffer (*see* Note 5).
7. Once separation of the bands is complete, photograph the gel on a UV trans-illuminator (Fig. 1) (*see* Notes 6 and 7).

3.1.2. SSCP/Heteroduplex Analysis (see Note 8)

3.1.2.1. PCR CONDITIONS

The final concentrations of the reaction components are: 67 mM Tris, pH 8.3, 16.6 mM NH$_4$SO$_4$, 3.7 mM MgCl$_2$, 85 μg/mL BSA, 0.5 μM each primer, 3 mM dNTPs, 20–50 ng of genomic DNA, and 0.5 U of *Taq* polymerase in a total volume of 10 μL.

1. Prepare a master mix of all the components, except the DNA (*see* Note 9). Aliquot 8 μL into a 0.5-mL Eppendorf tube.
2. Add 2 μL of DNA solution (10–25 ng/μL) (*see* Note 3).
3. Add one drop of light paraffin oil, and place on a PCR machine with a preheated block at 94°C.
4. PCR cycling conditions: Initial denaturation: 94°C for 3 min followed by 30 cycles of 94°C for 1 min, 60°C for 1 min, and 72°C for 2 min. Final synthesis: 72°C for 5 min.
5. After the PCR reaction, if using male DNA samples (*see* Note 10), mix 5 μL of two unrelated male samples together.
6. Heat at 95°C for 5 min, and then allow to cool slowly to room temperature to create heteroduplexes.
7. Add 15 μL of distilled water to the PCR reaction, and then add 25 μL of formamide loading buffer.
8. Load 2 μL of PCR product (double-stranded DNA) onto an 8% polyacrylamide (49:1) gel (*see* Note 11).
9. Heat the remaining sample at 95°C for 5 min. Snap cool on ice.
10. Load 6 μL of PCR product (single-stranded DNA) into the same well as the double-stranded DNA.
11. Run slowly overnight at 4°C, with a maximum current of 20 mA (*see* Notes 12 and 13). The precise electrophoretic conditions depend on the PCR products being analyzed.
12. When the DNA has migrated the desired distance, silver stain the gel.

3.1.2.2. SILVER STAINING (*SEE* NOTE 14)

1. Separate the gel plates, and carefully transfer the gel into a photographic staining tray.
2. Immerse the gel in 300 mL of solution A, shake gently for 3 min, pour off the solution, and immerse the gel in a further 300 mL of solution A.
3. Pour off solution A and add 400 mL of solution B. Shake gently for 15 min.
4. Pour off solution B (this can be reused), rinse the gel very briefly in distilled water, and add 300 mL of freshly made solution C. Shake gently. The gel should turn yellow after a few minutes, and dark staining bands should appear shortly after.
5. When the bands are sufficiently strong, pour off solution C, and add 300 mL of solution D. Leave for at least 10 min.
6. Dry the gel down between two sheets of cellophane in a drying frame at 37°C for 4–16 h.
7. Interpretation (*see* Notes 15–18).

3.2. Linked Markers

3.2.1. PCR Conditions

The final concentrations of the reaction components are: 67 mM Tris, pH 8.3, 16.6 mM NH$_4$SO$_4$, 3.7 mM MgCl$_2$, 85 μg/mL BSA, 0.5 μM each primer, 3 mM dNTPs, 20–50 ng of genomic DNA, and 0.3 U of *Taq* polymerase in a total volume of 10 μL.

1. Prepare a master mix of all the components except the DNA. Aliquot 8 μL into a 0.5-mL Eppendorf tube.
2. Add 2 μL of DNA solution (10–25 ng/μL).
3. Add one drop of light paraffin oil, and place on PCR machine with preheated block at 94°C.
4. PCR cycling conditions: All markers use an initial denaturation at 94°C for 3 min and final synthesis at 72°C for 5 min. Cycling conditions for all dystrophin markers are given in Table 3.

3.2.2. RFLPs (see Note 19)

1. After the PCR is complete digest the products by adding 1.5 μL of restriction enzyme buffer, 2.5 μL of distilled water, and 1 μL (5–10 U) of restriction enzyme.
2. Incubate at the appropriate temperature for 4–16 h.
3. Add 4 μL of 5X TBE loading buffer.
4. Load 10 μL of sample onto a 2% agarose gel (1% Nusieve/1% BCL agarose) containing ethidium bromide (5 μg/mL). Use 1% BCL agarose for products >500 bp.
5. Run at 100 mA for an appropriate time to resolve the fragments.
6. When separation is complete, photograph the gel under UV transillumination.

3.2.3. Microsatellites

1. When necessary (*see* Notes 20 and 21), digest the PCR products by adding 1.5 μL of restriction enzyme buffer (10X), 2.5 μL of distilled water, and 1 μL (5–10 U) of restriction enzyme.
2. Incubate at the appropriate temperature for 4–16 h.
3. If the PCR products are >120 bp, phenol-extract the sample (*see* Note 22).
4. Add an equal volume of phenol/chloroform (1:1) to the PCR sample, mix thoroughly, and spin in a microcentrifuge for 1 min.
5. Take 4 μL of PCR product (middle phase—paraffin oil is on the top and phenol/chloroform on the bottom—*see* Note 23), and add 1 μL of 5X sucrose loading buffer.
6. Load onto a polyacrylamide (19:1—*see* Note 24) gel, and run at 50 mA for 90–180 min (*see* Note 25). The strength of the gel depends on the size of the microsatellites to be resolved. A 10% gel is used for products <100 bp, an 8% gel for products in the range 100–160 bp, and a 6% gel for products 160–200 bp.
7. When DNA has traveled the desired distance, silver stain the gel (*see* Section 3.1.2.2.).
8. Interpretation (*see* Notes 26 and 27).

4. Notes

1. In all PCR assays, great care should be taken to avoid contamination of the reaction by external sources of DNA. The most common source of contamination is by amplimers from previous reactions. The most important precaution to avoid this is always to use separate pipets for setting up the reaction and for analyzing the prod-

Table 3
Dystrophin-Specific Markers Detectable Using PCR[a]

Marker	Location	Type	A/S/C	Fragment size, bp unless stated	Het	Notes
DYS I	Promoter	CA rpt	50/1/27	177–185	0.78	
DYS II	Promoter	CA rpt	52/1/30	~80–94	0.82	
pERT84 /MaeIII	Promoter	RFLP	60/1/27	236/128 + 108	0.38	
NM72/73	Intron 1	CA rpt	52/1/30	56–88	0.57	
pERT87-1/BstNI	Intron 12	RFLP	60/1/30	400/250 + 150	0.45	Cut with BstNI
pERT87-8/TaqI	Intron 13	RFLP	55/1/30	145/74 + 71	0.38	Cut with TaqI
pERT87-15/BamHI	Intron 17	RFLP	60/1/30	216/166 + 50	0.47	Cut with BamHI
pERT87-15/TaqI	Intron 17	RFLP	60/1/30	416/233 + 183	0.44	Cut with TaqI
pERT87-15/XmnI	Intron 17	RFLP	57/1/30	730/520 + 220	0.44	Cut with XmnI
Ca1a/PstI	Intron 24	RFLP	60/1.5/30	1.2/0.7 + 0.5 kb	0.40	Cut with PstI
Cf23a/TaqI	Intron 38	RFLP	58/2.5/30	2.1 + 0.3/1.6 + 0.5 + 0.3 kb	0.48	Cut with TaqI
Exon 43/TA	Intron 43	2-bp del	60/1/30	357	0.34	SSCP gel conditions
STR44	Intron 44	CA rpt	60/1/27	174–204	0.87	
Exon 45/SSCP	Intron 44	SSCP poly	60/1/30	307	0.35	SSCP gel conditions
STR45	Intron 45	CA rpt	60/1/27	156–184	0.89	
Exon 48/MaeI	Exon 48	RFLP	63/1/30	108/85 + 23	0.38	Plus constant bands
DXS997	Intron 48	CA rpt	58/1/27	109–117	0.64	
STR49	Intron 49	CA rpt	60/1/27	~110–140	0.93	Cut PCR product with AluI
STR50	Intron 50	CA rpt	60/1/27	~150–160	0.71	Cut PCR product with MseI
Exon 53/SSCP	Exon 53	SSCP poly	60/1/30	212	0.25	SSCP gel conditions
DMD I	Intron 55–57	CA rpt	55/1/27	~125–135	0.50	Cut PCR product with MseI
J66	Intron 60	VNTR	60/2/30	1.25/1.2/1.1 kb	0.57	Difficult to resolve
STR62/63	Intron 62/63	CA rpt	60/1/27	~190–200	0.38	
STRHI	Intron 64	TAA rpt	52/1/30	90–102	0.68	
MP1P	3' Untrans	4-bp del	55/1/30	82/78	0.20	
3' DYS	3' Untrans	CA rpt	60/1/25	127–135	0.34	

[a] Abbreviations: A/S/C, annealing temperature (°C)/synthesis time (min)/number of cycles; Het, heterozygosity.

ucts. If products are seen in the negative (no DNA) control, then the results are invalid, and all working stocks should be discarded and fresh solutions made up.

2. This buffer system gives more consistent results when using multiple primer pairs than the conventional buffer (*see* Section 2.2.) that is used for the majority of PCR applications. An ammonium sulfate-based buffer is essential for this and other multiplex PCR systems.

3. In addition to the obligatory no DNA control, always run a female sample as a positive control, and samples from patients with known deletions covering all the exons in the multiplex reaction as negative controls.

4. Loading the samples onto a preheated PCR block improves the efficiency of the reaction and is an easier and cheaper alternative to the conventional "hot start" system.

5. The bands can be resolved on a 10-cm gel. Use of ethidium bromide in the running buffer prevents fade-out of the smaller PCR products. Alternatively, the gel can be run without ethidium bromide and then stained when the resolution is complete.

6. The multiplex system was designed so that problems with the quality of the sample DNA owing to the degradation of high-mol-wt material or the presence of inhibitors in the sample would give rise to results consistent with non-contiguous deletions. False-negative results are still theoretically possible when amplification of an exon fails because of the presence of a polymorphism in the primer binding site. If a deletion of a single exon is observed, then ideally the result should be confirmed either by cDNA analysis using Southern blotting or by PCR analysis using an alternative primer pair.

7. If when using the multiplex system for a prenatal diagnosis a nondeleted male result is obtained, then the sample should be checked for maternal contamination by comparing the fetal and maternal DNA samples using an X chromosome-specific microsatellite marker for which the mother is heterozygous. Any sign of heterozygosity in the male fetus would invalidate the multiplex result.

8. Both SSCP analysis and heteroduplex analysis can be carried simultaneously using this system. This requires precise electrophoretic conditions so that the double-stranded DNA remains on the gel while there is sufficient resolution of single-stranded DNA.

9. The exons of the multiplex system can be analyzed in sets of three or four. Suggested sets are:

    a. Exons 1, 17, 19, 8.
    b. Exons 48, 51, 3, 43.
    c. Exons 45, 50, 13, 47.
    d. Exons 53, 60, 52.
    e. Exons 44, 6, 52.

These combinations can be changed, but some exons are incompatible, since their single strands comigrate. Incompatible exons are (45, 48), (17, 3), (45, 19), (45, 8), and (44, 53). Alternatively, PCR products from the multiplex reaction can be run directly on an SSCP gel. These are difficult to interpret, even with the use of single-exon controls. Any nonresolved exons can be reamplified and run on a second gel.

10. If female samples are used, then there are sufficient heteroduplexes produced during the 30 rounds of amplification. If male samples are used, two unrelated samples must be mixed to produce heteroduplexes. This increases the number of affected males that can be tested, but any positive result must be further analyzed to determine which of the two samples contained the putative mutation.

11. Loading double-stranded and single-stranded DNA in the same well means heteroduplex analysis and SSCP analysis both can be performed on the same gel. It is not always necessary to load any nondenatured sample, since there is always some double-stranded DNA present after the sample has been denatured and snap cooled. However, addition of nondenatured sample to the same well improves the efficiency of the heteroduplex analysis.

12. Temperature is a very important parameter in SSCP analysis. The gel system should be assembled and precooled at 4°C for at least 1 h before loading the samples. The gel should be run as slowly as possible, usually overnight, to avoid any increase in temperature. The exact running conditions depend on the products being analyzed and should be determined empirically.

13. If it is not possible to perform the analysis at 4°C, then the system can be run at room temperature with the addition of 10% glycerol to the gel. Again the gel should be run slowly, and resolution is improved by using buffer precooled to 4°C. Single-stranded DNA can show markedly different migration patterns using these two alternative approaches.

14. Detailed notes on silver staining are given in Chapter 3. This technique is only applicable to gels approx 1 mm thick. Handling a large gel for silver staining can be difficult. The gel should be gently rolled off the plate into the solution of fix. Staining is then straightforward. After staining, the gel can be trimmed to size before being transferred to the drying frame.

15. If a heteroduplex or a change in the migration of the single-stranded DNA is detected (*see* Fig. 2), then the rest of the family of the individual concerned should be analyzed to exclude the presence of a polymorphism rather than a genuine mutation. There are a number of polymorphisms described in the exon-specific products of the multiplex system (*see* Table 4).

16. If the change appears not to be the result of polymorphism the sample should be sequenced.

17. If a mutation is found, then an alternative test should be devised to confirm it in the original sample. This can be a restriction enzyme digestion if the mutation alters a recognition site, or a modified primer can be designed that creates a restriction site in the presence or absence of the mutation. Alternatively, an ARMS-based system may be used with primers designed for the normal and mutant sequences.

18. SSCP or heteroduplex analysis should not be used to screen other family members for the mutation, since the presence of polymorphisms in other members may alter the mutation-specific pattern seen on the original gel.

19. In addition to the obligatory no DNA control, always use samples that are heterozygous (+/–) and homozygous (+/+) for the restriction site as controls. The

1　　　　2　　　　3　　　　4　　　　5

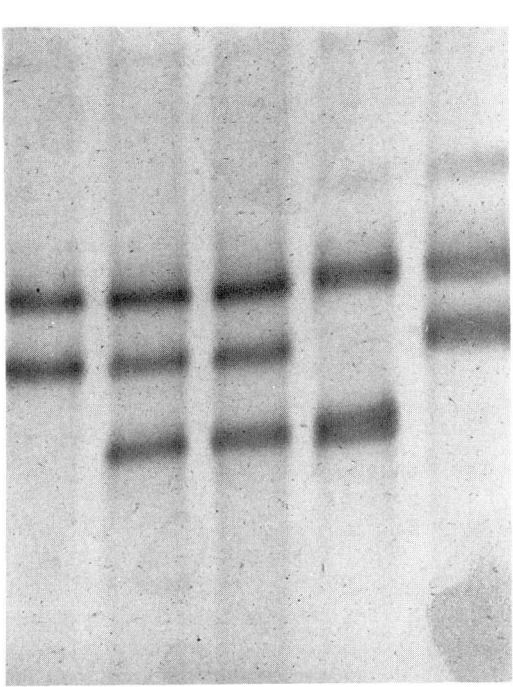

Fig. 2. Detection of dystrophin point mutations by SSCP analysis. Analysis of single-stranded PCR products containing exon 3 of the dystrophin gene. Tracks 1 and 5 show the normal pattern seen with this exon (two bands corresponding to the two single strands of DNA). Track 4 shows an abnormal pattern in an affected male. This is due to a point mutation (2-bp deletion at nucleotide 382). Tracks 2 and 3 are from the boy's mother and sister (both carriers of the mutation).

+/+ control sample should always be fully digested. If it is not, the results of the test are invalid. The fragment intensities should be constant in any +/− test samples compared to the +/− control. Any deviation is indicative of sample-specific partial digestion, and further enzyme should be added to the PCR products or the analysis should be repeated.

20. All of the dystrophin-specific microsatellite markers listed in Table 3 can be resolved on 14-cm nondenaturing polyacrylamide gels. This system is capable of resolving 2-bp differences in PCR products up to 200 bp in size. Above this size, a longer gel is required or the product can be predigested with a restriction enzyme (*see* Table 3) to give a smaller product containing the dinucleotide repeat unit.
21. The marker STR49 has alleles that only differ by 1 bp. This is on the limit of resolution of this system. If 1-bp differences are present and the alleles are unclear

Table 4
Polymorphisms Detectable Using SSCP Analysis
of the 18 Dystrophin Exon-Specific PCR Products
Used in the Multiplex Deletion Assay[a]

Exon	Polymorphism	Frequency
3	302-9 ins T	0.31
13	1539-68 A→T	0.12
13	1539-73 T→C	0.08
43	6326-60 ins TT	0.20
45	6647-143 G→A	0.21
45	6671 C→T	0.05
48	7121-113 A→T	0.08
48	7304 C→A	0.27
53	7936 T→C	0.15

[a]Adapted from ref. *13*.

on the above system, the products should run out on a 30-cm gel and be silver-stained as described.

22. The silver-staining method also stains proteins present in the PCR reaction. These migrate through the gel as a broad front corresponding to double-stranded DNA of mol wt 140 bp and above. If the microsatellite PCR product is >120 bp, the resolution will be disrupted by the protein. Therefore, it is necessary to remove the protein by phenol/chloroform extraction prior to electrophoresis.

23. It can be difficult to remove an aliquot of the middle phase after phenol/chloroform extraction. This can be made easier by increasing the volume of the reaction to 20 μL after amplification. An alternative method is to remove the PCR products to a new tube before phenol/chloroform extraction.

24. Nondenaturing gel conditions are used because the degree of resolution is greater over a shorter distance compared to a denaturing system. This has an effect on interpretation of dinucleotide repeats (*see* Note 26).

25. The electrophoresis time depends on the microsatellite in question. In an 8% polyacrylamide gel, xylene cyanole migrates at a rate equivalent to 80 bp of double-stranded DNA.

26. Interpretation of dinucleotide microsatellites (CA repeats) is not straightforward. The phenomenon of "stuttering" is seen where for reasons that are at present unknown, amplication of an allele of a CA repeat yields decreasing amounts of products that are 2 and 4 bp (and occasionally 6 bp) smaller than the expected size. In addition, when run on nondenaturing gels bands migrating behind the allele and its stutter bands are seen. These are due to the double-stranded DNA forming an alternative conformation with reduced mobility and are not seen under denaturing conditions. Therefore, the key to interpretation is first to distinguish the bands that represent the allele from the "stutter" and "conformational bands" (*see* Fig. 3). This can be difficult if the sample is heterozygous for alleles that differ by 2 bp.

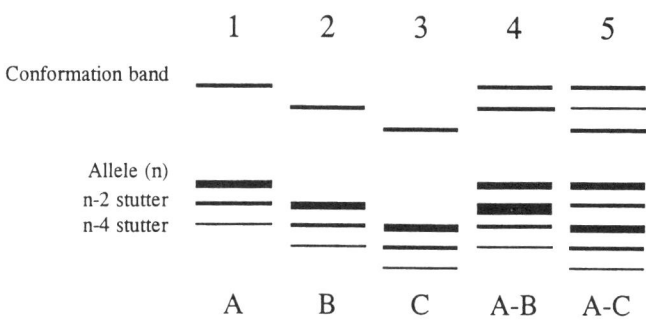

Fig. 3. Analysis of microsatellite markers on nondenaturing gels. Tracks 1 ,2, and 3 represent alleles A, B, and C that each differ by 2 bp. Track 4 is heterozygous for alleles A and B. Note the presence of two conformation bands and allele B is reinforced by the n-2 stutter from allele A. Track 5 is heterozygous for alleles A and C. Note that a third conformation band is sometimes seen between the two expected bands. The reason for this is unknown.

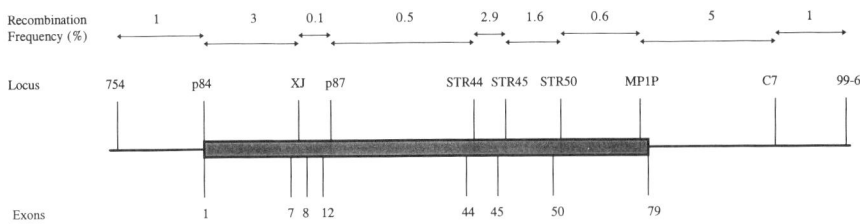

Fig. 4. Recombination frequencies across the dystrophin gene. Abbreviations: p84, pERT84; p87, pERT87.

27. Ideally, when performing DMD/BMD-linked marker analysis, a family should be made informative with three markers—one at either end of the gene plus one in an intermediate position. The intermediate marker should preferably be between the two recombination hot spots in introns 3 and 45 (*see* Fig. 4). The first choice of markers are DYSII, STR44, and 3'-DYS. The latter is often uninformative in which case STRHI, STR49, or STR50 should be used. If these are used, the error rate is increased, since there is a small chance of recombination between the marker and the 3' end of the gene.

References

1. Koenig, M., Monaco, A. P., and Kunkel, L. M. (1988) The complete sequence of dystrophin predicts a rod-shaped cytoskeletal protein. *Cell* **53,** 219–228.
2. Roberts, R. G., Coffey, A. J., Bobrow, M., and Bentley, D. R. (1993) Exon structure of the human dystrophin gene. *Genomics* **16,** 536–538.

3. Abbs, S., Roberts, R. G., Mathew, C. G., Bentley, D. R., and Bobrow, M. (1990) Accurate assessment of intragenic recombination frequency within the Duchenne muscular dystrophy gene. *Genomics* **7,** 602–606.

4. Oudet, C., Hanauer, H., Clemens, P., Caskey, T., and Mandel, J. L. (1992) Two hot spots of recombination in the DMD gene correlate with the deletion prone regions. *Hum. Mol. Genet.* **1,** 599–603.

5. Bakker, E., Veenema, H., Den Dunnen, J. T., van Broeckhoven, C., Grootscholten, P. M., Bonten, E. J., and van Ommen, G. J. B. (1989) Germinal mosaicism increases the recurrence risk for new DMD mutations. *J. Med. Genet.* **26,** 553–559.

6. van Essen, A. J., Abbs, S., Baiget, M., Bakker, E., Boileau, C., van Broeckhoven, C., et al. (1992) Parental origin and germline mosaicism of deletions and duplications of the dystrophin gene: a European study. *Hum Genet.* **88,** 249–257.

7. Den Dunnen, J. T., Grootscholten, P. M., Bakker, E., Blonden, L. A., Ginjaar, H. B., Wapenaar, M. C., et al. (1989) Topography of the DMD gene, FIGE and cDNA analysis of 194 cases reveals 115 deletions and 13 duplications. *Am. J. Hum. Genet.* **45,** 835–847.

8. Forrest, S., Cross, G. S., Speer, A., Gardner-Medwin, D., Burns, J., and Davies, K. E. (1987) Preferential deletion of exons in Duchenne and Becker muscular dystrophies. *Nature* **329,** 638–640.

9. Beggs, A. H., Koenig, M., Boyce, F. M., and Kunkel, L. M. (1990) Detection of 98% of DMD/BMD gene deletions by polymerase chain reaction. *Hum Genet.* **86,** 45–48.

10. Roberts, R. G., Barby, T. F. M., Manners, E., Bobrow, M., and Bentley, D. R. (1991) Direct detection of dystrophin gene rearrangements by analysis of dystrophin mRNA in peripheral lymphocytes. *Am. J. Hum. Genet.* **49,** 298–310.

11. Roest, P. A. M., Roberts, R. G., Sugino, S., van Ommen, G. J. B., and Den Dunnen, J. T. (1993) Protein truncation test (PTT) for rapid detection of translation terminating mutations. *Hum. Mol. Genet.* **2,** 1719–1721.

12. Roberts, R. G., Gardner, R. J., and Bobrow, M. (1994) Searching for the 1 in 2,400,000: a review of dystrophin gene point mutations. *Hum. Mutat.* **4,** 1–11.

13. Rinisland, F. and Reiss, J. (1994) Microlesions and polymorphisms in the DMD/BMD gene. *Hum Genet.* **94,** 111–116.

14. Clemens, P. R., Fenwick, R. G., Chamberlain, J. S., Gibbs, R. A., de Andrade, M., Chakraboty, R., and Caskey, C. T. (1991) Carrier detection and prenatal diagnosis in Duchenne and Becker muscular dystrophy families using dinucleotide repeat polymorphisms. *Am. J. Hum. Genet.* **49,** 951–960.

15. Reid, T., Mahler, V., Vogt, P., Blonden, L., van Ommen, G. J. B., Cremer, T., and Cremer, M. (1990) Direct carrier detection by in-situ hybridisation with cosmid clones of the Duchenne/Becker muscular dystrophy locus. *Hum Genet.* **85,** 581–586.

16. Kodaira, M., Hiyama, K., Karakawa, T., Kameo, H., and Satoh, C. (1993) Duplication detection in Japanese Duchenne muscular dystrophy patients and identification of carriers of partial gene deletions using pulsed-field gel electrophoresis. *Hum Genet.* **92,** 237–243.

17. Schwartz, L. S., Tarleton, J., Popovich, B., Seltzer, W. K., and Hoffman, E. P. (1992) Fluorescent multiplex linkage analysis and carrier detection for Duchenne/ Becker muscular dystrophy. *Am. J. Hum. Genet.* **51,** 721–729.
18. Mansfield, E. S., Robertson, J. M., Lebo, R. V., Lucero, M. Y., Mayrand, P. E., Rappaport, E., et al. (1993) Duchenne/Becker muscular dystrophy carrier detection using quantitative PCR and fluorescence based strategies. *Am. J. Med. Genet.* **48,** 200–208.
19. Lathrop, G. M. and Lalouel, J. M. (1984) Easy calculation of LOD scores and genetic risks on small computers. *Am. J. Hum. Genet.* **36,** 460–465.

3

Detection of Unstable Trinucleotide Repeats

Andrew J. Wallace

1. Introduction

Unstable trinucleotide repeats are a newly recognized class of disease mutation. Several major human single gene disorders are now attributed to expansions of these highly unstable sequences *(1–4)*. Their molecular analysis is particularly challenging, since:

1. Accurate allele sizing is essential;
2. Polymerase chain reaction (PCR) amplification across the repeat is hampered by extreme guanine cytosine (GC) content and strong secondary structure; and
3. Size differences between normal and mutated alleles may be great, for instance, in fragile X they can range from 6 to over 1000 repeats.

In this chapter the analysis of four important diseases for a service laboratory, fragile X syndrome, myotonic dystrophy (MD), Huntington disease (HD), and spinal bulbar muscular atrophy (SBMA) is detailed. All four diseases are amenable to analysis by a modified PCR reaction followed by polyacrylamide gel electrophoresis and visualization using a simple silver staining protocol. With the exception of SBMA, Southern blotting is necessary in at least some diagnostic cases to visualize the larger repeats.

A low magnesium buffer is used for PCR amplification; this maintains high levels of *Taq* polymerase activity while facilitating amplification of GC-rich templates. These are notoriously refractory to PCR because of a combination of high strand dissociation temperatures and strong secondary structure. Ten percent dimethyl sulfoxide (DMSO) is added to the reactions to lower the dissociation temperature of dsDNA and to reduce secondary structure effects. The nucleotide analog, 7-deaza-guanosine triphosphate (GTP), is also incorporated where the template is particularly GC-rich and the repeat length is large. Silver stain-

From: *Methods in Molecular Medicine: Molecular Diagnosis of Genetic Diseases*
Edited by: R. Elles Humana Press Inc., Totowa, NJ

ing is used to visualize the amplified PCR products. This is the method of choice since it is cheap, rapid, relatively safe, and 5–10 times more sensitive than ethidium bromide staining. Also it is capable of staining both ssDNA and dsDNA.

Southern blotting is employed to detect the presence of the largest trinucleotide repeats. Southern blotting is a form of direct genome analysis. Genomic DNA is cut by an appropriate Type II restriction endonuclease to yield the sequence of interest within a suitably sized DNA fragment (usually 500–12,000 bp). The DNA is size fractionated by electrophoresis on agarose gels and transferred as ssDNA from the gel onto an inert (usually nylon) membrane by capillary action, forming a faithful replica of the gel. The fragment of interest is revealed by probing the membrane with a radioactively labeled DNA fragment of complementary sequence. An adaptation of standard Southern blotting where PCR-amplified DNA is transferred from a gel is used to detect intermediate trinucleotide repeats in MD.

2. Materials

2.1. PCR Amplification, Polyacrylamide Gel Electrophoresis, and Silver Staining

Analytical grade reagents should be used at all stages unless otherwise indicated.

1. 20X PCR amplification buffer: $1.0M$ Tris-HCl, pH 9.0, 400 mM ammonium sulfate, 30 mM magnesium chloride. Filter sterilize and store as 1 mL-aliquots at $-20°C$.
2. Deoxynucleoside triphosphates (dNTPs): These can be purchased individually at 100 mM concentration, i.e., Boehringer Mannheim (Mannheim, Germany). Prepare for use by diluting down to 10 mM concentration in sterile dH$_2$O and mix together to form an equimolar mix of all four dNTPs (or dATP, dCTP, and dTTP if 7-deaza-GTP is to be used in the PCR reaction). Store frozen as aliquots at $-20°C$, avoid excessive freezing and thawing.
3. 7-deaza-GTP: Store at $-20°C$, aliquot to avoid excessive freeze–thaw cycles, do not use beyond expiration date, and do not store as a solution with other deoxynucleoside triphosphates.
4. *Taq* polymerase: The author recommends *Taq* polymerase from Perkin-Elmer Cetus (Buckinghamshire, UK), Boehringer Mannheim, or Life Technologies Inc. (Gaithersburg, MD). Store at $-20°C$. Quantities recommended for PCR assume a *Taq* polymerase activity of 5 U/μL.
5. DMSO.
6. Formamide loading buffer: 10 mL formamide, 200 μL $0.5M$ EDTA, pH 8.0, 15 mg xylene cyanole, 3 mg bromophenol blue.
7. Ammonium persulfate (AMPS): Prepare a 10% solution that can be stored at 4°C for up to 24 h.
8. Six and 8% (19:1) sequencing grade acrylamide, ready to use, i.e., Sequagel 6 and Sequagel 8 (National Diagnostics, Atlanta, GA).

9. Polyacrylamide minigel system. ATTO AE6210 slab gel system (Genetic Research Instrumentation, Essex, UK).

10. Electrophoresis power pack: This should be capable of maintaining a constant current of 50 mA and voltage 400 V.

11. Silver staining solution A: 10% ethanol (industrial grade) 0.5% acetic acid. Prepare on the day of use. Store at room temperature.

12. Silver staining solution B: 0.1% $AgNO_3$. Prepare a 10X stock solution of 1% $AgNO_3$ and store at room temperature in a brown bottle. 1X solution should be stored in clear bottles at room temperature but away from light. The 1X solution may be reused to stain up to five gels.

13. Silver staining solution C: 1.5% NaOH, 0.15% formaldehyde. This solution is labile, add the formaldehyde immediately (i.e., within 3 min) before use (*see* Note 1).

14. Silver staining solution D: 0.75% Na_2CO_3. Prepare a 10X stock of 7.5% Na_2CO_3. Store at room temperature.

15. Cellophane sheets (i.e., part no. SE1202 Hoefer Scientific Instruments, San Francisco, CA).

16. Drying frame and platform (i.e., part nos. SE1210 and SE1214 Hoefer Scientific Instruments).

17. Flat capillary gel loading tips, i.e., Stratatips (Stratagene Cloning Systems, La Jolla, CA).

2.2. Southern Blotting

Purity of reagents is of utmost importance for success, ensure that analytical grade reagents are used for the preparation of all solutions.

1. A 20 × 20-cm submarine gel electrophoresis tank suitable for running agarose gels is essential, i.e., Horizon 20.25 system (Life Technologies). Buffer recirculation is a very helpful feature because of the long electrophoresis times involved, although in tanks without this facility the electrophoresis buffer may be changed during the run.

2. An electrophoresis power pack: Most cheaper basic models should be adequate, i.e., model 400L (Life Technologies).

3. A temperature controlled rotisserie style hybridization oven, i.e., midihybridization oven (Hybaid, Middlesex, UK) (*see* Note 2).

4. Agarose: This is available from many manufacturers but should be electrophoresis grade.

5. Restriction enzymes: *Eco*RI and *Ecl*XI are needed for fragile X analysis. *Eco*RI alone is used for MD analysis, whereas *Pst*I is used for HD. The author has experience with enzymes supplied by Boehringer Mannheim, Life Technologies, and New England Biolabs (Beverley, MA). Restriction enzymes are supplied with their own reaction buffers. Store at –20°C.

6. Probes: OX1.9, fragile X *(5)*, pGB2.6, MD *(6)* (*see* Note 3), 4g6P1.8, HD.

7. TBE electrophoresis buffer: Make as a 10X stock solution, 0.89M Tris, 0.89M boric acid, 0.02M EDTA, pH 8.0. Store at room temperature.

8. 5X TBE gel loading buffer: 5 mL 10X TBE, 4.9 mL glycerol, 0.1% SDS, 3 mg bromophenol blue, and 15 mg xylene cyanol. Store at room temperature.

9. Phosphate prehybridization/hybridization solution (PPH): Prepare prehybridization solution as a 2X stock, $0.5M$ NaH$_2$PO$_4$, $0.5M$ NaCl, and 1 mM EDTA, adjust pH to 7.5 with $5M$ NaOH. Store 2X stock solution at room temperature. When ready to use, dilute with dH$_2$O and add SDS to 0.5%. For hybridization solution add polyethylene glycol (PEG 6000) to 6%. The probes PGB2.6 and 4g6P1.8 require further blocking with Denhardt's solution and herring sperm (HS) DNA (*see* Notes 4 and 5).

10. 50X Denhardt's solution: 0.5% ficoll, 0.5% polyvinylpyrrolidone, 0.5% bovine serum albumin (BSA) (Pentax fraction V). Filter sterilize and store as aliquots frozen at $-20°C$.

11. HS DNA: Prepare as a 5 mg/mL stock solution, shear by repeatedly syringing the solution through a fine-gage needle. Store frozen in aliquots at $-20°C$.

12. Random primer labeling kit: A commercially manufactured kit is the easiest option, ones based on random hexanucleotide primers are adequate, i.e., Multiprime (Amersham International, Buckinghamshire, UK). There are others on the market that use random nonanucleotides as primers.

13. α^{32}PdCTP radioisotope label (Amersham International). Store at $-20°C$. Note that storage and use of radioactive materials is governed by national and local safety regulations.

14. Denaturing solution: $1.5M$ NaCl, $0.5M$ NaOH. Store at room temperature.

15. 20X SSC: $3M$ NaCl, $0.3M$ Na-citrate. Store at room temperature.

16. Positively charged nylon membrane for DNA transfer, i.e., Hybond N$^+$ (Amersham International).

17. 500-Gage polythene layflat tubing (P&B Plastics, Stockport, UK).

18. Autoradiograph cassettes fitted with blue emitting intensifying screens, i.e., High Speed X (X-Ograph, Wiltshire, UK).

19. X-ray film: Fuji RX (Fuji Photo Film Co., Tokyo, Japan).

20. A $-70°C$ freezer.

21. A slow orbital shaker, i.e., The Swirler (Hybaid, Middlesex, UK).

22. A shortwave UV transilluminator.

2.3. 5' End Labeling of a (CTG)$_5$ Oligonucleotide Probe for Detection of Intermediate MD Trinucleotide Expansions

1. A synthetic oligonucleotide (CTG)$_5$ probe. Dilute down to 10 ng/µL in sterile dH$_2$O and store at $-20°C$.

2. 20X SSPE: $3M$ NaCl, $0.2M$ NaH$_2$PO$_4$, $0.02M$ EDTA. Adjust pH to 7.6 with $5M$ NaOH. Store at room temperature.

3. T4 polynucleotide kinase (Amersham International). Store at $-20°C$.

4. 10X Polynucleotide kinase buffer: $0.5M$ Tris-HCl, pH 7.6, 100 mM MgCl$_2$, 100 mM dithiothreitol, 500 µg/mL BSA (fraction V). Filter sterilize and store as 1-mL aliquots at $-20°C$.

5. γ^{32}PdATP radioisotope label (Amersham International). Note that use and storage of radioactive materials is governed by national and local safety regulations.

6. 100 mM EDTA, pH 8.0 stop solution. Store at room temperature.

3. Methods

3.1. PCR Amplification, Polyacrylamide Gel Electrophoresis, and Silver Staining of Trinucleotide Repeats

3.1.1. PCR Amplification

1. This has been covered in detail in Chapter 2. The components of the PCR reaction, however, do differ for optimal amplification of trinucleotide repeats. For amplifications not requiring 7-deaza-GTP (*see* Table 1) reactions should be prepared as follows: 0.5 μL 20 × PCR buffer, 1.0 μL forward and reverse primer (5 μ*M* each), 1.0 μL 10 m*M* dNTPs (2.5 m*M* dATP, dCTP, dGTP, dTTP), 0.1 μL *Taq* polymerase (0.5 U), 1.0 μL genomic DNA (5–25 ng), and 6.4 μL dH$_2$O.
2. The following mastermix substituting 7-deaza-GTP for GTP is recommended for GC-rich trinucleotide repeat templates (*see* Table 1): 0.5 μL 20X PCR buffer, 1.0 μL forward and reverse primer (5 μ*M* each), 0.75 μL 10 m*M* dNTPs (3.3 m*M* dATP, dCTP, dTTP), 0.25 μL 7-deaza-GTP (10 m*M*), 1.0 μL DMSO, 0.1 μL *Taq* polymerase (0.5 U), 1.0 μL genomic DNA (5–25 ng), and 5.4 μL dH$_2$O.
3. "Hot Start" PCR gives optimal amplification with the Huntington primers A and B (Table 1). This can be done cheaply by omitting *Taq* polymerase and dH$_2$O from the reactions and adding them to the PCR reactions while they are passing through the initial denaturation at 95°C on the thermal cycler. Alternatively, proprietary wax plugs may be purchased for this purpose.
4. When thermal cycling is complete, samples should be electrophoresed on the same day, or, if this is not possible, stored frozen at –20°C. Prior to electrophoresis, the samples should be removed to a fresh microcentrifuge tube and mixed with an equal volume of formamide loading buffer.

3.1.2. Polyacrylamide Gel Electrophoresis

1. Assemble a clean set of glass plates with gasket in the casting tray. No siliconizing treatment is necessary.
2. Pour 30 mL of the appropriate concentration Sequagel acrylamide into a clean beaker.
3. Add 240 μL of freshly made 10% ammonium persulfate solution to the Sequagel and swirl gently to mix.
4. Draw the acrylamide solution carefully into a 50-mL disposable syringe. Try to avoid introducing air bubbles.
5. Place the assembled glass plates and casting tray vertically on the bench and slowly pour the acrylamide between the glass plates. Any air bubbles introduced while pouring can be removed by carefully tilting the meniscus of the acrylamide solution down to the level of the bubbles.
6. Insert an appropriate comb, taking care not to trap any air bubbles and leave to polymerize horizontally for 1 h (*see* Notes 6 and 7).
7. Dismantle the casting tray and carefully pull the silicone rubber gasket from between the edges of the glass plates.

Table 1
Conditions for PCR Amplification and Polyacrylamide Gel Electrophoresis

Disease	Primer sequences	PCR amplification conditions	Product size with no repeats, bp	Acrylamide concentration, %	7-deaza-GTP or dGTP
Fragile X	5'-TCCGGTGGAGAGGGCCGCCTCTGACC-3' 5'-TTCAGCCCTGCTAGCGCCGGGAGC-3'	95°C: 1 min 65°C: 1 min 72°C: 2 min 35 cycles	159	6	7-deaza-GTP
MD	5'-CTTCCCAGGCCTGCAGTTTGCCCATC-3' 5'-GAACGGGGCTCGAAGGGTCCTTGTAGC-3'	95°C: 1 min 62°C: 1 min 72°C: 2 min 30 cycles	113	6	Either
HD	Primer A 5'-GCCTTCGAGTCCCTCAAGTCCTTC-3' Primer B 5'-GGCGGTGGCGGGCTGTTGCTGCTGC-3' Primer C 5'-AAACTCACGGTCGGTGCAGCGGCTC-3'	95°C: 1 min 60°C: 1 min 72°C: 2 min 30 cycles	(A + B) 42 (A + C) 188	8 (A + B) 6 (A + C)	7-deaza-GTP
SBMA	5'-TCCAGAATCTGTTCCAGAGCGTGC-3' 5'-GCTGTGAAGGTTGCTGTTCCTCAT-3'	95°C: 1 min 60°C: 1 min 72°C: 2 min 30 cycles	218	6	dGTP

8. Make 800 mL of 1X TBE electrophoresis buffer from the 10X TBE stock solution and pour into the bottom of an electrophoresis tank until its level just reaches the gasket that forms the upper buffer chamber when compressed by the gel plates.
9. Place the gel plates in the electrophoresis tank taking care not to introduce any bubbles along the bottom edge of the plates, insert the wedge/compressor in the appropriate orientation for 1-mm gels.
10. Place the remaining electrophoresis buffer in a large conical flask and heat in a microwave oven until it reaches a temperature of approx 60°C. Fill the top buffer tank with hot electrophoresis buffer. (This has the effect of heating the gel obviating the need for pre-running.) Remove the comb and flush urea and unpolymerized acrylamide from the wells with a disposable syringe and hypodermic needle.
11. Place the samples on a heated block or thermal cycler set at 95°C for 5 min and cool on ice to quench reannealing of the ssDNA. Load 6–10 µL of the sample in each well (depending on the size of the wells and amplification efficiency) using thin gel loading tips. Place the cover and leads on the electrophoresis tank and electrophorese at 50 mA constant current. *See* Table 1 for details of expected molecular weights of DNA fragments.

3.1.3. Silver Staining

1. Gently prize the glass plates apart, avoiding using metal instruments that may cause the plates to chip. Mark the orientation of the gel by cutting the corner adjacent to lane no. 1. Place in a plastic tray containing 300 mL of solution A, leave on a slow orbital shaker for 3 min, pour off, and reimmerse in a further 300 mL of solution A (*see* Note 8).
2. Pour off solution A and add 400 mL of solution B and gently shake for 15 min. Pour off solution B (remember to recover and reuse solution B until staining efficiency declines). Rinse the gel quickly with two changes of distilled water (*see* Note 9).
3. Add 300 mL of *freshly made* solution C and leave the gel to develop, shaking gently, in a fume cupboard for 20 min. A small amount of powdery metallic silver precipitate should be observed when this solution is added to the gel. Brown/black bands on a yellow background slowly appear on the gel during this stage.
4. Pour off solution C and add 300 mL of solution D and leave for 15 min.

3.1.4. Drying and Storing Gels

1. Cut two sheets of cellophane to size and soak in a sink or tray of tap water for a few seconds. The sheets will become heavy and pliable when wetted. Ensure that the whole sheet is thoroughly wetted.
2. Place one moistened cellophane sheet flat over an assembled platform and drying frame inner section. Ensure that the inner section is facing correctly upward.
3. Carefully transfer the gel onto the surface of the cellophane sheet and trim away any unwanted areas using a ruler pressed hard onto the gel surface. Thoroughly wet the gel and cellophane by spraying with a wash bottle.

4. Lay the second cellophane sheet on top of the gel and frame, taking care to exclude air bubbles. Place the outer section of the drying frame firmly in over the inner frame's rubber gasket, drawing the cellophane/gel sandwich taut.

5. Lift the drying frame off the platform and turn the retaining screws to hold the cellophane/gel sandwich in place. Sponge excess water from the cellophane surface using a tissue and place to dry in a 37°C incubator for approx 6 h or alternatively on a benchtop in a warm room for approx 20 h.

6. When the gel is thoroughly dry, dismantle the frame and cut the gel from the excess cellophane with scissors, leaving a border of 1–2 cm around the gel. Seal the perimeter of the cellophane by folding strips of adhesive tape over all the edges. This prevents peeling of the dried gel.

7. Do not bend or fold the dried gels and store flat away from moisture, avoid abrading the surface of the cellophane (*see* Note 10).

3.2. Southern Blotting for Analysis of Large Trinucleotide Expansions

3.2.1. Restriction Digestion and Gel Electrophoresis

1. The genomic DNA samples need to be cut with restriction enzymes prior to electrophoresis. The restriction enzyme(s) used depends on the disease being studied (*see* Table 2). Prepare restriction digests of all the samples to be analyzed in either 0.6- or 1.6-mL microcentrifuge tubes as follows: 5 μg of genomic DNA, 3 μL of 10X restriction enzyme buffer, 10 U of each restriction enzyme (typically, 1 μL), add sterile dH_2O to 30 μL, and incubate in a water bath at 37°C for *at least* 4 h.

2. While the samples are digesting, prepare an agarose gel for electrophoresis of the samples (*see* Table 2). For a typical 20 × 20-cm format, the following amounts should be sufficient: 35 mL of 10X TBE, 315 mL of dH_2O, 2.8 g (0.8% gel), 3.15g (0.9% gel) or 4.2 g (1.2% gel) of agarose. The gel should be heated gently to dissolve the agarose either in a microwave oven or on a hotplate with a magnetic stirrer bar. Once the agarose has completely dissolved add 17.5 μL of a 10 mg/mL solution of ethidium bromide, swirl gently to mix, and allow the gel solution to cool to 65°C.

3. Place an appropriate comb in the gel former and seal the open ends with plastic tape. When the gel has cooled down pour carefully into the former. Check for air bubbles, especially around the comb. These can be removed using a Pasteur pipet. Allow the gel to set for at least 1 h before running; if the gel is not required immediately it may be wrapped in cling film and stored in a refrigerator at 4°C for up to 48 h. When ready to run remove the tape and immerse in 1X TBE buffer to a depth over the gel surface of approx 1.5 mm. Only remove the comb once the gel is fully submerged in the running buffer.

4. The samples should be monitored for complete digestion before running. Take 3 μL of each restriction digest and mix with 1 μL of 5X TBE loading buffer and run for 30 min at 60 mA on a 0.8–1.0% agarose monitor gel (monitor gels can

Table 2
Conditions for Southern Analysis

Disease	Agarose, %	Restriction enzyme(s)	Size of fragment containing repeats, kb	Electrophoresis distance	Probe	Prehybridization solution	Hybridization solution	Stringent wash
Fragile X	0.9	EcoRI and EclXI	2.8–10	2 kb–20 cm	OX1.9	1X PPH, 0.5% SDS	1X PPH, 0.6% PEG, 0.5% SDS	1–0.5X SSC
MD	0.8	EcoRI	9–14	3 kb–20 cm	pGB2.6	1X PPH, 5X Denhardt's 100 µg/mL denatured HS DNA, 0.5% SDS	1X PPH, 0.6% PEG, 5X Denhardt's 100 µg/mL denatured HS DNA, 0.5%SDS	0.5X SSC
HD	1.2	PstI	1.2–1.6	0.5 kb–20 cm	4g6P1.8	1X PPH, 5X Denhardt's, 100 µg/mL denatured HS DNA, 0.5% SDS	1X PPH, 0.6% PEG, 5X Denhardt's 100 µg/mL denatured HS DNA, 0.5%SDS	0.2X SSC

either be minigels made specifically for monitoring purposes or alternatively simply use two combs at opposite ends of your main gel and run the main samples in the opposite direction to the monitor samples). The digested samples should then be visualized on a UV transilluminator. Undigested or partially digested samples have a characteristic streaky appearance. Add an additional 10 U of restriction enzyme to any uncut samples and reincubate for at least 2 h (*see* Note 11).

5. Once the samples are completely digested, mix each with 9 μL of dH$_2$O and 9 μL of 5X TBE loading buffer. Load the whole sample onto the gel using a fresh micropipetor tip for each sample. A mol-wt standard, i.e., 1-kb ladder (Life Technologies) should also be loaded in one of the outer wells. Set the gel to run at 55 mA in constant current mode for at least 16 h (*see* Table 2 for details of the distance the gels should be electrophoresed).

3.2.2. Southern Blotting

1. When the gel has electrophoresed the correct distance (*see* Table 2), place the gel on a UV transilluminator. Cut off the mol-wt marker, the wells, and any waste agarose. Remember to slice off a corner of the gel to allow it to be orientated and note the dimensions of the trimmed gel. Transfer the gel into a plastic tray and submerge in denaturing solution. Denature on a slow orbital shaker for 1 h.

2. While the gel is denaturing, cut a piece of charged Nylon membrane and two pieces of Whatman (Maidstone, UK) 3MM filter paper to a size slightly larger than the gel. Mark or cut one corner of the membrane to correspond to the cut corner of the gel. Transfer the gel onto an inverted gel casting tray and carefully place the nylon membrane onto the gel avoiding introducing air bubbles. Briefly wet the sheets of filter paper in denaturing solution and place on top of the membrane. Complete the blot by adding a stack of paper towels to a depth of approx 6 cm and compress with a suitable weight (approx 500 g). Leave to blot for 12–16 h (*see* Note 12).

3. Dismantle the blot and discard any damp paper towels. Place the membrane into a tray containing 200 mL of 3X SSC and shake gently for 2 min, pour off the 3X SSC and repeat twice. The filter should now be of neutral pH and may be probed immediately or sealed in plastic while still damp and stored at 4°C.

3.2.3. Probe Labeling and Hybridization

1. The instructions supplied with the labeling kit need to be followed with care for successful labeling. You will be handling dangerous radioisotopes and need to use adequate protection in the form of perspex shields. Remember to monitor both the working area and yourself adequately after handling radioisotopes. Between 50 and 100 ng of probe should be labeled for each Southern blot and most kits recommend that 2.5 to 5 μCi of α^{32}PdCTP be used per labeling reaction. Remember that single-stranded DNA is needed as a template for the labeling reaction so you must denature the probe by heating to 100°C in a dry block or water bath before adding to the rest of the reaction. For safety reasons labeling reactions should always be carried out in screw-capped microcentrifuge tubes.

2. Make up 100 mL of prehybridization solution per filter by diluting down the 2X stock to 1X and adding SDS to a final concentration of 0.5%. Place each filter in a separate hybridization bottle from the rotisserie oven, add the prehybridization solution, and seal the lid tightly. Place in the rotisserie oven, which should be equilibrated at 65°C. Set to rotate, and leave for at least 1 h to prehybridize.
3. Make up 10 mL of hybridization solution per filter by adding 0.6 g (0.6%) PEG 6000 to 10 mL of prehybridization solution in a clean Universal tube. Place in the rotisserie oven for 1 h to allow the PEG to fully dissolve. The probes pGB2.6 and 4g6P1.8 require extra blocking (*see* Note 4).
4. After the required labeling time check that the PEG has dissolved fully in the hybridization solution before pouring the prehybridization solution away and adding 10 mL of hybridization solution. (Take care not to allow the filter to dry out at this stage.) Add 500 μL of hybridization solution *without SDS* to the labeled probe and mix. Heat the probe to 100°C for 6 min, then cool for 3 min in a water bath at 37°C (this quenches reannealing of the probe). Quickly add the cooled probe to the hybridization solution in the bottle avoiding splashing the filter. Replace the cap firmly and place in the rotisserie oven to rotate at 65°C overnight.

3.2.4. Filter Washing and Autoradiography

1. Prepare 1 L of a wash solution for each filter comprising SSC of the appropriate concentration and 0.1% SDS and equilibrate at 65°C. The strength of SSC used varies with probe (*see* Table 1).
2. Pour off the hybridization solution down a sink designated for the disposal of radioactive waste and add about 100 mL of wash solution. Replace in the rotisserie oven for approx 30 min.
3. Remove the filter after the first wash with a pair of forceps and place on a clean surface. Monitor the radioactivity using a Geiger counter, if this is >10 counts per second (cps) (with the plastic shield left over the Geiger detection window) wash in fresh solution for another 30 min. Keep repeating this step until the activity is between 5 and 10 cps or until no drop in activity is observed between washes.
4. Either heat seal the filter in 500-gage plastic or wrap in cling film. Place with a sheet of X-ray film inside an autoradiograph cassette fitted with intensifying screens in a darkroom. Remember to mark the film in some way to allow it to be properly orientated, i.e., by folding a corner.
5. Leave to expose at −70°C for 1–5 d before developing. The film is usually developed after an overnight exposure to judge the length of time needed for a good result (*see* Note 13).

3.3. 5' End Labeling of a (CTG)₅ Oligonucleotide Probe for Detection of Intermediate MD Trinucleotide Expansions

3.3.1. Gel Electrophoresis and Southern Blotting

1. PCR amplify target DNAs in a 10-μL volume as described in Section 3.1.1.
2. Pour a 1.2% 20 × 20 cm agarose gel as described in Section 3.2.1

3. Mix samples with 2.5 μL of 5X TBE loading buffer and electrophorese at 100 mA (*see* Section 3.2.1.) until 100 bp reaches the end of the gel.
4. Blot the whole gel onto a sheet of positively charged nylon membrane as described in Section 3.2.2.

3.3.2. 5' End Labeling
and Hybridization of an Oligonucleotide Probe

1. Prehybridize the filter by placing in a hybridization bottle and adding 50 mL of a solution comprising 5X SSPE, 5X Denhardt's, and 0.5% SDS. Prehybridize for 1 h in a rotating hybridization oven set at 42°C.
2. Prepare a labeling reaction in a 1.5-mL screwcapped microcentrifuge tube as follows: 1 μL 10X polynucleotide kinase buffer, 1 μL (CTG)$_5$ oligonucleotide probe (10 ng/μL), 2 μL γ^{32}PdATP label, 5 μL sterile dH$_2$O, and 1 μL T4 polynucleotide kinase (10 U).
3. Mix the labeling reaction, briefly spin down, and incubate at 37°C for 30 min.
4. After 30 min stop the reaction by adding 10 μL of 100 m*M* EDTA stop solution.
5. Pour away the prehybridizing solution and add an additional 10 mL of 5X SSPE, 5X Denhardt's, and 0.5% SDS solution. Carefully add the labeling reaction to this solution at the bottom of the bottle, avoiding touching the filter. Firmly seal the bottle and hybridize for at least 1 h while rotating in the oven at 42°C (*see* Note 14).
6. Pour off the hybridization solution down a sink designated for disposal of radio-isotopes. Wash away the unbound probe with 3 × 100 mL room temperature rinses with 2X SSPE, 0.1% SDS. For the stringent wash add 50 mL of 2X SSPE, 0.1% SDS, and incubate while rotating at 42°C for 20 min.
7. Pour off the stringent wash and carefully remove the filter from the hybridization bottle. (Protective screens must still be used since the filter should still be radio-active.) Seal the filter while still damp in plastic.
8. In a darkroom place the filter with a sheet of X-ray film in an autoradiograph cassette. The first autoradiograph can be developed after a 1-h incubation at room temperature. Further exposures can then be judged depending on the initial result.

3.4. Interpretation of Results

3.4.1. Appearance of Trinucleotide Repeat Alleles
on Silver-Stained Gels

Trinucleotide repeat alleles do not appear as single discrete DNA bands on polyacrylamide gels but as an allelic band accompanied by one to several "stutter" bands. This is owing to an artifact originating during PCR. Most *Taq* polymerases do not have proofreading activity and occasionally slippage occurs during replication of the trinucleotide repeat. This leads to omission of multiples of the repeat unit. The allelic band should be interpreted as the strongest band (e.g., mol-wt n bp) the accompanying stutter bands are progressively weaker at multiples of n minus the length of the repeat unit (for trinucleotides, 3 bp). The number of stutter bands does not remain constant but increases with increasing repeat length. Furthermore, once a certain limit is reached this pattern breaks down and stutter bands at multiples of n plus 3 also occur. When determining the size of these larger alleles the strongest band should still be used. Given these circumstances identifying heterozygotes for closely spaced alleles is difficult but with experience they can be reliably recognized (*see* Fig. 1 for examples).

3.4.2. Allele Sizing

Alleles can be sized provided a suitable mol-wt marker is also run on each gel. The $\log_{10}$ bp of each fragment of the marker should be plotted against the distance migrated from the origin (the wells) to create a calibration curve specific to the gel. The molecular weights of the alleles can then be calculated by interpolation on the calibration curve. Provided care is taken at all stages, this method of sizing is usually reproducible to one repeat unit (± 3 bp). Allele sizing is usually not necessary since most alleles clearly fall into either the normal or the expanded range.

3.4.3. Fragile X Interpretation

3.4.3.1. Fragile X Repeat Size Range

The common fragile X mutation is an expanding $(CGG)_n$ repeat located in the 5' untranslated region (UTR) of the FMR-1 gene. The FMR-1 gene is located on the long arm of the X-chromosome at location Xq27.3. The normal size of the FMR-1 trinucleotide repeat is considered to lie between 6 and 54 repeats (7). The most common alleles are between 28 and 30 repeats and over 98% of all normal alleles are below 46 repeats. Some alleles within the transitional range, from 46–54 repeats, are unstable. However, there is no evidence to suggest that these alleles are capable of expansion into the full mutation range with a single transmission (8). Unstable alleles within the intermediate range are thought to lack interspersed AGG repeats within the CGG repeat array (9). In families with fragile X syndrome the allele is larger than 54 repeats and is unstable when transmitted from parent to offspring. More than 95% of mutations of these alleles result in an increase in size. Alleles are considered to be premutations up to a size of 200 repeats since up to this size they are not hypermethylated and have no phenotypic effects in both sexes. Above this length hypermethylation occurs and the allele is referred to as a full mutation. Full mutations are almost always accompanied by mental retardation in males and significant but milder symptoms in about one-half of females.

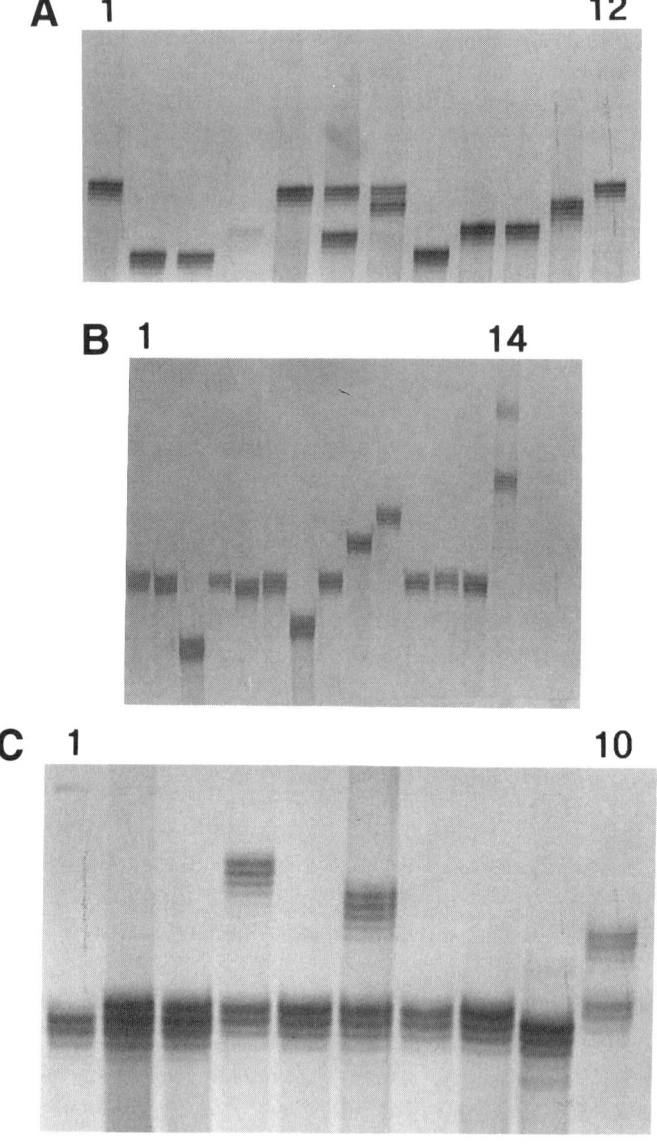

Fig. 1. PCR amplification and silver staining of the fragile X CGG repeat: **(A)** Lanes 6 and 7 are heterozygous female samples. The remaining samples are from normal males, although amplification in lane 4 is weak. **(B)** Lane 14 is a female sample with an allele within the transitional range (50 repeats) and a premutation allele (74 repeats). Note how the premutation allele appears as a smear, this is owing to the presence of stutter bands of higher molecular weight than the allele. **(C)** Lanes 2, 3, 4, 6, and 10 are all female heterozygotes. Lanes 2 and 3 are heterozygous for alleles differing by one repeat unit. The remaining samples are all normal males.

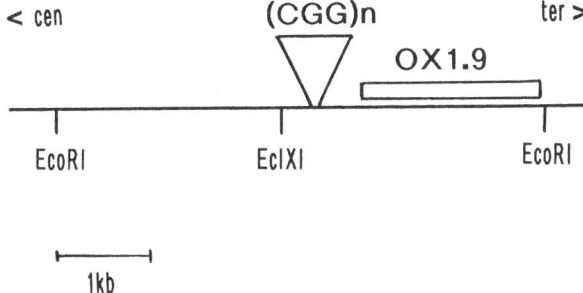

Fig. 2. Genomic restriction map of the region flanking the expanding CGG repeat that causes fragile X syndrome. The position of the probe OX1.9 is indicated by an open bar. The *Ecl*XI site immediately adjacent to the CGG repeat is subject to methylation on the lyonized X in normal females and on chromosomes carrying a full mutation.

3.4.3.2. HYBRIDIZATION PATTERN OF PROBE OX1.9

The probe OX1.9 hybridizes to a 5.2 kb *Eco*RI fragment encompassing the CGG repeat that undergoes expansion in the majority of fragile X cases. Within this fragment lies an *Ecl*XI site centromeric of the FMR-1 gene and the CGG repeat (Fig. 2). *Ecl*XI is sensitive to methylation and only cuts at an unmethylated recognition sequence. Consequently, normal male and female DNA samples give rise to different hybridization patterns with this probe. Males giving rise to a single 2.8-kb band, whereas females give a 2.8- and 5.2-kb band corresponding to the active and lyonized X-chromosomes, respectively. Variations within the normal range can often be discerned in the 2.8-kb band and expansions into the premutation range up to 200 repeats are clearly associated with this band. Interpretation of premutation carrying females can be compounded by skewed methylation, especially so when the expanded allele is preferentially methylated. Great care should be taken to ensure that the 5.2-kb band is clearly in line with the neighboring tracks to exclude this possibility. Since expansions above 200 repeats (full mutations) are accompanied by hypermethylation, the signal from these large alleles is associated with the 5.2-kb band. Full mutations are highly unstable and often exist as mosaics within the peripheral lymphocytes, giving rise to a diffuse, smear-like signal (Fig. 3). Other forms of mosaicism can occur, for instance, a typical diffuse methylated full mutation may be accompanied by an unmethylated premutation repeat sequence. Very rarely a full expansion can be accompanied by a small population of cells with alleles in the normal range. This would lead to a false-negative result if PCR alone was used to exclude fragile X. Preliminary data from a collaborative study in the UK has estimated that 1% of full mutation males have PCR amplifiable alleles within the normal range (G. Cross, personal communication).

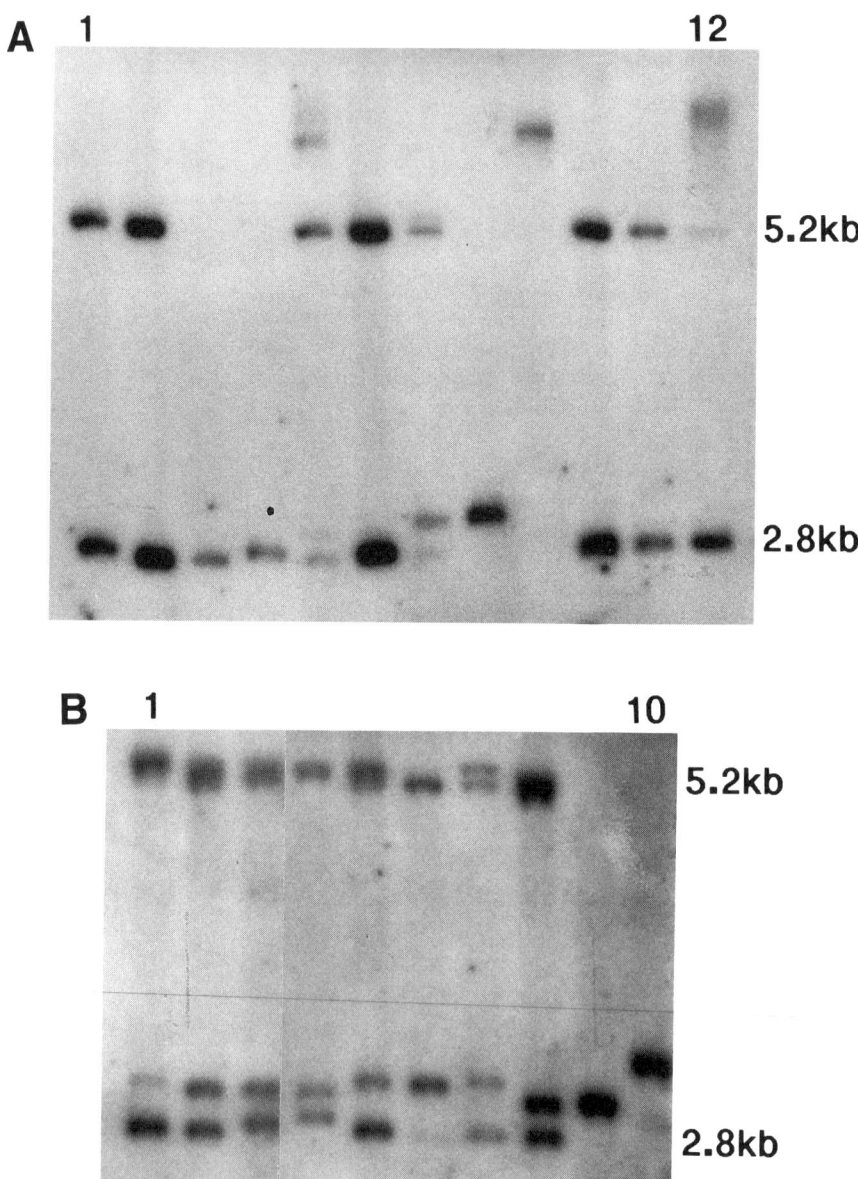

Fig. 3. Autoradiographs produced by probing Southern blots from *Eco*RI/*Ecl*XI digests with OX1.9: **(A)** Lanes 1, 2, 5, 6, 10, and 11 are all from normal females (note the 5.2-kb fragment originating from the lyonized X chromosome). Lanes 3 and 4 are from normal males (note the slight variation in mobility owing to normal variation in CGG repeat size). Lane 7 is weak but is from a premutation carrier female with a

3.4.3.3. DIAGNOSIS IN FRAGILE X

PCR and Southern blotting complement each other in the diagnosis of fragile X. Only alleles in the normal range and those at the lower end of the premutation range can be detected reliably by PCR and silver staining, whereas all premutation and full mutation alleles can be detected using Southern blotting. For the purposes of excluding a diagnosis of fragile X, the normal range must be considered to lie below 46 repeats because of the possibility of mutational instability of alleles above this size (unless there is clear evidence from other family members of stable transmission of an allele 46–54 repeats in size).

In samples at low prior risk of being affected by fragile X syndrome, it is acceptable to exclude fragile X by demonstrating the presence of a single allele in the normal range in males or heterozygosity within the normal range in females. In order to eliminate the possibility of mosaicism it is still essential to screen by Southern blot all samples with a family history of the disease. Extreme care must be taken when interpreting female heterozygotes with closely spaced alleles by PCR and if there is any doubt, exclusion by Southern blot is essential. The absence of PCR amplification never should be interpreted as confirming the presence of a full mutation, confirmation by Southern blot should always be carried out.

3.4.3.4. CONTROL SAMPLES

The following control samples should be run alongside all diagnostic cases:

1. Polyacrylamide gels:
   a. A mol-wt standard against which alleles can be sized;
   b. A male sample with a full mutation, in which no amplification should occur;
   c. A female carrier with an expansion at the lower end of the premutation range; the expanded allele should be visible; and
   d. A distilled water control containing all other elements of the PCR reaction except target DNA; no amplification should be observed.
2. Southern blots:
   a. A sample with an allele at the transitional range (46–54 repeats); and
   b. A sample with a diffuse full mutation.

Fig. 3 *(continued)* degree of skewed methylation. Lane 8 is a premutation carrying male (often referred to as a normal transmitting male). Lane 10 is from a male with a full mutation (note that the *Ecl*XI site is now methylated in this sample). Lane 12 is a full mutation carrying female. (Note that the normal allele in this case remains largely unmethylated.) **(B)** a selection of premutation carrying males and females. Lanes 9 and 10 are both premutation carrying males, the remaining samples are premutation carrying females. Lane 1 shows skewed methylation of the premutation allele whereas track 6 shows skewed methylation of the normal allele. Skewed methylation as demonstrated by lane 1 can be misleading and lead to diagnostic error.

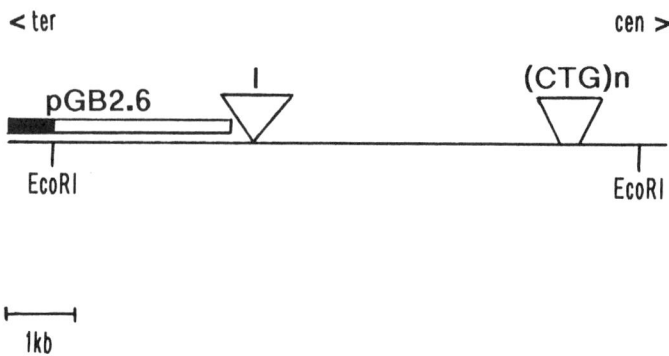

Fig. 4. Genomic restriction map of the region encompassing the expanding CTG repeat that causes MD. The position of the 1-kb insertion polymorphism (I) is indicated. The region to which probe pGB2.6 is complementary is also indicated by a bar. The shaded region of pGB2.6 is removed when the insert is released from the plasmid vector by digestion with both *Bam*HI and *Eco*RI (*see* Note 3).

3.4.4. MD Interpretation

3.4.4.1. MD Repeat Size Range

MD is an autosomal dominant disease that causes myotonia and progressive muscular weakness, other associated symptoms also frequently occur. The mutation causing MD is an expanding $(CTG)_n$ repeat located in the 3' UTR of a gene encoding a protein kinase *(2)*. The MD gene is located on the long arm of chromosome 19 at 19q13.3. The normal range of the MD repeat is considered to lie between 3 and 37 repeats *(10)*. The most common alleles are those with 5, 11–14, and 18–22 CTGs *(2)*. In nonmanifesting or mildly affected myotonic patients the repeat size varies between 42 and 150 *(11)*. Expansions in severely and congenitally affected patients can be up to 2000 repeats *(2)*.

3.4.4.2. Hybridization Pattern of Probe pGB2.6

The probe pGB2.6 hybridizes to a 9.0- or 10.0-kb *Eco*RI fragment containing the MD CTG repeat. The size variation is due to a 1-kb insertional polymorphism, the larger allele occurring at a frequency of 0.6 in the normal population *(6)* (Fig. 4). The 10-kb allele is associated with virtually all MD chromosomes. Consequently expansions are almost exclusively greater than 10 kb in size. Only the larger expansions, from approx 130 repeats upward, are discernible with this probe–enzyme combination. Mosaicism is also present with the larger MD expansions but this is usually less pronounced than the smearing experienced with fragile X and probe OX1.9 (Fig. 5).

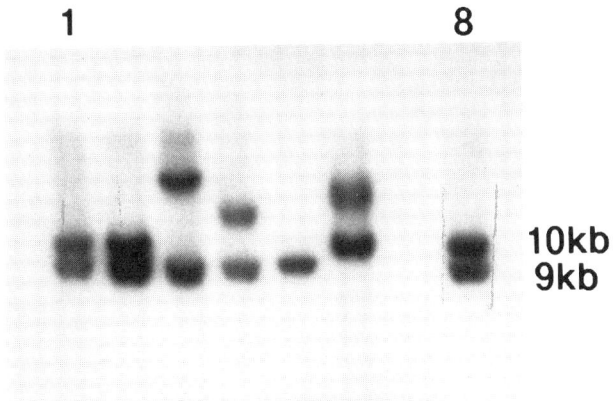

Fig. 5. Autoradiograph produced by probing a Southern blot from *Eco*RI digests with pGB2.6. Lanes 1, 2, and 8 are from samples heterozygous for the 1-kb insertion polymorphism. Lane 7 is blank. Track 5 is homozygous for the 9-kb allele. Lanes 3, 4, and 6 all carry large expansions and are thus affected by MD.

3.4.4.3. SOUTHERN BLOT ANALYSIS OF PCR-AMPLIFIED MD EXPANSIONS

A series of exposures is usually necessary to properly interpret these gels. The signal from the normal alleles will be very strong and typically will be visualized after an exposure of 1 or 2 h. Longer exposures are required to properly visualize the larger normal and small disease-causing expansions. Disease-causing expansions tend to smear heavily on the autoradiograph (*see* Fig. 6). This is an effect of secondary structure, owing to the DNA fragment's high GC content, rather than reflecting extreme mosaicism. Samples negative for MD expansions in the intermediate range show no in-track hybridization outside the normal range.

3.4.4.4. DIAGNOSIS IN MD

For accurate diagnosis of MD the three complementary techniques of direct PCR, Southern blotting of PCR products, and Southern blotting of genomic DNA need to be employed. Direct PCR detection on polyacrylamide gels will only reliably detect the smallest disease-causing expansions. Whereas the probe–enzyme combination described here only detects larger expansions. Southern blotting of PCR-amplified products is necessary to cover intermediate expansions. MD can be excluded using the direct PCR approach only if the sample is heterozygous for alleles within the normal range (3–37 repeats). Southern blotting can exclude MD in those cases homozygous for the 9 kb pGB2.6 (*Eco*RI digest) allele. Samples that do not fall into either of these categories must show no expansion after Southern blotting of PCR products to

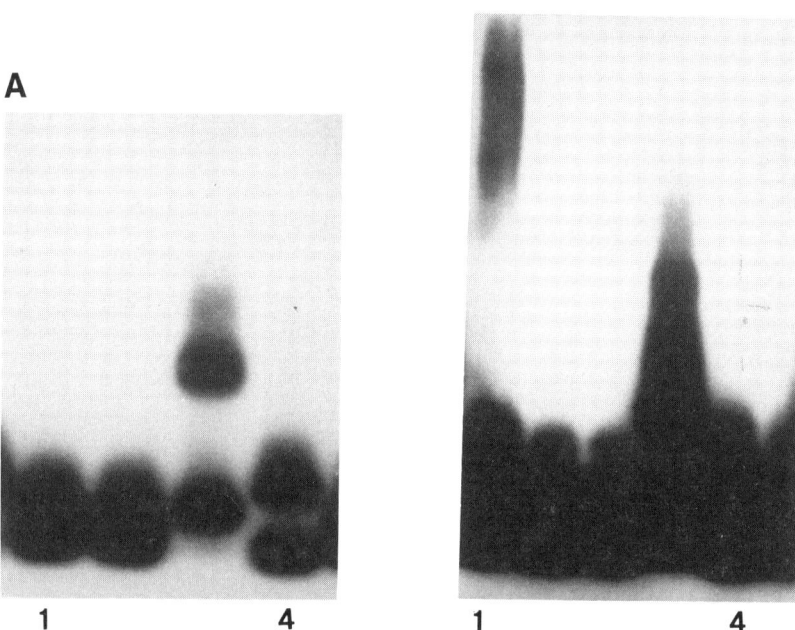

Fig. 6. Autoradiographs produced by Southern blotting MD repeat PCRs and probing with a $(CTG)_5$ oligonucleotide. Different exposures of the same four samples.
Lanes 1 and 4 both have expansions too large to be visualized by PCR and silver
staining but too small to be reliably detected on Southern blot with probe pGB2.6. **(A)**
A short exposure. Note the strong hybridization to the normal alleles and that the
smaller expansion in lane 3 is picked out clearly. **(B)** A five times longer exposure.
The normal alleles and the small expansion in lane 3 are now overexposed; however,
the larger expansion in lane 1 is now visualized as an in-track smear. The smearing is
an effect of secondary structure, not mosaicism.

exclude MD. Positive diagnosis of MD rests on detecting an allele exceeding
the normal range of 37 repeats using any of these techniques. Although there is
good evidence that the size of expansion is related to the severity of clinical
features, this should never be used as a prognostic indicator.

3.4.4.5. Control Samples

The following control samples should be run alongside all diagnostic cases:

1. Polyacrylamide gels:
   a. A mol-wt standard for sizing alleles;
   b. A sample with an allele at the upper end of the normal range; the large normal
      allele should be clearly visible;

    c. A sample with a small disease-causing expansion; the expanded allele should be visible; and

    d. A distilled water control containing all other elements of the PCR reaction except target DNA; no amplification should be observed.

2. Southern blots of PCR products:

    a. A sample with an allele at the upper end of the normal range; strong probe hybridization should be observed;

    b. A sample with a small disease-causing expansion just detectable on Southern blots with probe pGB2.6; probe hybridization should be observed on longer exposures; and

    c. A distilled water control containing all other elements of the PCR reaction except target DNA; no hybridization with the probe should occur in this lane.

3. Southern blots of genomic DNA:

    a. Samples heterozygous for the insertion polymorphism in every fifth lane; and

    b. A sample with an expansion small enough to be detectable on Southern blots of PCR products, a clear difference should be observed in the mobility of the expansion and the 10.0-kb allele in neighboring tracks.

3.4.5. HD Interpretation

3.4.5.1. HD REPEAT SIZE RANGE

HD is a progressive neurodegenerative disorder of late onset. It is inherited as a fully penetrant autosomal dominant condition. The HD mutation is an expanding $(CAG)_n$ repeat located within the coding sequence of the Huntingtin gene *(3)* located on 4p16.3. The range of the HD CAG repeat varies from 10–37 repeats in unaffected individuals and over 97% of normal alleles have <28 repeats *(12)*. Alleles found in HD affected individuals range in size from 37–121 repeats, with the size of allele related to age of onset *(12)*. Alleles in the range 30–38 repeats are considered to be intermediate alleles and appear to be at raised probability of undergoing expansion into the HD range *(13,14)*. Taking this factor into account, the normal range of the HD repeat can only be considered to extend to 32 repeats for diagnostic purposes, although those alleles in the intermediate range are unlikely to cause HD.

3.4.5.2. HYBRIDIZATION PATTERN OF 4G6P1.8

The probe 4G6P1.8 hybridizes to a *Pst*I fragment encompassing the HD CAG repeat. It detects a fragment of approx 1.8 kb in HD normal alleles that becomes larger on HD-affected chromosomes (up to 2.2 kb). 4g6P1.8 also shows strong secondary hybridization at an unknown locus, however this fragment is much larger and does not interfere with interpretation.

3.4.5.3. DIAGNOSIS IN HD

Diagnosis of HD rests heavily on PCR, although Southern blotting of genomic DNA is necessary when dealing with the largest expansions or in the small proportion of suspected cases that are homozygous after PCR. Most cases will

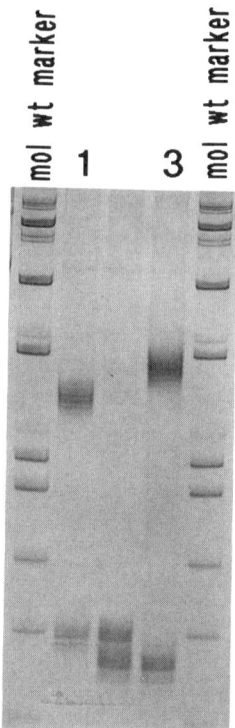

Fig. 7. PCR amplification and silver staining of the HD CAG repeat using primer pair A + B. Lanes 1 and 3 are from samples with expansions into the HD affected range. The sample in lane 2 is from an unaffected heterozygote in which HD can now be excluded.

be amenable to analysis with the primer pair A + B (*see* Table 1). HD can be excluded for those samples that are heterozygous in the normal range and the vast majority of HD expansions will amplify. A positive diagnosis of HD can be made providing there is an allele of >38 repeats (Fig. 7). Those cases that appear homozygous with A + B can be amplified with A + C, which produces a larger fragment containing a polymorphic CCG repeat immediately 3' of the HD CAG repeat *(15)*. The size of this polymorphic CCG repeat has no effect on HD but can be useful in detecting heterozygosity in the normal range at the HD locus. Primer pair A + C should not routinely be used for sizing HD alleles since the variability of the CCG repeat may confound HD CAG sizing causing errors of up to 15 bp *(15)*. Any remaining cases that are still homozygous should be Southern blotted and probed with 4g6P1.8. HD may be excluded if only a single band in the normal range is present. At present HD cannot be excluded in patients with an allele in the range 32–38 repeats, although the probability of them being affected is small. A multicenter study is presently underway in the United Kingdom to determine the HD risk to individuals with alleles in this range (D. C. Rubinsztein, personal communication). Although the correlation between HD CAG repeat size and age of onset is strong *(12)*, this should not be used as a prognostic indicator.

3.4.5.4. CONTROL SAMPLES

The following control samples should be run alongside all diagnostic cases:

1. Polyacrylamide gels:
   a. A mol-wt standard for sizing alleles;
   b. A sample with an allele at the upper end of the normal range; the large normal allele should amplify clearly;
   c. A sample with a large HD expansion; the HD allele should be visible; and
   d. A distilled water control containing all elements of the PCR reaction except target DNA; no amplification should be observed.
2. Southern blots:
   a. A sample with an allele at the top of the normal range (over 30 repeats); and
   b. A sample with a large HD expansion.

3.4.6. SBMA

3.4.6.1. SBMA REPEAT SIZE RANGE

SBMA is caused by an expanding $(CAG)_n$ repeat in the coding sequence of the androgen receptor gene situated on the long arm of the X-chromosome at location Xq11-12 *(4)*. The normal range of the SBMA repeat is 13–30 repeats and its heterozygosity exceeds 90% *(16)*. The SBMA repeat size in affected males and carrier females lies within a narrow range of 40–62 repeats. Large expansions and intermediate alleles have not been observed *(16)*. SBMA is inherited as an X-linked recessive disorder, males with expansions show progressive muscle weakness and atrophy that may be accompanied by gynecomastia and infertility.

3.4.6.2. DIAGNOSIS IN SBMA

Since SBMA expansions are small diagnosis can be carried out solely using PCR. A male sample with an allele in the normal range excludes SBMA. Female samples ideally should be heterozygous to exclude the carrier state. However, provided amplification is efficient and the relevant controls are run alongside the test sample, the absence of an expansion can be taken as excluding SBMA.

3.4.6.3. CONTROL SAMPLES

The following control samples should be run alongside all diagnostic cases:

1. A mol-wt standard against which alleles can be sized;
2. A female carrier with an expansion at the upper end of the range; the expansion should amplify clearly; and
3. A distilled water control containing all other elements of the PCR reaction except target DNA; no amplification should be observed.

4. Notes

1. Remember that formaldehyde usually is supplied as a 37% aqueous solution (formalin). Take this into account when calculating amounts for silver staining solution C. The formaldehyde concentration is critical.

2. A rotisserie style hybridization oven is not essential for Southern hybridization. The hybridization steps can be carried out in heat sealed plastic bags in a temperature controlled oven.

3. When probe pGB2.6 is used on *Eco*RI digests without modification, a constant fragment is visualized that coincides with the range of MD expansions. In order to overcome this problem, pGB2.6 insert should be released from the plasmid vector by digesting with both *Bam*HI and *Eco*RI. The larger of the two insert fragments released (approx 2.2 kb) no longer hybridizes to the constant fragment.

4. The prehybridization and hybridization solutions described here are suitable for most probes; however, the probes pGB2.6 and 4g6P1.8 contain repetitive elements and need further blocking to prevent cross-hybridization to other related genomic sequences. Both prehybridization and hybridization solutions should contain 5X Denhardt's solution and 100 µg/mL of denatured HS DNA for extra blocking. The HS DNA can be denatured by standing in a boiling water bath for 10 min prior to use.

5. If the ambient temperature falls, crystals may precipitate out in the prehybridization solution used for Southern blotting. These may be dispersed by gentle reheating.

6. Sometimes polyacrylamide gels may not polymerize fully, especially if the 10% AMPS solution was not fresh. Since the well dividers are usually the last parts of the gel to polymerize, this can lead to the loss of the gel. A partly polymerized gel can usually be saved by incubating for 20 min at 37°C provided this is done before the gel has been poured for too long.

7. Polyacrylamide gels can be poured the day before use provided they are prevented from drying out. Place the polymerized gel inside the electrophoresis tank with running buffer before leaving overnight. Alternatively, cover the comb end of the gel with damp paper towels and wrap in cling film.

8. Pouring away solutions without losing the polyacrylamide gel during silver staining can be difficult. The gel can be held in place with gloved hands while pouring away solutions. However, the talc on some brands of disposable gloves can mark the gels and gloves must be changed once they have come into contact with any alkaline solution (especially solution C). A good tip is to use an old piece of X-ray film to hold the gel in place while changing solutions.

9. Sometimes while a gel is in silver staining solution 2 (0.1% $AgNO_3$) if it comes into accidental contact with a strong salt or alkali solution it may turn a milky white color as silver chloride precipitates. Continuing to stain a gel such as this is bound to fail. The gel can be saved by washing the gel twice briefly in dH_2O, immersing in a 2.5% solution of ammonia followed by rinsing twice in dH_2O. Silver staining should then be restarted using solution A (*see* Section 3.1.3.).

10. Silver-stained gels need not necessarily be dried down for long-term storage, they store quite adequately when sealed damp between plastic. Beware of damaging them by crushing with heavy objects (especially elbows!).

11. Care must be taken to ensure that genomic DNA is fully digested before Southern blotting. The distribution of DNA within partially digested tracks will be skewed to higher mol-wt fragments. Some DNA samples are consistently difficult to digest, probably because of carry-over of contaminating reagents from the DNA extraction. This problem can often be overcome by adding Spermidine to a concentration of 4 m*M* in the restriction digest. If this does not overcome the problem, a second phenol:chloroform extraction and precipitation is the only remedy.

12. Southern transfer of DNA from a gel to nylon membrane need not be an overnight step if there is some urgency. If the paper towels are changed every half hour for the first 2 h and subsequently every hour, transfer of fragments up to 12 kb can be achieved in 5 h. Consequently the membrane can be probed the same day.

13. If a membrane binds probe nonspecifically, as occasionally happens, it can usually be stripped and reprobed successfully. To strip a membrane, place in a plastic tray and boil 200 mL of dH$_2$O. Once the water has boiled, remove from the heat source, add SDS to a concentration of 0.5%, and pour onto the membrane. Leave on an orbital shaker for 10 min and repeat. Monitor the membrane with a Geiger counter, if radiation is now down to background level the membrane can be reprobed.

14. The oligonucleotide hybridization step described in Section 3.3.2. can be left overnight without any deterioration in quality of results. Short hybridization times are often quoted for this technique. This is because the kinetics of hybridization are much faster owing to the small probe size.

15. Some DNA samples are refractory to PCR amplification. Diluting out the inhibiting contaminant is the best way of circumventing this problem. Make a dilution series of genomic DNA, i.e., 1:20, 1:40, 1:80, 1:160 and try amplifying each separately. It is surprising how well these samples amplify once the contaminant is diluted out.

16. Great care must be taken to avoid cross contamination of PCR reactions. The most potent source of contaminating DNA are old PCR reactions. These should always be disposed of carefully. Pipets are a major medium of contamination and a set of pipets should be dedicated to the setting up of PCR reactions alone. Another set can then be used solely for post-PCR manipulations. Setting aside a special area of benching for setting up PCRs along with other dedicated items, such as racks, is good practice and further reduces the chances of PCR contamination. If primer stocks do become contaminated, placing the primers in a microcentrifuge tube on a shortwave UV transilluminator for 5–10 min will cure all but the most severe cases. UV irradiation nicks the contaminating DNA making it refractory to PCR amplification.

References

1. Verkerk, A. J. M. H., Pieretti, M., Sutcliffe, J. S., Fu, Y.-H., Kuhl, D. P. A, Pizzuti, A., et al. (1991) Identification of a gene (FMR-1) containing a CGG repeat coincident with a breakpoint cluster region exhibiting length variation in fragile X syndrome. *Cell* **65,** 905–914.

2. Brook, D. J., McCurrach, M. E., Harley, H. G., Buckler, A. J., Churh, D., Aburatani, H., et al. (1992) Molecular basis of myotonic dystrophy: expansion of a trinucleotide (CTG) repeat at the 3' end of a transcript encoding a protein kinase family member. *Cell* **68,** 799–808.

3. Huntington's Disease Collaborative Research Group (1993) A novel gene containing a trinucleotide repeat that is expanded and unstable on Huntington's disease chromosomes. *Cell* **72,** 971–983.

4. La Spada A. R., Wilson, E. M., Lubahn, D. B., Harding, A. E., and Fischbeck, K. H. (1991) Androgen receptor mutations in X-linked spinal and bulbar muscular atrophy. *Nature* **352,** 77–79.

5. Hirst, M. C., Nakahori, Y., Knight, S. J. L., Schwartz, C., Thibodeau, S. N., Roche, A., et al. (1991) Genotype prediction in the fragile X syndrome. *J. Med. Genet.* **28,** 824–829.

6. Mahadevan, M., Tsilfidis, C., Sabourin, L., Shutler, G., Amemiya, C., Jansen, G., et al. (1992) Myotonic dystrophy mutation: an unstable CTG repeat in the 3' untranslated region of the gene. *Science* **255,** 1253–1255.

7. Fu, Y.-H., Kuhl, D. P. A., Pizzuti, A., Pieretti, M., Sutcliffe, J. S., Richards, S., et al. (1991) Variation of the p(CGG)n repeat at the fragile X site results in genetic instability: resolution of the Sherman paradox. *Cell* **67,** 1047–1058.

8. Reiss, A. L., Kazazian, H. H., Krebs, C. M., McAughan, A., Boehm, C. D., Abrams, M. T., and Nelson, D. L. (1994) Frequency and stability of the fragile X premutation. *Hum. Mol. Genet.* **3,** 393–398.

9. Hirst, M. C., Prabjhit, K. G., and Davies, K. E. (1994) Precursor arrays for triplet repeat expansion at the fragile X locus. *Hum. Mol. Genet.* **3,** 1553–1560.

10. Brunner, H. G., Nillesen, W., vanOost, B. A., Jansen, G., Wieringa, B., Ropers, H.-H., and Smeets, H. J. M. (1992) Presymptomatic diagnosis of myotonic dystrophy. *J. Med. Genet.* **29,** 780–784.

11. Hunter, A., Tsilfidis, C., Mettler, G., Jacob, P., Mahadevan, M., and Korneluk, R. G. (1992) The correlation of age at onset with CTG trinucleotide repeat amplification in myotonic dystrophy. *J. Med. Genet.* **29,** 774–779.

12. Andrew, S. E., Goldberg, Y. P., Kremer, B., Telenius, H., Theilmann, J., Adam, S., et al. (1993) The relationship between (CAG) repeat length and clinical features of Huntington's disease. *Nature Genet.* **4,** 398–403.

13. Myers, R. H., MacDonald, M. E., Koroshetz, W. J., Duyao, M. P., Ambrose, C. M., Taylor, S. A. M., et al. (1993) *De novo* expansion of a $(CAG)_n$ repeat in sporadic Huntington's disease. *Nature Genet.* **5,** 168–173.

14. Goldberg, Y. P., Kremer, B., Andrew, S. E., Theilmann, J., Graham, R. K., Squitieri, F., et al. (1993) Molecular analysis of new mutations for Huntington's disease: intermediate alleles and sex of origin effects. *Nature Genet.* **5,** 174–179.

15. Andrew, S. E., Goldberg, Y. P., Theilmann, J., Zeisler, J., and Hayden, M. R. (1994) A CCG repeat polymorphism adjacent to the CAG repeat in the Huntington disease gene: implications for diagnostic accuracy and predictive testing. *Hum. Mol. Genet.* **3,** 65–67.

16. La Spada, A. R., Roling, D. B., Harding, A. E., Warner, C. L., Spiegel, R., Hausmanowa-Petrusewicz, I., et al. (1992) Meiotic stability and genotype-phenotype correlation of the trinucleotide repeat in X-linked spinal and bulbar muscular atrophy. *Nature Genet.* **2,** 301–304.

4

Searching for Mutations

Familial Adenomatous Polyposis as a Case Study

Ian M. Frayling and Andrew J. Rowan

1. Introduction

1.1. Overview

   The molecular diagnosis of a genetic disease can be made by demonstrating linkage of suitable markers to the disease allele. However, it is generally agreed that it is better to define the mutation responsible. There is a plethora of techniques available for the detection of mutations within genes. No one method is predominant, although single-stranded conformational polymorphism (SSCP) may be the single most widely used technique. The choice in any given situation is a complex function of a particular method's efficiency (i.e., the proportion of all mutations in a given set that are detected), reproducibility, ease, speed, and cost, coupled with local considerations, such as the equipment, expertise, and budget available. Factors specific to the disease and gene(s) concerned also play an important part: genes can vary greatly in size; mutations may be clustered in regions or occur in "hot spots"; some specific mutations may occur at a high frequency in a particular population; mutations may be mostly either mis-sense or non-sense; some diseases may have a high new mutation rate. In addition, the nature of the material available for diagnosis (e.g., stored DNA or lymphoblastoid cell line, formalin-fixed, or frozen tissue) may be a deciding factor. The priorities of providing a clinical service may be somewhat different from those of a research laboratory, but any laboratory's decision on the methods it employs will be governed by the cost-to-benefit ratio. All these points are illustrated when considering the molecular diagnosis of familial adenomatous polyposis (FAP). For service laboratories,

From: *Methods in Molecular Medicine: Molecular Diagnosis of Genetic Diseases*
Edited by: R. Elles Humana Press Inc., Totowa, NJ

however, there is the special consideration regarding whether the expense of mutation detection can be justified by the clinical benefit, but a discussion on the assessment of this is beyond the scope of this chapter.

Clinically, FAP is characterized by the development of multiple gastrointestinal (GI) adenomas, usually hundreds to thousands, one or more of which if left untreated inevitably progress to carcinomas. FAP may be one of the first inherited predispositions to cancer to have been described given the reports of Cripps and Bickersteth over a century ago (1,2). This propensity to develop GI adenomas is inherited in an autosomal dominant fashion, a characteristic of germline mutations in tumor suppressor genes (3–5). The adenomas are generally thought of as sited in the colorectum, but they also occur in the upper GI tract, where they are a source of considerable morbidity and mortality now that most patients are treated by prophylactic colectomy (6,7). There is, in addition, a wide spectrum of extraintestinal manifestations, including desmoid tumors, retinal hamartomas (congenital hypertrophy of the retinal pigment epithelium; CHRPE), sebaceous adenomas, osteomas, and dentiginous cysts. Gardner and Richards (8) first described a syndrome comprising the latter three features occurring in individuals with colonic polyposis from the same family, but most patients with FAP exhibit at least one of the extraintestinal features of Gardner's syndrome (9).

Germline mutations of the APC gene are responsible for FAP; the gene was first localized to 5q22 by exploiting a combination of serendipitous chromosomal deletions and linked genetic markers, which subsequently enabled it to be identified, the cDNA cloned, and its intron/exon structure determined (10–16). The early, restriction fragment length polymorphism (RFLP)-based, linked markers inevitably suffered from being mostly dimorphic, sited at some distance from the gene and requiring Southern analysis. There are now several more closely linked highly polymorphic polymerase chain reaction (PCR)-based microsatellite markers in the region, and diagnosis based on linkage is thus nowadays easier and more secure (17–19). However, successful linkage analysis is dependent on a suitable pedigree structure and material being available from as many family members as possible, including those unaffected and/or only related by marriage; conditions that often cannot be fulfilled. In any event, in those families where the disease has arisen owing to a so-called new mutation, linkage analysis is of no help: It is estimated that between 10 and 30% of FAP cases arise as such (20–23).

The APC gene, and the spectrum and site of germline mutations within it responsible for FAP, show certain features that both assist and complicate mutation detection. The APC gene has a protein-coding region approx 8.5-kb long spread over 15 exons. These in turn are spread over some 100–150 kb of genomic DNA (gDNA), and the full-length mature APC protein is predicted to be 2843 amino acids long with, assuming no posttranslational modifications, an M_r of 311, 658 *(14)*. The *APC* mRNA shows alternate splicing of some exons, e.g., exons 7 and 9/9a *(14,24)*. Exons 1–14 vary in size from 78 (exon 12) to 379 bp (exon 9/9a). Together they account for 23% of the protein-coding region of the gene. Exon 15, however, is remarkable for its size. At some 7.5 kb long, it is one of the largest, if not the largest, eukaryotic exon yet described. On the basis of the sites of the various PCR primers, which they used to amplify exon 15 piecemeal, Groden et al. *(14)* divided it into 23 overlapping regions, viz. 15A–15W. The 5' untranslated region (UTR) of the *APC* mRNA is encoded by a number of alternately spliced exons; some are subject to alternate splicing in conjunction with exon 1; one is sited close to a candidate promoter region *(24–26)*. The full significance of these findings is as yet unclear, but the alternate splicing appears, at least to some extent, to be tissue specific. It may be that reports of unequal expression of *APC* alleles in association with FAP are owing to mutations in promoter or related regions, but these are rare and only likely to account for a small proportion of FAP families *(27)*.

What is evident, however, is that the majority of *APC* germline mutations responsible for FAP are non-sense or frame-shift in nature and result in premature termination of the APC protein *(28–31)*. Of 174 published mutations reviewed by Nagase et al. *(32)*, only six were mis-sense. The siting within the gene of mutations associated with FAP is also of interest. FAP-associated mutations have been described between codons 168 (3' end of exon 4) and 2839 (3' end of exon 15) inclusive. However, most are found in the region between codons 168 (exon 4) and codon 1640 (exon 15), with a particular concentration in a 2-kb region of exon 15 between codons 900 and 1600 *(32)*. Two mutations, at codons 1061 and 1309 (both 5-bp deletions), are the most commonly observed, together accounting for maybe one-fifth of all FAP mutations, and they probably represent germline mutational "hot spots" *(28)*. It should be borne in mind that all present estimates of the prevalence, and even types, of individual mutations are biased. The direction and extent of the bias depend on the particular mutation detection method(s) used and/or the proportion of the gene searched.

Some clues to the site of a family's mutation may be gained from phenotype. Olschwang et al. *(33)* found that the likelihood of finding CHRPE in a family was related to the position of the mutation with respect to exon 9 (codons 312–412): CHRPE was associated with mutations located 3' to exon 9 (although by no means all mutations 3' of exon 9 were associated with CHRPE), and mutations 5' to exon 9 had a low probability of association, whereas those within exon 9 had an intermediate likelihood. Mutation in exon 6 has been found to be associated with late age-of-onset of colorectal polyps *(34)*, whereas a variant of FAP in which the number of colorectal adenomas is much reduced, known as attenuated adenomatous polyposis coli (AAPC), seems to be associated with mutations located 5' of codon 160 (exon 4), at least as far as codon 83 (exon 3) *(35,36)*. However, the question of attenuated disease is complicated by some interpreting it as necessarily late onset, which may not be a valid distinction *(37)*. The phenotype associated with complete absence of the *APC* gene is still the subject of debate. It would be reasonable to predict that loss of one *APC* allele, in the absence of any other hemizygosity in the surrounding area, will be associated with an AAPC or AAPC-like phenotype. Almost all reported cases to date have a visible cytogenetic deletion involving 5q22 and, as might be expected, are associated with some degree of intellectual impairment *(38)*. It is interesting that the intellectual handicap in these individuals seems to be an impairment of communication of abstract concepts. Hence, an assessment of the level of handicap based on purely verbal criteria results in these individuals being considered more handicapped than they actually are.

All these different correlations are by no means absolute, but may be useful in deciding where or how to start looking for an individual family's mutation. The fact remains that for the majority of FAP cases, there is only the balance of probability to go on, i.e., that the mutation probably lies between codons 168 and 1600, most likely at codons 1309 or 1061, but could be anywhere between codons 1 and 2843, or even outside of this. Finally, it should be noted that there may be genetic heterogeneity in FAP *(39–41)*.

1.2. Choice of Methods

The methods described later in this chapter, which we have used and adapted to screen for germline mutations responsible for FAP, will be, we hope, of use to those also working in this area or who wish to apply the techniques to other genes. The two methods that we initially decided to use were chemical cleavage of mismatch (CCM; Fig. 1) *(42–45)* and DNA heteroduplex analysis (HDA) *(46,47)*. Lately, we have started to screen for mutations with the protein truncation test (PTT; Fig. 2) *(27,48)*. If we were starting again now, PTT would be our first choice, but as will be seen, the other methods have their merits and have not been completely supplanted. All these techniques are dependent on the amplification of DNA by means of PCR, using as a template either gDNA or complementary DNA (cDNA), the latter synthesized by reverse transcription from mRNA. A major consideration in the initial choice of CCM was the desire to use the most efficient (and inherently least biased) method available *(49)*. As is seen later, although this might involve using a technique that takes longer to perform, there is a payoff when screening the *APC* gene in being able to screen large DNA fragments, thus requiring rather fewer PCRs than if using the simpler, but less efficient method of SSCP. The methods are used in a complementary fashion, usually depending on the material available from affected members of a particular family, i.e., DNA or RNA. DNA is

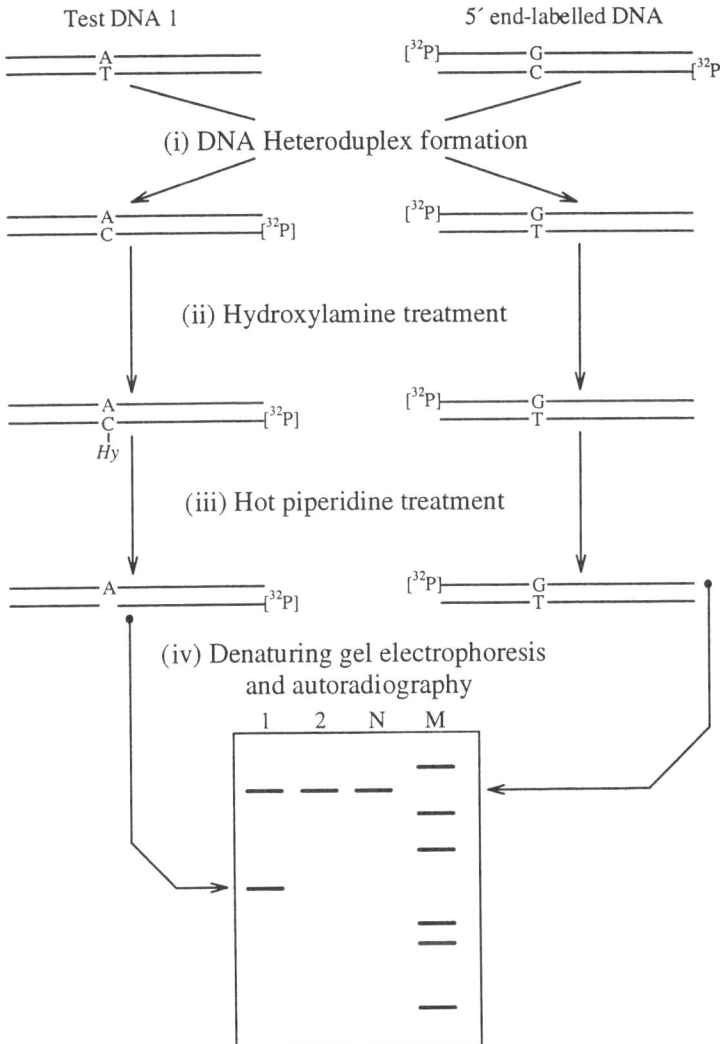

Fig. 1. Diagram showing the principal steps in CCM: (i) [^{32}P]-End-labeled probe DNA is annealed with test DNA; (ii) the resulting heteroduplexes are treated with either osmium tetroxide or, as in this example, hydroxylamine, which reacts with mis- or unmatched cytosine residues (osmium reacts similarly with thymine residues); (iii) hot piperidine treatment cleaves the DNA at those sites where bases have reacted; and (iv) the cleavage products are then separated by PAGE under denaturing conditions and their positions determined by autoradiography. Note that homoduplexes that form in step (i) are not shown; normally an excess of test DNA over probe is used to minimize their formation. From a comparison between the positions of [^{32}P]-labeled DNA size markers and the cleaved products, an accurate estimate of the distance of the mutation from the end of the DNA fragment can be obtained.

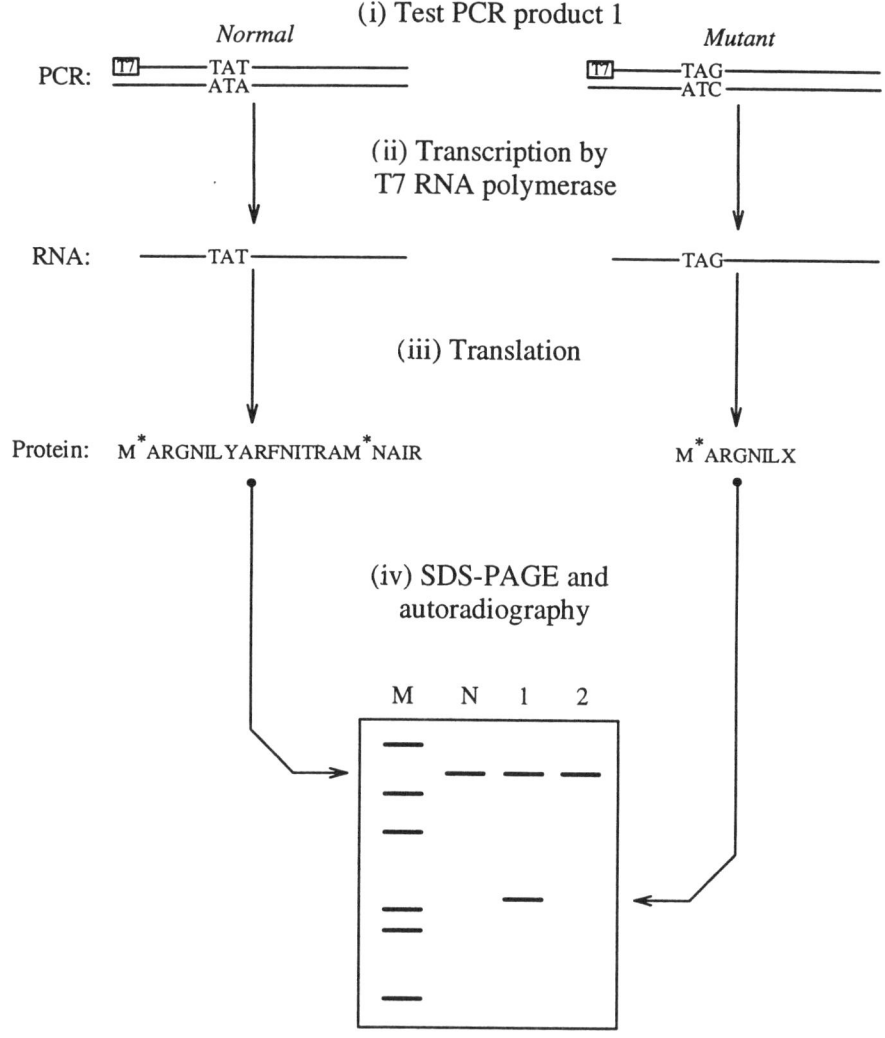

Fig. 2. Diagram showing the principle steps in the PTT: (i) the DNA sequence of interest is amplified by PCR using a sense-strand primer, including a T7 RNA polymerase (transcription start) site and in-frame start codon (ATG); (ii) RNA is synthesized by T7 RNA polymerase using the PCR product as the template; (iii) which is then simultaneously translated into protein in the presence of a labeled amino acid (in this example [^{35}S]-methionine, but [^{3}H]-leucine or biotin-labeled lysine can be used); and (iv) the labeled polypeptide reaction products are separated by SDS-PAGE and detected by autoradiography. Mutant DNAs containing premature stop codons give rise to smaller-sized products, the precise size of which can be used to give an estimate of the site of the mutation (bearing in mind that the stop codon generated by some frame-shifting mutations can be downstream of the mutation itself).

obtained, whenever possible, by purification from blood (Nucleon™ Genomic DNA Extraction Kit; Scotlab, Strathclyde, UK), but in those instances where a living affected member of the family is not available, it is extracted from the wax-embedded histologically normal tissue of a deceased affected relative *(50)*. RNA is usually extracted from a lymphoblastoid cell line, but could be from fresh blood or snap-frozen normal tissue, e.g., colonic mucosa *(51)*.

For PCR amplification of exons 1–14, we use the oligonucleotide primers given in Groden et al. *(14)*, but omitting the M13 universal primer sequence tags. These are mostly sited within the introns, the exceptions being the forward primers for exons 1 (immediately adjacent to the start codon), 3, 4, and 9a, and the reverse primer for exon 9, all sited within the exons themselves. However, Groden et al. *(52)* subsequently published replacements for two of these, that for exon 1 sited well upstream of the start codon and that for exon 3 sited within the intron (Table 1). Exon 9/9a we amplify in a single PCR, utilizing the forward primer for exon 9 and the reverse primer for exon 9a, and using the same conditions as the exon 15 PCRs. The primers Groden et al. *(14)* originally described for exon 15 amplify the exon as a series of 23 overlapping regions (15A–W), which were screened for mutations by SSCP and of necessity had to be no longer than about 250 bp. One of the advantages of CCM is that it can screen DNA fragments as large as 1.5 kb. For this reason, we amplify exon 15 in only six overlapping PCRs, of up to 1.4 kb at a time, which we term 15.1–15.6 (Table 2). This compares most favorably with the number of PCRs originally deemed necessary, especially in view of the concentration of mutations between codons 900 and 1600 (covered by our regions 15.1–15.3). Thus, we screen 99.78% of the protein-coding region of the gene in 20 (14 + 6) PCRs rather than the 38 that Groden et al. *(14)* described. The 0.22% that is not screened corresponds to basepairs 423–442 (codons 141–147) at the 5' end of exon 4, because of the forward primer being sited partially within the exon (Table 1). The order in which we screen PCR products has evolved in response to the likelihood of finding mutations: we screen 15.1–15.3 first, followed by exons 6–14 and then 5–1 (in that order), finally analyzing 15.4–15.6.

Before carrying out CCM analysis of the exon 15 PCR-amplified fragments, we have found it convenient to screen them first by HDA on MDE™ gels, a quick and simple method with acceptable efficiency *(53,54)*. Although the size of these fragments might be thought to be too large for efficient mutation detection by this method, we are able to detect a worthwhile proportion of mutations, not surprisingly deletions and insertions rather than point mutations. We routinely detect the common 5-bp deletions at codons 1061 and 1309 by this method (Fig. 3, p. 73). It ideally requires some form of low-temperature-controlled vertical electrophoresis equipment, but this does not need to be sophisticated. Samples screening negative by HDA are subsequently analyzed by CCM.

Table 1
The *APC* Gene: Exons 1–14[a]

Exon	Length, bp[b]	Position[c]	Codons[d]	PCR primer[e], 5'–3'
1	>135	−33–135	1–45	1F: ATTAACACAATTCTTCTTAAACGTC[f]
				1R: TAAAAATGGATAAACTACAATTAAAAG
2	85	136–220	46–74	2F: AAATACAGAATCATGTCTTGAAGT
				2R: ACACCTAAAGATGACAATTTGAG
3	202	221–422	74–141	3F: GACCCAAGTGGACTTTTCAGG[f]
				3R: ACAATAAACTGGAGTACACAAGG
4	109	442–531	148–177[g]	4F: ATAGGTCATTGCTTCTGCTGAT[h]
				4R: TGAATTTAATGGATTACCTAGGT
5	114	532–645	178–215	5F: CTTTTTTTGCTTTTACTGATTAACG
				5R: TGTAATTCATTTTATTCCTAATAGCTC
6	84	646–729	216–243	6F: GGTAGCCATAGTATGATTATTTCT
				6R: CTACCTATTTTTATACCCACAAAC
7	105	730–834	244–278	7F: AAGAAAGCCTACACACATTTTGC
				7R: GATCATTCTTAGAACCATCTTGC
8	99	835–933	279–311	8F: ACCTATAGTCTAAATTATACCATC
				8R: GTCATGGCATTAGTGACCAG
9/9a	379	934–1312	312–438	9F: AGTCGTAATTTGTTTCTAAACTC
				9aR: GCTTTGAAACATGCACTACGAT
10	96	1313–1408	438–470	10F: AAACATCATTGCTCTTCAAATAAC
				10R: TACCATGATTAAAAATCCACCAG
11	140	1409–1548	470–516	11F: GATGATTGTCTTTTCCTCTTGC
				11R: CTGAGCTATCTTAAGAAATACATG
12	78	1549–1626	517–542	12F: TTTTAAATGATCCTCTTATTCTGTAT
				12R: ACAGAGTCAGACCCTGCCTCAAAG

13	117	1627–1743	543–581	13F: TTTCTATTCTTACTGCTAGCATT
				13R: ATACACAGGTAAGAAATTAGGA
14	215	1744–1958	582–653	14F: TAGATGACCCATATTCTGTTTC
				14R: CAATTAGGTCTTTTGAGAGTA

aAs described in Groden et al. (14).
bLength of the exons themselves, not the PCR products.
cThose basepairs within each exon that are screened, numbered according to the sequence in Joslyn et al. (15).
dThose codons partially or wholly screened.
eAs given in Groden et al. (14).
fAs in Groden et al. (52), but omitting the M13 universal primer sequences.
gExon 4 comprises codons 141–177.
hThe only primer not sited wholly within an intron, showing underlined the region sited in exon 4.

Table 2
The *APC* Gene: Exon 15 Regions and PCR Primers

Region	Length, bp[a]	Position[b]	Codons[c]	PCR primers, 5'–3'
15.1	1018	(1959–14)–2916	653–972	15.1F: GTGACCTTAATTTTGTGATCTCT
				15.1R: TTCATTTGACCTCTTTACCATA
15.2	992	2874–3819	959–1273	15.2F: TATGCCAAATTAGAATACAAGAG
				15.2R: GACAAAGATGATAATGAACTACA
15.3	1152	3784–4886	1262–1628	15.3F: TTAACCAAGAAACAATACAGACT
				15.3R: CATCCCCGGTGTAAAACTAACA
15.4	1197	4867–6017	1623–2005	15.4F: ACAAACTTCTACCATCACAAAAC
				15.4R: CATGAAATGATTAGGAGCATAG
15.5	1329	6005–7287	2003–2429	15.5F: CTCACAGGGAGAACCAAGTAAAC
				15.5R: AATACAGGTCTTTCTGATCTATC
15.6	1415	7247–8615	2417–2843	15.6F: TGGAGCCAATAAAAAGGTAGAAC
				15.6R: CCTATTTACAAAATTTTTCAGTC

[a]Length of the PCR products.
[b]Those bases between the primer pairs, numbered according to Joslyn et al. (15).
[c]Those complete codons between the primers.

APC Region: 15.1   15.2   15.3

N 1 n N 2 n N 3 4 M

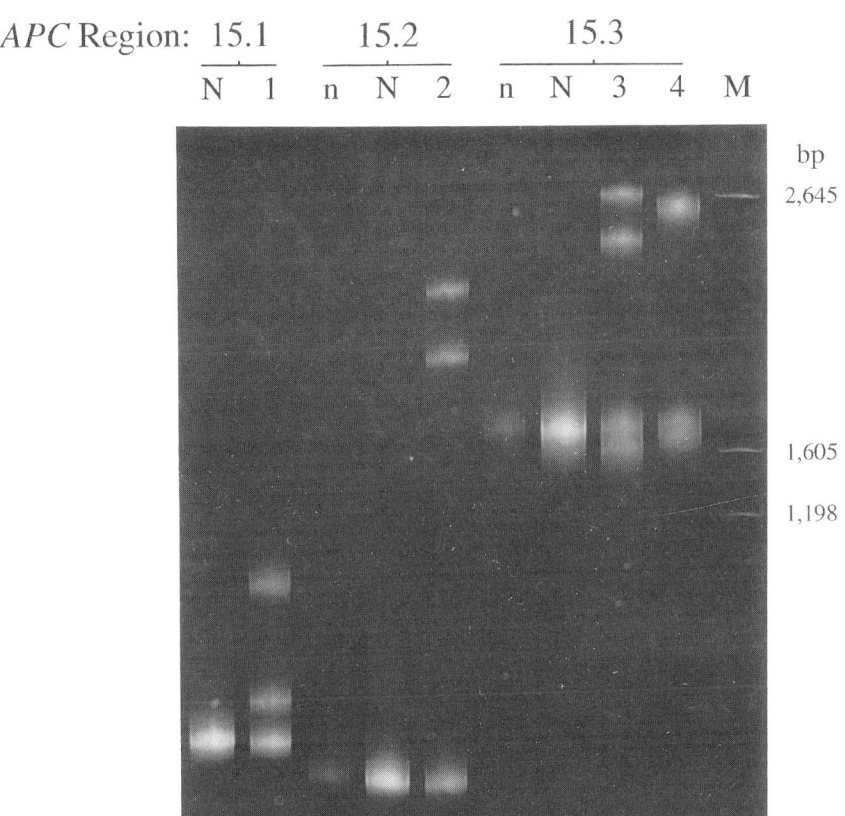

bp
2,645

1,605

1,198

Fig. 3. Analysis of DNA heteroduplexes of *APC* mutants by MDE gel electrophoresis. PCR products from four individuals known to have a mutation in exon 15 (regions 15.1–15.3) of the *APC* gene were heat denatured and then allowed to reanneal, forming heteroduplexes between the wild-type and mutant alleles. These were then subjected to electrophoresis under native conditions (1X MDE gel, 0.6X TBE, 150 g/L urea; 20 cm gel run at 20 V/cm for 16 h). The gel was stained after running with ethidium bromide and then photographed with UV transillumination. All lanes were loaded with 10 μL of purified PCR product (equivalent to 20 μL of raw PCR), except for lane "n," which was loaded with 2 μL. The various DNA fragments do not run strictly according to size, because this is a native gel run without ethidium bromide. Heteroduplexes are evident, which have retarded migration with respect to the wild-type homoduplexes, in the samples containing mutant product. Two homoduplex bands are seen in mutant samples 3 and 4 corresponding to wild-type:wild-type and mutant:mutant duplexes. M, pGEM™ DNA markers (Promega); N and n, PCR product from normal individual; 1, 2-bp deletion at codon 796 (CTATGCTG); 2, 5-bp deletion at codon 1061 (AACAAAGAG); 3, 5-bp deletion at codon 1309 (AAAAGATAT); and 4, 3-bp deletion at codon 1396 (GAGAGGG).

Chemical cleavage of mismatch exploits the fact that hydroxylamine (Hy) and osmium tetroxide (Os) will react with un- or mismatched bases in heteroduplexed DNA, which can then be cleaved at these sites with hot piperidine (Fig. 1) *(42,55,56)*. If the DNA was end-labeled with [^{32}P] before heteroduplex formation, then autoradiography after gel electrophoresis will reveal those DNA fragments that have been shortened, i.e., cleaved at a mismatch. If labeled size markers are included on the gel, then the site of the mismatch can be deduced. Because hydroxylamine is specific for mis- or unmatched C residues, and osmium tetroxide is specific for mis- or unmatched T-residues, then additional information regarding the nature of the mismatch is gained. As a way of screening for mutations, CCM has been overshadowed by superficially quicker and simpler methods, such as SSCP. This is understandable since CCM requires the use of toxic and carcinogenic chemicals, although the amounts involved are very small, as well as radioactivity. What may be a greater disincentive is the requirement for a fume-hood suitable for use with toxic reagents, carcinogens, and [^{32}P], which could involve considerable expense if a laboratory does not already have one. On paper, CCM appears more time consuming than many other mutation detection methods, but some steps can be semiautomated or circumvented, and it is possible to use fluorescently labeled primers and analyze the reaction products on an automated sequencer *(57)*. Where larger DNAs can be screened (as with exon 15 of *APC*), CCM compares favorably with other methods. Chemical cleavage of mismatch also gives precise information on the position and nature of the possible mutation detected, which is often most useful during subsequent sequencing.

Mutation detection methods based on biochemical or functional tests of gene products are also being developed, and are likely to prove to be of increasing utility. One of these, the PTT, is an application of the technique of in vitro-coupled transcription and translation (IVTT), which exploits the protein-truncating nature of some mutations (Fig. 2) *(27,48,58)*. There are two features of FAP and the *APC* gene that make PTT a particularly attractive method in this instance. First, most FAP mutations result in either novel stop codons or frame shifts, which lead to premature termination of the APC protein. Second, the large size of exon 15, where a high proportion of mutations happen to be located, means that gDNA can be used as the PCR template, rather than having to use cDNA. A major feature of PTT, which is more generally useful, is that it can be used to screen a number of exons simultaneously, although this does necessitate a source of mRNA; for *APC*, this allows screening of exons 1–14 in just two tests. When performed using cDNA, the PTT is also potentially capable of detecting abnormalities of message splicing, which may not be picked up using other techniques, but it is not, at present, capable of detecting mis-sense mutations. It should also be mentioned that PTT does not detect all those mutations, which would be predicted from the genomic sequence to cause premature termination of the protein. The reasons for this are not apparent, but may involve message stability in vivo or in vitro, or close proximity of the mutation to one end of the PCR fragment.

In a small minority of cases in which a mutation is not apparent within the protein-coding region, other techniques will need to be employed, e.g., studies of allele-specific expression. Gross cytogenetic deletions involving 5q22 will probably have been picked up in cases with intellectual impairment. Otherwise chromosomal microdeletions should be suspected in cases where linked markers show unexpected apparent homozygosity. Chromosomal deletions also might be found by pulsed-field gel electrophoresis or fluorescence *in situ* hybridization.

1.3. Linkage Analysis

In those instances when mutation detection is not possible, not successful, or is limited in extent and does not find the mutation responsible, then linkage analysis can be carried out. It also can be of use when a mis-sense mutation has been found and additional evidence is needed that it is pathogenic, i.e., responsible for FAP in a particular family. Chromosomal microdeletions are a rare cause of FAP. They should be suspected when the linked marker pattern suggests nonpaternity or nonmaternity, but analysis of markers on other chromosomes has excluded these hypotheses. If an individual has not inherited a chromosomal marker allele from a parent, this almost certainly means that he or she is hemizygous and has a deletion involving one copy of the *APC* gene. Although it is possible to use the Southern analysis-based RFLPs, the PCR-based microsatellites are far more convenient and more likely to be informative. We would advocate the use of flanking markers, e.g., the distal markers LNS *(D5S346 [DP-1] [59])* and/or MBC *(MCC [60])*, together with the proximal markers CB26 *(D5S299 [60])* and/or CA83A *(D5S122 [61])*. It is possible to multiplex these *(see* Chapter 10). There are a number of intragenic polymorphisms *(62–65)*, but they are in linkage disequilibrium, which reduces their utility (Bodmer, W. F. and Cottrell, S., personal communication, 1995). However, they can be of use, for example, in studying allele-specific expression.

2. Materials

2.1. PCR

1. *Taq* DNA-polymerase (5 U/μL), store at –20°C.
2. 10X *Taq* DNA-polymerase buffer: 100 mM Tris-HCl, 500 mM KCl, 15 mM MgCl$_2$, 1% (v/v) Triton-X 100, pH 9.0 (20°C), store at –20°C.
3. dNTP Mix (100 mM total dNTPs): 25 mM each of dATP, dCTP, dGTP, and TTP, make from equal amounts of 100 mM stock dNTPs (Pharmacia, Milwaukee, WI), and store at –20°C.

4. Oligonucleotide primers: For CCM and HDA, *see* Tables 1 and 2, and for PTT, *see* Table 3. Stock 250-μ*M* solutions of primers, in 20 m*M* Tris-HCl, 1 m*M* Na$_2$EDTA, pH 8.0, are stored at –20°C. Each primer pair is diluted with water in a forward and reverse primer mix, with each primer at 10 μ*M*.

5. Water: water for injections, 10-mL polyethylene ampules, store at room temperature.

6. Mineral oil (Sigma, St. Louis, MO), store at room temperature.

7. Loading dye: 0.1% (w/v) bromophenol blue, 0.1% (w/v) xylene cyanole, 25 m*M* Na$_2$EDTA (pH 8.0), 80% (w/v) sucrose, make by adding dyes to the boiled syrup, and store at room temperature.

8. Electrophoresis buffer (TBE): 89 m*M* Tris-borate, 1 m*M* Na$_2$EDTA (pH 8.0). Make as 5X stock and dilute prior to use with addition of 300 μg/L of ethidium bromide (using 10 g/L stock ethidium bromide [Sigma]), and store at room temperature.

9. Agarose: 1.5% (w/v) solution of LE Seakem® Agarose (FMC Bioproducts, Rockland, ME) in 1X TBE containing 300 μg/L of ethidium bromide.

10. Wizard™ PCR Preps DNA Purification System (Promega, Madison, WI).

2.2. Heteroduplex Analysis (HDA) on MDE (Hydrolink™) Gels

1. 2X MDE™ gel concentrate (FMC Bioproducts), store at room temperature.

2. 0.5*M* Na$_2$EDTA, pH 8.0.

3. Ammonium persulfate (Sigma): 10% (w/v) solution in distilled water, store at 4°C. Keep for 1 wk only.

4. *N,N,N',N'*-tetramethylethylenediamine (TEMED) (Sigma), store in the dark at 4°C.

5. Urea (UltraPure enzyme-grade; Gibco BRL, Paisley, UK).

6. Electrophoresis buffer (TBE) (*see* Section 2.1., item 8).

7. Loading dye (*see* Section 2.1., item 7).

8. Ethidium bromide solution: 1 mg/L ethidium bromide in 0.6X TBE, make using 10 g/L stock ethidium bromide (Sigma). Store at room temperature, either in the dark or a dark glass bottle.

2.3. CCM

1. T4 Polynucleotide kinase, 10 U/μL (Promega), store at –20°C.

2. 10X T4 Polynucleotide kinase buffer (Promega), store at –20°C.

3. Redivue™ [γ-^{32}P]-ATP (3000 Ci/mmol; Amersham, Little Chalfont, UK), store at 4°C.

4. TE buffer: 10 m*M* Tris-HCl, 1 m*M* Na$_2$EDTA, pH 7.5, autoclave and store at room temperature.

5. Sephadex® G-50 (Pharmacia): make up in TE buffer as per manufacturer's instructions, and store at 4°C.

6. 2X Annealing buffer: 0.6*M* NaCl, 7 m*M* MgCl$_2$, 6 m*M* Tris-HCl, pH 7.7, store at 4°C.

7. Hydroxylammonium chloride (HO · NH$_3$Cl; BDH) or hydroxylamine hydrochloride (Sigma), store at room temperature.

8. Diethylamine (Sigma), store at room temperature.

9. Pyridine (Sigma), store at room temperature.

Table 3
The APC Gene: PTT Primers

Region	Length, bp[a]	Position[b]	Codons[c]	PCR primers, 5'-3'
Exons 1-6	707	25-731	9-243 (28,000)	114pF: T7[d]-GCTGCAGCTTCATATGATCAG 7Re: ATGCTTGTTCTGAGATGAC
Exons 1-15.2	2383	25-2326	9-775 (86,000)	114pF: T7-GCTGCAGCTTCATATGATCAG 114pR: CCTTGGGACTTAAATTGTCTA
15p1	1922	1979-3819	661-1273 (70,000)	15p1F: T7-CAAATCCTAAGAGAGAAACA 15.2R: GACAAAGATGATAATGAACTACA[e]
15p2	2655	3385-5955	1129-1985 (95,000)	15p2F: T7-AATCAAAATGTAAGCCAGTCT 15p2R: GGGCTCAGTCTCTTTGATAGG
15p3	3049	5680-8645	1894-2843 (103,000)	15p3F: T7-AATAAGGAATCAGAGGCTAAA 15p3R: CAGAACAAAAACCCTCTAACAAG

[a]Length of the PCR products.
[b]Those bases between the primer pairs, numbered according to Joslyn et al. (15).
[c]Those complete codons between the primers, with (in parentheses) the M_r of the predicted full-size polypeptide product (calculated from the sequence).
[d]T7-, GGATCCTAATACGACTCACTATAGGAACAGACCACCATG.
[e]As used for region 15.2; see Table 2.

10. Osmium tetroxide, 4% (w/v) solution (Sigma), store at room temperature. This is supplied in glass ampules that are opened and the contents aliquoted into small (4-mL) glass bottles with polypropylene lids, which are then wrapped in aluminum foil (to exclude light) and stored in a sealed plastic box at 4°C. For waste disposal, *see* Note 21.
11. Stannous chloride solution: 100 g/L $SnCl_2$ (BDH, Poole, UK) in $1M$ HCl.
12. Mussel glycogen, 20 mg/mL (Boehringer Mannheim GmbH, Mannheim, Germany), store at –20°C.
13. Precipitation solution: $0.3M$ sodium acetate, 0.1 mM Na_2EDTA, make from $3M$ sodium acetate (pH 5.0) and $0.5M$ Na_2EDTA (pH 8.0), store at 4°C.
14. Ethanol, store at room temperature.
15. Piperidine (Sigma), store at room temperature.
16. Formamide loading buffer: 96% (v/v) formamide (Sigma), 20 mM Na_2EDTA (pH 8.0), 0.05% (w/v) each bromophenol blue and xylene cyanole, store at 4°C.
17. Electrophoresis buffer (TBE) (*see* Section 2.1., item 8).
18. Sigmacote® (Sigma), store at 4°C.
19. Sequagel™ Sequencing System (National Diagnostics, Atlanta, GA).
20. Ammonium persulfate (*see* Section 2.2., item 3).
21. TEMED (*see* Section 2.2., item 4).

2.4. Reverse Transcription of RNA

1. Oligonucleotide primer 15.1R, stock solution of 250 μM, as in Section 2.1., item 4, dilute to 10 μM in sterile water, and store at –20°C.
2. M-MLV Reverse transcriptase, RNase H Minus (Promega).
3. 5X Reverse transcription buffer (Promega).
4. Dithiothreitol (DTT): $0.1M$ solution in sterile water, store at –20°C.
5. RNasin ribonuclease inhibitor (Promega), store at –20°C.
6. dNTP Mix (100 mM total dNTPs) (*see* Section 2.1., item 4).
7. Water (*see* Section 2.1., item 5).
8. First-Strand cDNA Synthesis Kit (Pharmacia; *see* Note 33).

2.5. PTT

1. TNT® T7 Coupled Reticulocyte Lysate System (Promega), store per manufacturer's instructions.
2. L-[^{35}S]-Methionine in vivo cell labeling grade (>1000 Ci/mmol; Amersham), store at –20°C.
3. RNasin™ ribonuclease inhibitor (Promega), store at –20°C.
4. TE buffer (*see* Section 2.3., item 4).
5. 2X SDS-PAGE loading buffer: 20% (v/v) glycerol, 6% w/v SDS, $0.1M$ DTT, 0.05% (w/v) bromophenol blue, store at –20°C.
6. Tris buffer (for resolving gel): $1.5M$ Tris-HCl, 0.4% (w/v) SDS, pH 8.8, store at room temperature.
7. Tris buffer (for stacking gel): $0.5M$ Tris-HCl, 0.4% (w/v) SDS, pH 6.8, store at room temperature.

8. Stock acrylamide solution: 30% (w/v) acrylamide, 0.8% (w/v) bis-acrylamide (BDH), store at 4°C.
9. Ammonium persulfate solution (10% [w/v]) (*see* Section 2.2., item 3).
10. TEMED (*see* Section 2.2., item 4).
11. Rainbow™ Protein markers: high range (Amersham), store at –20°C.
12. SDS-PAGE running buffer: 25 mM Tris base (3.0 g/L), 192 mM glycine (14.4 g/L), 0.1% (w/v) SDS (5 mL of 20% [w/v] SDS/L), store at room temperature.
13. SDS-PAGE gel fix solution: aqueous 10% (v/v) methanol, 10% (v/v) acetic acid.

3. Methods

3.1. PCR

1. Prepare a master PCR mix, referring to Table 4 for the volume of each reagent per sample to be amplified. Keep on ice until dispensed. Add the *Taq* DNA-polymerase immediately before use (*see* Note 1).
2. To 0.6-mL microcentrifuge tubes, add 2 μL of each DNA solution to be amplified (equivalent to 200–1000 ng DNA) or, for PTT from cDNA, add 10 μL of a cDNA reaction (Section 3.4.).
3. Add the appropriate volume of the master PCR mix to each tube, ensuring thorough mixing with the DNA. Add sufficient mineral oil to overlay the reaction mix. Cap the tubes and store on ice until ready to place in the thermal cycler (*see* Note 2).
4. Place the tubes in the thermal cycler, and perform the PCR. For conditions, *see* Table 5 (and Note 3).
5. When finished, check for satisfactory amplification by agarose gel electrophoresis. Include a suitable DNA size marker, e.g., ϕX174 *Hin*f I digest or pGEM™ (Promega) (*see* Notes 4 and 5).
6. It is necessary to purify the PCR products for use in CCM, using the Wizard™ PCR Preps DNA Purification System (Promega) and following the manufacturer's instructions. Elute from the resin with 50 μL of TE buffer, and store at 4°C or lower (*see* Note 6).

3.2. HDA on MDE Gels

1. Pipet 20 μL of each unpurified PCR (Section 3.1., step 5) into 0.6 mL-microcentrifuge tubes containing 1 μL of 0.5M Na$_2$EDTA, ensuring thorough mixing. Cover the reactions with some mineral oil, which can conveniently be taken from the original PCR (*see* Note 7).
2. Form DNA heteroduplexes by heating the tubes to 95°C for 3 min and then cooling to 37°C over approx 30 min (e.g., 30 s/°C). This reaction is best carried out using a thermal cycler.
3. Add 4 μL of loading dye, and mix thoroughly.
4. Cast an MDE gel in a suitable vertical electrophoresis system (e.g., Bio-Rad [Richmond, CA] Protean IIxi, using 20-cm plates and 1-mm spacers), with 1X MDE gel concentration, 0.6X TBE, and 150 g/L urea, as per manufacturer's instructions (*see* Note 8).
5. Wash out the wells and load the samples. Keep the tank cool with a suitable supply of cold water (*see* Note 9). Run the gel at 20 V/cm. An 18–20 h run is

Table 4
Master PCR Mixes: Reagent Volumes/Sample

Reagent	CCM/HDA Exons 1–15[a], µL	PTT From cDNA[b], µL	PTT From gDNA[c], µL
Water	76.7	29.1	37.1
10X PCR buffer	10.0	5.0	5.0
250 mM MgCl$_2$	—	—	—
dNTP mix[d]	0.8	0.4	0.4
Forward and reverse primer mix[e]	10.0	5.0	5.0
Taq DNA-polymerase (5 U/µL)	0.5	0.5	0.5
Total volume (per sample)	98	40	48

[a]Exons 1–14 (*see* Table 1) and regions 15.1–15.6 of exon 15 (*see* Table 2).
[b]Exons 1–6 and 1–15.2 (*see* Table 3).
[c]Exon 15, regions 15p1–15p3 (*see* Table 3).
[d]25 mM each dNTP.
[e]2.5 µM each.

Table 5
PCR Conditions for the *APC* Gene[a]

Region	Denaturing	Annealing	Extension
Exons 1, 2, 3, 5, 7, 8 and 10–14	94°C × 60 s	55°C × 60 s	72°C × 60 s
Exons 4 and 6	94°C × 60 s	58°C × 60 s	72°C × 60 s
Exons 9 and 15.1–15.6[b]	94°C × 60 s	52°C × 60 s	72°C × 120 s
PTT	94°C × 60 s	52°C × 80 s	72°C × 180 s

[a]All PCRs should be performed with a single initial denaturation step of 94°C × 120 s, followed by 34 cycles of denaturing, annealing, and extension, followed by a single final extension step of 72°C × 300 s.
[b]The PCRs for exon 9 and regions 15.1–15.6 can be carried out using the PTT conditions, i.e., an extension time of 180 s (*see* Note 3).

needed for the exon 15 regions 15.1–15.6, but only 6–8 h for the smaller exons: Refer to the manufacturer's instructions.

6. When finished, separate the glass plates, and stain the gels by immersing them in the ethidium bromide solution (1 mg/L in 0.6X TBE) for 15–20 min (*see* Note 10). Destain in 0.6X TBE for 20–30 min. View the stained gel on a UV-transilluminator.

7. Wild-type homoduplex DNAs usually migrate as a single band, but occasionally as a doublet. Heteroduplex DNAs give an additional doublet of bands (which may be close together appearing as one), almost always migrating more slowly than the wild-type homoduplex (Fig. 4, pp. 82,83). Sequencing is necessary to determine whether the sequence difference is a polymorphism or mutation.

3.3. CCM

There are essentially five steps in CCM (not including the preliminary PCR and purification):

1. Labeling of the probe DNA (usually wild type).
2. Formation of heteroduplexes between the probe and test samples.
3. Reaction of the heteroduplexes with hydroxylamine or osmium tetroxide.
4. Reaction with hot piperidine (to cleave sites of mismatch).
5. Separation of the reaction products by DNA-denaturing polyacrylamide gel electrophoresis followed by autoradiography (Fig. 1).

3.3.1. Labeling DNA for Use as the Probe

1. In a 0.6-mL microcentrifuge tube on ice and using the PCR product amplified from wild-type DNA, set up the following labeling reaction: 2 μL purified PCR product (50–100 ng), 1 μL 10X polynucleotide kinase buffer, 6 μL γ-^{32}P-ATP (3000 Ci/mmol; 60 μCi), and 1 μL T4 polynucleotide kinase (10 U/μL) (*see* Notes 11 and 12).
2. Incubate at 37°C for 30–60 min.
3. Add 50 μL of TE buffer to stop the reaction, and place the tube on ice.
4. Remove unincorporated γ-^{32}P-ATP by gel filtration through Sephadex G-50. This is conveniently performed by filling a 0.45-μm pore-size Ultrafree®-MC filter-spin column (Millipore, Bedford, MA) with the Sephadex, washing three times with 0.2 mL of TE buffer, each time spinning the column in a microcentrifuge for 10 s. The labeling reaction is then put onto the column and spun for 20 s at full speed in the microfuge (*see* Note 13).
5. Make up the volume of the eluate (typically 70–80 μL) to 100 μL with water. If not used immediately, the probe should be stored at –20°C or lower (for up to 2 wk depending on the labeling efficiency).

3.3.2. DNA Heteroduplex Formation

Each test DNA is now heteroduplexed with the labeled wild-type DNA (*see* Note 14).

1. In 0.6-mL microcentrifuge tubes, mix: 3 μL purified PCR product (100–200 ng), 8 μL 2X annealing buffer, and 5 μL [^{32}P]-labeled probe. The probe and annealing buffer can be premixed and dispensed in 13-μL aliquots, prior to addition of the PCR product. Ensure the tubes are tightly capped (*see* Note 15).
2. Form heteroduplexes by heating the tubes to 95°C for 5 min and then annealing at 42°C for 100–120 min (*see* Note 16). This is best carried out using a thermal cycler.
3. Briefly spin the tubes in a microcentrifuge to bring down any condensation from the inside of the lids (*see* Note 17).

3.3.3. Hydroxylamine Treatment

Either this step, *or* the next (Section 3.3.4.), is carried out on each heteroduplexed sample (*but see* Note 14).

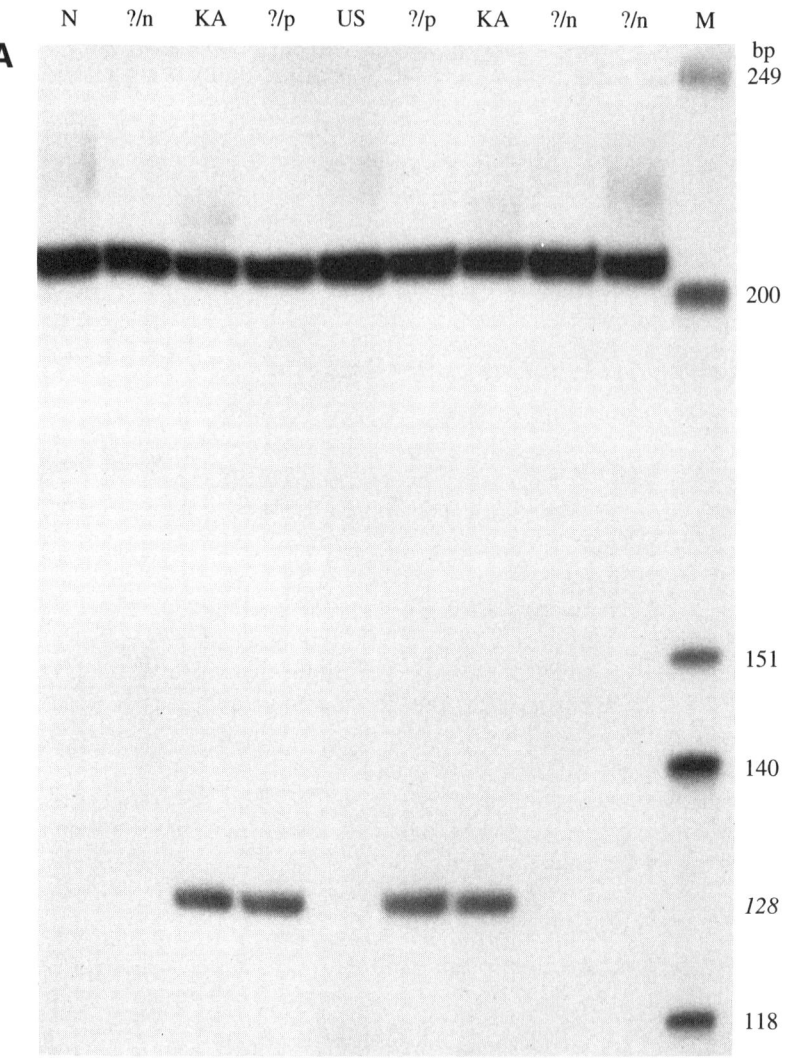

Fig. 4. CCM analysis of FAP families with *APC* exon 6 mutations. Autoradiographs of CCM gels. Testing carried out on members of two FAP families with mutations in *APC* exon 6: **(A)** a Q233X mutation (CAG→TAG), and **(B)** an R216X mutation (CGA→TGA). All reactions with hydroxylamine, and products run out on 6% denaturing polyacrylamide gels. Note the full-size PCR product at 204 bp and the cleavage products in (A) at 128 bp, and (B) at 76, 77, and 78 bp. Autoradiograph (B) also shows the generally consistent pattern of background bands, which is more obvious in films exposed for longer periods. Subsequent sequencing has shown the mutation in (B) to be at 77 bp, indicating that cleavage also took place at the guanine residues flanking

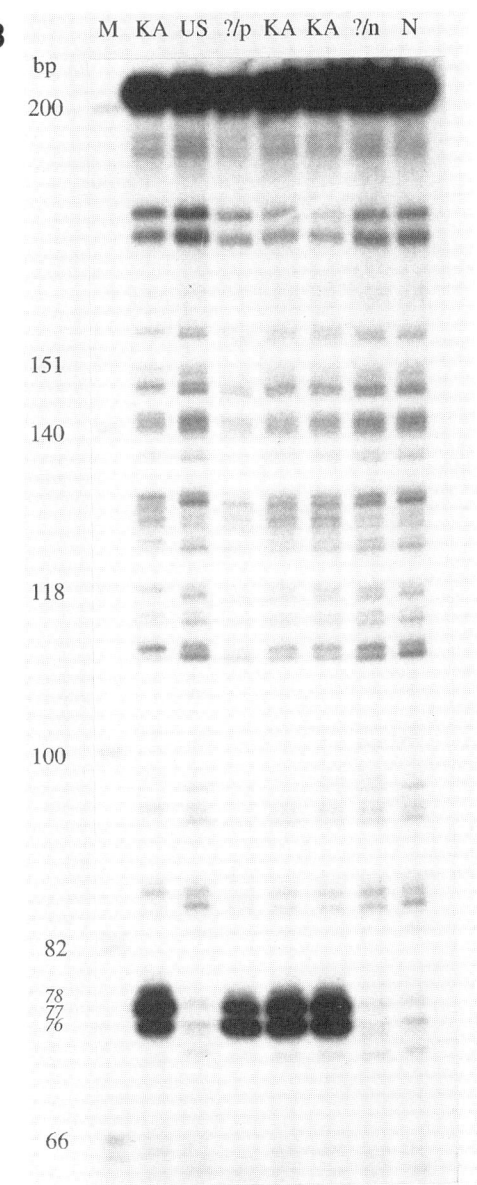

Fig. 4 *(continued)* the mutation. M, [^{32}P]-labeled markers; N, normal DNA (from which [^{32}P]-labeled probe was made); KA, sample from individual known to be affected with FAP; US, sample from unaffected spouse; ?/n, sample from individual at risk of inheriting the mutant allele testing negative; and ?/p, sample from individual at risk of inheriting the mutant allele testing positive.

1. Make a solution of hydroxylamine (approx 5*M*) by dissolving 1.4 g of hydroxyl-ammonium chloride in 1.6 mL of distilled water, and adjust to pH 6.0 with diethylamine (between 2 and 2.4 mL, depending on the batch of hydroxylam-monium chloride) (*see* Note 18).
2. To each 16-µL heteroduplex reaction, add 55 µL of the hydroxylamine solution.
3. Incubate at 37°C for 90 min. Proceed immediately to the cleavage step (Section 3.3.5.).

3.3.4. Osmium Tetroxide Treatment

1. In a 1.5-mL microcentrifuge tube, mix 1 mL of TE buffer (pH 8.0), 45 µL of pyridine, and 1 µL of osmium tetroxide (4% w/v), taking appropriate precautions. This mixture should be used immediately after mixing. It cannot be stored.
2. Add 40 µL of the osmium/pyridine mix to each 16-µL heteroduplex reaction. Ensure each tube is capped tightly, and then incubate at 37°C for 90 min (*see* Note 19). Proceed immediately to the cleavage step (Section 3.3.5.).

3.3.5. Heteroduplex Cleavage

1. Add 60 µL of mussel glycogen (20 g/L) to 2 mL of precipitation solution (Section 2.3., item 12).
2. To each heteroduplex reaction, which has been treated with *either* hydroxylamine (Section 3.3.3.) *or* osmium tetroxide (Section 3.3.4.), add 100 µL of the precipitation solution containing mussel glycogen. Then add 400 µL of ethanol, cap the tubes, and mix well. Cool to −20°C or lower for at least 15 min (*see* Note 20).
3. Spin the tubes at full speed in a microcentrifuge for 10 min at 4°C. Tip off the supernatant into a glass beaker, and, while keeping the tube inverted, touch it on some paper tissue to blot off the excess and prevent contamination of the outside of the tube (*see* Note 21).
4. Add 250 µL of 70% (v/v) ethanol, cap, and spin for 10 min at 4°C (*see* Note 22).
5. Carefully remove the 70% ethanol with a pipet, and allow the tubes to dry for a few minutes at room temperature with their lids open.
6. Make up a 1*M* solution of piperidine by adding 110 µL of the pure liquid to 1 mL of distilled water, and add 50 µL to each tube, ensuring that each tube is tightly capped.
7. Vortex mix each tube for at least 30 s to ensure that the pellets are completely dissolved. This is most important.
8. Heat the tubes to 90°C for 30 min. Use a heavy block to prevent any tube lids from opening, or else carry out the reaction in a thermal cycler with a lid.
9. Remove the tubes from the heating block and allow to cool briefly before adding 100 µL of precipitation solution (without glycogen), followed by 400 µL of ethanol, to each tube. Place at −20°C or colder for at least 15 min.
10. Repeat step 3, and then wash twice with 70% ethanol as in steps 4 and 5.
11. Now dissolve the pellets in 5 µL of TE buffer. It is critical to ensure that the pellets are dissolved *before* the final addition of 3 µL of formamide loading buffer to each tube (*see* Note 23).

3.3.6. Electrophoresis

The chemically cleaved end-labeled heteroduplex DNAs are now separated by electrophoresis under denaturing conditions, and their positions are revealed by autoradiography of the gel.

1. Scrupulously clean the glass plates of the sequencing apparatus (e.g., Bio-Rad Sequi-Gen). A suggested procedure is to clean the plates with dilute (3–5% v/v) Decon90™ (BDH), followed by thorough rinsing in hot tap water, and then a final wash with 70% ethanol, wiping with lint-free paper tissue. When completely dry and dust-free, the back plate is silanized with Sigmacote® so that the gel will separate cleanly off after electrophoresis, but adhere to the front plate. The back plate is then given a final wipe clean with 70% ethanol to remove the residues from the silanization.

2. Assemble the sequencing apparatus, and cast a 0.4-mm thick denaturing 6% poly-acrylamide gel in 1X TBE (*see* Note 24). Use a suitable comb to form discrete wells in the gel for loading individual samples (*see* Note 25). Before the pre-run, the wells must be flushed out thoroughly (*see* Note 26).

3. Pre-run the gel at 1.7 kV (equivalent to approx 60 W for a 40 cm wide × 50 cm high gel) for about 30 min or until the gel has reached a temperature of 50°C (*see* Note 27).

4. While the gel is pre-running, the samples are denatured by heating them to 95°C for 5 min in a hot block or thermal cycler. They are then snap-chilled by transfer-ring them from the block at 95°C straight into an ice-water bath, and leaving them for 5 min or until the gel is ready for loading (*see* Note 28).

5. Dilute some [^{32}P]-labeled DNA size marker, so that in a volume of around 5 μL (including 3 μL of formamide loading buffer), there is approx 0.5–1× the radio-activity in a sample, as assessed by holding the tube up to a β-monitor. *Do not* denature the size marker, since it results in multiple uninterpretable bands on the autoradiographs!

6. After the pre-run, the wells must be flushed out again, before loading the samples and size marker; it is convenient to flush and load three or four wells at a time.

7. When all wells are loaded, start the electrophoresis (*see* Note 29).

8. When the electrophoresis has finished, separate the plates and transfer the gel to an X-ray film cassette with intensifying screens. This can be achieved without resorting to having to fix and dry the gel. Cut two pieces from sheets of 3MM paper (Whatman, Maidstone, UK): 40 × 26 and 26 × 15 cm. Apply the short edge of the larger sheet to the lower edge of the gel (adherent to the front glass plate), and smooth it out over the rest of the gel. Cut across the gel with a scalpel along the top edge of the sheet (usually about 10 cm from the top of the gel). Now, by carefully lifting the *long* edge of the sheet, the gel will peel away from the glass adherent to the paper. This is then wrapped in a single layer of Saran Wrap™ (Dow-Corning, Midland, MI) and placed in the X-ray cassette, gel uppermost. The smaller sheet can then be used to pick up the top piece of the gel, and after wrapping it is placed in the cassette next to the larger sheet (*see* Note 30).

9. After ensuring that the inside of the cassette is completely dry, load it with X-ray film (e.g., Kodak X-OMAT AR, Hemel Hempstead, UK), and place it *without delay* in a freezer at −70°C. This is essential to prevent diffusion of the bands in the gel, but it also enhances the effect of the intensifying screens (*see* Note 31).

3.3.7. Interpretation

1. The usual banding pattern seen on CCM autoradiographs is one or two major bands, together with a background of relatively low-intensity bands, present in all samples. The background pattern is probably the result of cleavage at sites of DNA damage that has occurred in vitro during sample processing, such as oxidative lesions and depurination *(66)*. When a mismatch has been cleaved, it results in an extra smaller band (Figs. 1 and 4A). A plot of migration distance, from a suitable datum line against $\log_{10}$ (marker size in bp) should be made. The size of this smaller fragment gives an estimate of the distance from one end or the other of the PCR product that the mismatch occurred; because *both* strands of the DNA were labeled, it is not possible to say which end the mismatch was closest to. Sequencing is always necessary to determine the exact nature of any mismatch, and decide whether it represents a mutation or polymorphism.

2. If the cleavage occurs in the hydroxylamine reaction, then the mismatch involves a mis- or unpaired C (i.e., C:A, C:T, C:C or C:–). If cleavage occurs in the osmium tetroxide reaction then the mismatch involves a mis- or unpaired T (i.e., T:C, T:G, T:T or T:–). Unpaired bases result from the looping out of a short stretch of ssDNA in heteroduplexes formed between wild-type and deletion/insertion mutants. Indeed, cleavage in both reactions is usually good evidence that such a mutation has been found (the alternative possibility is a C:T mismatch). With end labeling it is theoretically possible for two separate mismatches (e.g., a polymorphism and a mutation) to be observed in different parts of the same DNA fragment if they result in cleavage of opposite strands. Two sites sensitive to the same agent on the same strand should appear as a single site, i.e., that of the mismatch nearer to the label, assuming 100% cleavage.

3. Occasionally, a variant pattern is seen, in which two or more short bands are seen close together. This probably represents cleavage at and around the site of the mismatch (Fig. 4B), not necessarily following the "rules" in Section 2.

3.4. Reverse Transcription of RNA

To carry out a PCR using an mRNA template, the RNA must first be used to direct synthesis of cDNA. This is achieved with reverse transcriptase, because *Taq*-DNA-polymerase does not have RNA-directed DNA-polymerase activity. As with all work involving RNA, the greatest possible care should be taken to avoid contamination with RNases. Wear gloves at all times (and change them frequently), and use clean disposable plasticware whenever possible. The method described below uses separately sourced components. However, we have achieved satisfactory results using the First-Strand cDNA Synthesis Kit (Pharmacia); *see* Note 33.

1. Mix in a 0.6 mL microcentrifuge tube: 12.0 µL 5X reverse transcriptase buffer, 4.0 µL RNasin (40 U), 6.0 µL oligonucleotide 15.1R (10 µ*M*), 0.6 µL dNTP mix, *x* µL RNA (2–5 µg), *y* µL M-MLV reverse transcriptase (600 U), and water to 60.0 µL. Incubate at 37°C for 1 h.
2. Use immediately in PCR (Section 3.1.), or store at –20°C until needed.

3.5. PTT

Using suitable oligonucleotide primers, i.e., a forward primer containing a T7 RNA-polymerase binding site and an in-frame start codon, together with a compatible reverse primer, the PCR is used to amplify the required sequence, either from gDNA (for exon 15) or cDNA (for exons 1–14).

1. Thaw the reagents and place on ice.
2. Combine in a 0.6-mL microcentrifuge tube (this is sufficient for 12 reactions): 125 µL T~NT~ rabbit reticulocyte lysate, 10 µL T~NT~ reaction buffer, 5 µL RNasin (50 U), 10 µL [^{35}S]-methionine (1000 Ci/mmol), 5 µL amino acid mix (minus methionine), 40 µL TE buffer, pH 7.5, 5 µL T~NT~ T7 RNA-polymerase (50 U). Mix gently but thoroughly. Distribute 15 µL to each 0.6-mL microcentrifuge tube.
3. Add 4 µL of unpurified PCR product (*see* Note 34), mix, and incubate at 30°C for 1 h.
4. Add 20 µL of 2X SDS-PAGE loading buffer.
5. Cast two 15% polyacrylamide gels using the following: resolving gel mix (lower): 7.5 mL 1.5*M* Tris-HCl buffer, pH 8.8, 15 mL stock acrylamide solution, 7.5 mL distilled water, 40 µL TEMED, 100 µL 10% (w/v) ammonium persulfate. Overlay with distilled water (to exclude oxygen), and when set, cast the upper stacking gels. Stacking gel mix (upper) consists of: 2.5 mL 0.5*M* Tris-HCl buffer, pH 6.8, 2.5 mL stock acrylamide solution, 8.5 mL distilled water, 40 µL TEMED, 100 µL 10% (w/v) ammonium persulfate (*see* Note 35).
6. Assemble the gel apparatus, remove the combs, and flush the wells out with SDS-PAGE running buffer.
7. Denature the samples by heating them to 99°C for 2 min (conveniently achieved in a thermal cycler). In the meantime, mix 10 µL of 2X SDS-PAGE loading buffer with 10 µL of the Rainbow™ protein markers, and load 10 µL into each "Marker" lane (*do not* heat denature this mix, since it bleaches the dye-labeled proteins). Finally, load the denatured samples into the wells (*see* Note 36).
8. Run the gels at constant current (40 mA each for 100 × 100 × 0.8 mm Bio-Rad MiniProtean™ gels), until the bromophenol blue reaches the bottom of the gel (*see* Note 37).
9. Separate the glass plates and fix the gels in gel fixing solution for 10 min, with occasional gentle agitation.
10. Dry down the gels on 3MM paper (Whatman, Maidstone, UK), using a heated vacuum gel dryer (e.g., Model 853, Bio-Rad). Place the dried gels in an X-ray film cassette, and load it with film (e.g., Kodak X-OMAT AR). Expose for 12–24 h (e.g., overnight) at room temperature.
11. Interpretation depends first on estimating the sizes of any prematurely terminated polypeptides (Fig. 5). A very approximate idea can be gained by visual

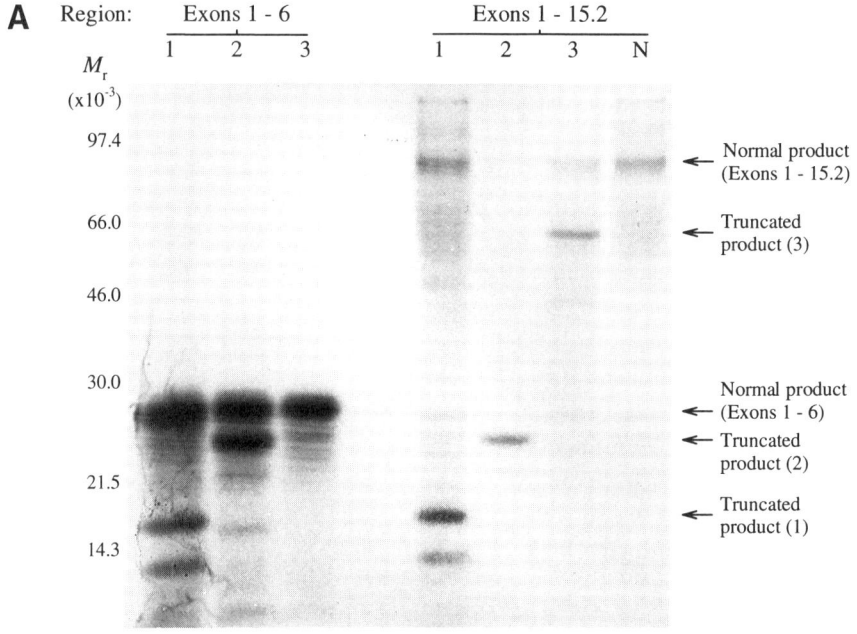

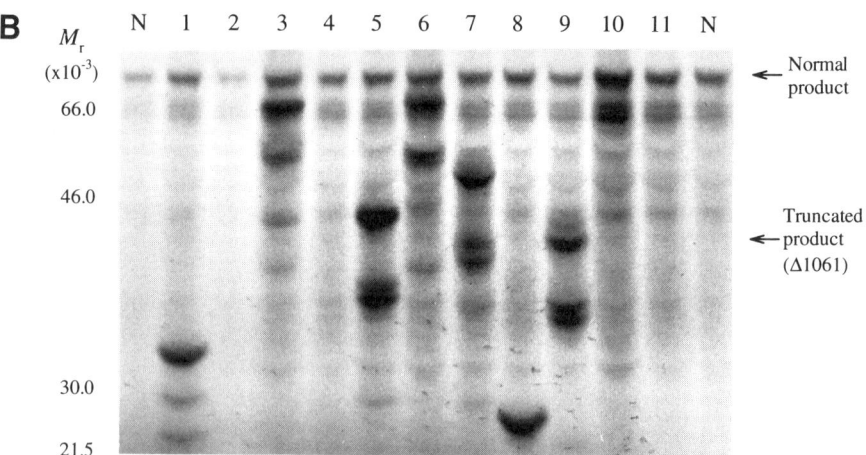

Fig. 5. PTT analysis of individuals with FAP. **(A)** Mutations in exons 1–14; and **(B)** mutations in exon 15 (PCR region 15p1). Autoradiographs of PTT gels. Testing carried out on FAP patients, and showing [^{35}S]-methionine-labeled products from (A) cDNA PCRs (spanning exons 1–6 and 1–15.2; *see* Table 3), and (B) products from gDNA PCR region 15p1 (codons 661–1273; *see* Table 3), analyzed by SDS-PAGE on 10% gels. Note in gel (A) that samples truncated in exons 1–6 give more strongly labeled products

interpolation between the marker proteins, but it is better to calibrate the gels by plotting the migration distances of the Rainbow protein markers (from a suitable datum line) against their $\log_{10}(M_r)$. By then measuring the migration distance of candidate bands, their M_r can be determined with reasonable accuracy, and by then assuming that each amino acid has an average M_r of 110 (*see* Note 38), the position of the termination codon can be estimated. It is strongly recommended to include some defined mutants on the gels, e.g., the 5-bp deletions at codons 1061 and/or 1309 depending on the PCR region, which will give products of known size as well as acting as positive controls (Fig. 5B). Note that the stop codon generated by many frame-shifting mutations can be some way downstream of the mutation itself. These would be predicted to produce mutant truncated versions of the APC protein with a novel stretch of amino acids at the carboxyl terminal. As an example, the stop codon generated by a single base deletion at position 3573 (in codon 1191; CAGA→CAA) is predicted to create a novel carboxyl terminal 73 amino acids long *(30)*.

4. Notes

4.1. PCR

1. Include a sample from a known normal individual (which will be necessary for subsequent labeling in CCM analysis) and a "no DNA" control. It is highly recommended to include a sample or samples from known mutants. In any event, this is essential if performing predictive testing.
2. The use of mechanical (e.g., Eppendorf Multipette; Eppendorf, Hamburg, Germany) or electronic (e.g., Gilson EDP-2; Gilson, Villiers-le-Bel, France) pipets allows considerable savings in time, for this and many other steps, particularly in CCM. Electronic pipets are recommended because the volume dispensed is not restricted to preset values and the dispensing velocity can be varied.

Fig. 5 *(continued)* when tested by the shorter cDNA PCR, but that the same mutant products are detectable in the 1–15.2 PCR. In gel (A) sample 1, and all lanes in gel (B), note that in addition to the full-sized normal product, there are shorter bands present. These arise owing to translation initiation at "internal" methionine codons (and to a lesser extent translation of RNAs present in the reticulocyte lysate). The doublet of bands immediately below the normal product in gel (B) is due to initiation at internal sites, and in most of those samples with a truncated product, an equivalent pair of truncated internally initiated products is evident below the mutant product (i.e., samples 1, 3, 5–7, and 9). (A): N, sample from normal individual; 1, 2, and 3, samples from affected individuals in different FAP pedigrees—their mutations have yet to be defined by sequencing. (B): N, sample from normal individual; test samples with known mutations: 1, codon 969; 3, codon 1204; 4, codon 1309; 9, codon 1061 (truncated product with M_r 44,000); and 11, codon 1407. Samples 2 and 10 have not yet had an *APC* mutation detected and the mutations in samples 5–8 have yet to be defined by sequencing.

3. The PCR thermal cycling parameters have been determined with standard thickness 0.6-mL microcentrifuge tubes (Treff, Scotlab, Strathclyde, UK) in OmniGene thermal cyclers (Hybaid™, Teddington, UK), using the "Simulated Tube" control option. The conditions may need adjusting if other tubes, machines, and/or control options are used.

4. Using small (28-mL) gels in suitable apparatus (HE33 Submarine Agarose Gel Units; Hoefer Scientific Instruments, San Francisco, CA), only 2–3 μL of PCR product are needed, plus 2 μL of loading buffer. These can be conveniently mixed in V- or U-well 96-well assay plates (e.g., Falcon® 3911; Becton Dickinson, Oxnard, CA).

5. It is recommended that the PCRs be stored at 4°C overnight, or −20°C for longer periods, until purification or use in HDA/PTT.

6. Purification is necessary to remove the oligonucleotide primers and dNTPs, which would otherwise interfere with the subsequent labeling and CCM reactions. This step can be semiautomated with the Vac-Man™ Laboratory Vacuum Manifold (Promega), which then enables up to 20 samples to be processed in 30–40 min (with minimal handling).

4.2. HDA on MDE (Hydrolink™) Gels

7. The instructions provided with the MDE gel concentrate by the manufacturer (AT Biochem) are most comprehensive and should be read before using the product.

8. The use of 150 g/L urea in the MDE gel mix is optional, but excluding it causes band broadening.

9. We use ordinary cold tap water to cool the electrophoresis tank. This keeps the gel between 10 and 12°C, depending on the time of year. The precise temperature does not appear to be critical. It might be worth experimenting with different temperatures if a suitable apparatus is available.

10. The 0.6X TBE from the electrophoresis tank can be used to stain the gel, after addition of ethidium bromide. Destaining, like staining, can be carried out with water or 0.6X TBE. Either causes the gels to swell, but the effect is greater with water, which may be a problem. The staining solution can be kept for several weeks if stored in the dark (or a dark glass bottle).

4.3. CCM

11. All the quantities quoted for CCM analysis are sufficient for up to 20 samples, using either osmium tetroxide *or* hydroxylamine. They can be scaled *pro rata*.

12. T4 polynucleotide kinase is labile at temperatures above −20°C. Therefore, keep it on ice at all times when out of the freezer. Alternatively, use a cold block, e.g., Stratacooler (Stratagene, La Jolla, CA).

13. Other methods, such as differential precipitation, can be used to purify end-labeled probes.

14. Double-size heteroduplex reactions can be carried out and then divided into two separate tubes, if it is desirable to carry out both the hydroxylamine and osmium reactions on the same samples with the same batch of probe.

15. The mass ratio of labeled:test DNA is approx 1:5–20. This biases the mutant DNA into taking part in heteroduplexes and thus helps to maximize the efficiency of the procedure.

16. DNAs larger than 1 kb only need 60 min to anneal. The tubes can be left to cool to room temperature after the 42°C step.

17. Heteroduplexes can be stored at 4°C, overnight if convenient, before the hydroxylamine or osmium treatment.

18. The pH should be measured with a pH electrode, and adjusted to within ±0.1 pH units. The solution should be stored at 4°C, but for no longer than 1 wk. Tubes containing 1.4 g of hydroxylamine can be conveniently weighed out in batches, taking appropriate precautions, and stored at room temperature for up to 3 mo.

19. Some batches of microcentrifuge tubes turn a gray color during the osmium tetroxide treatment. This does not affect the reaction and is a useful indicator that osmium was added to all the tubes.

20. Cooling can be achieved by using a suitable freezer or a dry-ice/methanol bath. However, if using the latter, the tubes must be labeled with a suitable pen, e.g., Securiline Biotech Marker™ (Radleys, Saffron Walden, UK), which has alcohol-resistant ink.

21. Waste containing osmium tetroxide, e.g., glass vials and supernatants, can be neutralized with the acid stannous chloride solution, but local disposal regulations should always be followed.

22. The precise volume used for the ethanol wash is not critical, but it is important to remove as much as possible before proceeding to the next step. Care should be taken to avoid disturbing the DNA/glycogen pellet, which should be just visible. In any event, the tubes can be quickly and easily checked by holding in front of a β-monitor. The pellets can be stored in the second wash overnight at –20°C.

23. Failure to dissolve the pellets in TE buffer first, before adding the formamide loading buffer, results in a sticky mass in the bottom of the tubes, which blocks the fine pipet tips used to load the samples onto the gel.

24. The range of Sequagel™ concentrates (National Diagnostics) is ideal and most convenient for this purpose. We use 22 × 50 cm (w × h) plates for running up to 20 samples, and 40 × 50-cm plates for running up to 36 samples.

25. The use of "sharkstooth" combs is not recommended. The lack of a gap between lanes when using these makes the interpretation of the subsequent autoradiographs rather difficult.

26. Wells can be flushed using a fine needle (e.g., 21-gage or smaller) on a 50-mL syringe filled with 1X TBE.

27. Pre-running time can be considerably reduced by filling the top electrophoresis tank with 1X TBE buffer which has been preheated (e.g., in a microwave oven) to 55–60°C.

28. If after denaturing the condensation in the lids is excessive, then the tubes can be briefly spun in a refrigerated microfuge. Otherwise it is usually found that the volume of the samples has conveniently reduced itself to about 5 µL. Loading volumes much greater than this causes excessive band broadening.

29. Electrophoresis conditions will vary depending on the size of the DNAs concerned. For regions 15.1–15.6 run on a 50-cm long gel at 1.7 kV, then 2.5–3.5 h (or until 15 min after the bromophenol blue runs out of the gel) are suitable. Shorter regions only need 1.5–1.75 h, but these parameters need to be decided by some trial and error depending on the fragment size(s), apparatus, ambient air temperatures, and other local factors. If a temperature-controlled electrophoresis power-pack is available (e.g., Bio-Rad PowerPack 3000), try with a set temperature of 45°C as a starting point.

30. With 50 × 40-cm gels, leave some wells unloaded in the center, use two 40 × 26-cm sheets side by side, and cut the gel down the middle and across the top (in a "T" shape). Finally, use a third sheet to pick up the top section of the gel.

31. Depending on the efficiency of the labeling and amount of probe used, we usually make three exposures: one overnight, another the next day for a few hours (in case there are any cleavage bands close to the main band, which are "swamped" by it at longer exposures), and a third for a few/several days (to reveal any products cleaved with reduced efficiency).

4.4. Reverse Transcription of RNA

32. RNA can be purified from lymphocytes extracted from fresh blood, lympho-blastoid cell lines, or tissue samples snap-frozen in liquid nitrogen *(51)*.

33. We have achieved equally good results using either separately sourced components or the First-Strand cDNA Synthesis Kit (Pharmacia). The choice comes down to one of cost and/or availability.

4.5. PTT

34. Best results are obtained with PCRs that have given a specific product in high yield (i.e., without spurious bands owing to mis-priming); poor-quality PCR products encourage the synthesis of spurious polypeptides and, hence, result in poor-quality protein gels. We design oligonucleotide primers with the aid of the software package OLIGO™ (MedProbe AS, Oslo, Norway); good design of primers is essential for good results in PCR.

35. The mix volumes given are for casting two Bio-Rad MiniProtean gels (100 × 100 × 0.8 mm). They should be scaled *pro rata* if using other apparatus. It is recommended that PTT products are analyzed on a 10 as well as a 15% polyacrylamide gel. The lower strength gel gives better resolution of higher mol-wt polypeptides assisting in detecting mutations close to the 3' end of the PCR product. The volumes of stock polyacrylamide solution and water in the resolving mix should simply be adjusted accordingly.

36. There will be condensation in the tube lids, but unless it is excessive, there is no need to centrifuge the tubes. It will usually be found that the volume of the PTT reaction has been conveniently reduced to about 35 µL. Load all of it on the gel.

37. Bio-Rad MiniProtean gels typically take about 90 min to run at a constant 40 mA.

38. This value of 110 for the average M_r of an amino acid is calculated from the predicted M_r of the full-length APC protein (311,658) divided by the number of amino acids (2843). It is in contrast to the "weighted mean" figure of 126.7 given in Sambrook et al. *(67)*.

4.6. DNA Sequencing

When a possible mutation has been localized to a particular exon or region, it is necessary to sequence the DNA involved to determine the precise nature of the putative lesion.

39. If localized to a region, e.g., exon 15.3, then further screening tests (HDA or CCM) can be carried out first on subregions to narrow down the area. The size of a truncated protein on PTT analysis can also be used to localize the region containing the mutation. However, it should be remembered that some frame-shift mutations can be quite a distance upstream of the site of premature termination and not necessarily in the same exon.

40. The exon/region is reamplified by PCR (as in Section 3.1.), but this time using a 5'-biotinylated primer in place of one of the ordinary primers. After checking the PCR on a small agarose gel, streptavidin-coated paramagnetic beads (e.g., Dynabeads® M-280; Dynal AS, Oslo, Norway) are used to purify the PCR product. There is no need to isolate the product from the excess biotinylated primer first.

41. After washing, as per the bead manufacturer's instructions, the biotinylated PCR product can be strand-separated, and by further manipulation if necessary, both strands can be used in a sequencing reaction, e.g., Sequenase™ (USB, Cleveland, OH). We have found results with $[\alpha\text{-}^{33}P]dCTP$ (Amersham) to be better than with $[\alpha\text{-}^{35}S]dCTP$. It also has the advantage of speeding up the process, because the gel-fixing and drying stages can be eliminated and the gels handled just like CCM gels (Section 3.3.6.).

42. For those with access to a fluorescent DNA analyzer (e.g., ABI 373, Applied Biosystems, Foster City, CA), it is not necessary to re-PCR with a biotinylated primer, but it is recommended to LMP-agarose gel-purify the PCR product, particularly if using the ABI Prism™ Dye-Deoxy Sequencing Kit. The accuracy with which CCM gives the site of a mismatch is extremely useful for calling heterozygotes with such systems. It is in fact possible to combine CCM with fluorescent DNA analysis, with the advantage that using a different dye on each strand (by the use of appropriate PCR primers) allows any mismatches to be located unambiguously, minimizing subsequent sequencing *(57)*.

Acknowledgments

The authors thank David Bicknell, Sally Cottrell, Victoria Johnson, Juliette Smith-Ravin, and Kevin Pack for their help in setting up the CCM and HDA methods, discussions about them, and performing some of the analyses seen in the various figures. We also thank Sir Walter Bodmer (Director General of the Imperial Cancer Research Fund, and Head of the ICRF Cancer Genetics Laboratory) for his original suggestions regarding the methods and his most helpful critical comments. Thanks are also due to Rob B. van der Luijt (Department of Human Genetics, Leiden University, The Netherlands), for giving us prepublication access to his method for PTT analysis, and John Burn (Division of Medical Genetics, University of Newcastle upon Tyne, UK) for helpful discussion about *APC* gene deletions. We also give thanks to Nigel Webb (Medical Illustrator at St. Mark's Hospital) and Bill Bessant (Photographic Unit, Imperial Cancer Research Fund) for their help in preparing the various autoradiographs and gel photographs for publication.

Note Added in Proof

Two laboratories have discovered an additional 54-bp exon located between exons 10 and 11, termed Exon X *(68)* or Exon 10A *(69)*.

References

1. Cripps, W. H. (1882) Two cases of disseminated polypus of the rectum. *Trans. Pathol. Soc. Lond.* **33,** 165–168.
2. Bickersteth, R. A. (1890) Multiple polypi of the rectum occurring in a mother and child. *St Bartholomew's Hosp. Rep.* **26,** 299–301.
3. Knudson, A. G., Jr. (1971) Mutation and cancer: statistical study of retinoblastoma. *Proc. Natl. Acad. Sci. USA* **68,** 820–823.
4. Fearon, E. R. (1992) Genetic alterations underlying colorectal tumorigenesis. *Cancer Surveys* **12,** 119–136.
5. Koorey, D. J. and McCaughan, G. W. (1993) Tumour suppressor genes and colorectal neoplasia. *J. Gastroenterol. Hepatol.* **8,** 174–184.
6. Jagelman, D. G., DeCosse, J. J., and Bussey, H. J. (1988) Upper gastrointestinal cancer in familial adenomatous polyposis. *Lancet* **1,** 1149–1151.
7. Nugent, K. P., Spigelman, A. D., and Phillips, R. K. (1993) Life expectancy after colectomy and ileorectal anastomosis for familial adenomatous polyposis. *Dis. Colon Rectum* **36,** 1059–1162.
8. Gardner, E. J. and Richards, R. C. (1953) Multiple cutaneous and subcutaneous lesions occurring simultaneously with hereditary polyposis and osteomatosis. *Am. J. Hum. Genet.* **5,** 139–147.
9. Brett, C. A. M., Hershman, M. J., and Glazer, G. (1994) Other manifestations of familial polyposis, in *Familial Adenomatous Polyposis and Other Polyposis Syndromes* (Phillips, R. K. S., Spigelman, A. D., and Thomson, P. S., eds.), Edward Arnold, London, pp. 143–158.
10. Herera, L., Kakatis, S., and Gibas, L. (1986) Gardner syndrome in a man with an interstitial deletion of 5q. *Am. J. Med. Genet.* **25,** 473–476.
11. Bodmer, W. F., Bailey, C. J., Bodmer, J., Bussey, H. J., Ellis, A., Gorman, P., et al. (1987) Localization of the gene for familial adenomatous polyposis on chromosome 5. *Nature* **328,** 614–616.
12. Leppert, M., Dobbs, M., Scambler, P., O'Connell, P., Nakamura, Y., Stauffer, D., et al. (1987) The gene for familial polyposis coli maps to the long arm of chromosome 5. *Science* **238,** 1411–1413.

13. Nakamura, Y., Nishisho, I., Kinzler, K. W., Vogelstein, B., Miyoshi, Y., Miki, Y., et al. (1991) Mutations of the adenomatous polyposis coli gene in familial polyposis coli patients and sporadic colorectal tumors. *Princess Takamatsu Symp.* **22,** 285–292.

14. Groden, J., Thliveris, A., Samowitz, W., Carlson, M., Gelbert, L., Albertsen, H., et al. (1991) Identification and characterization of the familial adenomatous polyposis coli gene. *Cell* **66,** 589–600.

15. Joslyn, G., Carlson, M., Thliveris, A., Albertsen, H., Gelbert, L., Samowitz, W., et al. (1991) Identification of deletion mutations and three new genes at the familial polyposis locus. *Cell* **66,** 601–613.

16. Kinzler, K. W., Nilbert, M. C., Su, L. K., Vogelstein, B., Bryan, T. M., Levy, D. B., et al. (1991) Identification of FAP locus genes from chromosome 5q21. *Science* **253,** 661–665.

17. Tops, C. M., Wijnen, J. T., Griffioen, G., von-Leeuwen, I. S., Vasen, H. F., den-Hartog-Jager, F. C., et al. (1989) Presymptomatic diagnosis of familial adenomatous polyposis by bridging DNA markers. *Lancet* **2,** 1361–1363.

18. MacDonald, F., Morton, D. G., Rindl, P. M., Haydon, J., Cullen, R., Gibson, J., et al. (1992) Predictive diagnosis of familial adenomatous polyposis with linked DNA markers: population based study. *Br. Med. J.* **304,** 869–872.

19. Dunlop, M. G., Wyllie, A. H., Steel, C. M., Piris, J., and Evans, H. J. (1991) Linked DNA markers for presymptomatic diagnosis of familial adenomatous polyposis. *Lancet* **337,** 313–316.

20. Bisgaard, M. L., Fenger, K., Bulow, S., Niebuhr, E., and Mohr, J. (1994) Familial adenomatous polyposis (FAP): frequency, penetrance, and mutation rate. *Hum. Mutat.* **3,** 121–125.

21. Hodgson, S. V. and Spigelman, A. D. (1994) Genetics, in *Familial Adenomatous Polyposis and Other Polyposis Syndromes* (Phillips, R. K. S., Spigelman, A. D., and Thomson, J. P. S., eds.), Edward Arnold, London, pp. 26–35.

22. Maher, E. R., Barton, D. E., Slatter, R., Koch, D. J., Jones, M. H., Nagase, H., et al. (1993) Evaluation of molecular genetic diagnosis in the management of familial adenomatous polyposis coli: a population based study. *J. Med. Genet.* **30,** 675–678.

23. Rustin, R. B., Jagelman, D. G., McGannon, E., Fazio, V. W., Lavery, I. C., and Weakley, F. L. (1990) Spontaneous mutation in familial adenomatous polyposis. *Dis. Colon Rectum* **33,** 52–55.

24. Horii, A., Nakatsuru, S., Ichii, S., Nagase, H., and Nakamura, Y. (1993) Multiple forms of the *APC* gene transcripts and their tissue-specific expression. *Hum. Mol. Genet.* **2,** 283–287.

25. Lambertz, S. and Ballhausen, W. G. (1993) Identification of an alternative 5' untranslated region of the adenomatous polyposis coli gene. *Hum. Genet.* **90,** 650–652.

26. Thliveris, A., Samowitz, W., Matsunami, N., Groden, J., and White, R. (1994) Demonstration of promoter activity and alternative splicing in the region 5' to exon 1 of the *APC* gene. *Cancer Res.* **54,** 2991–2995.

27. Powell, S. M., Petersen, G. M., Krush, A. J., Booker, S., Jen, J., Giardiello, F. M., et al. (1993) Molecular diagnosis of familial adenomatous polyposis. *N. Engl. J. Med.* **329,** 1982–1987.

28. Mandl, M., Paffenholz, R., Friedl, W., Caspari, R., Sengteller, M., and Propping, P. (1994) Frequency of common and novel inactivating *APC* mutations in 202 families with familial adenomatous polyposis. *Hum. Mol. Genet.* **3,** 181–184.

29. Cottrell, S., Bicknell, D., Kaklamanis, L., and Bodmer, W. F. (1992) Molecular analysis of *APC* mutations in familial adenomatous polyposis and sporadic colon carcinomas. *Lancet* **340,** 626–630.

30. Miyoshi, Y., Ando, H., Nagase, H., Nishisho, I., Horii, A., Miki, Y., et al. (1992) Germ-line mutations of the *APC* gene in 53 familial adenomatous polyposis patients. *Proc. Natl. Acad. Sci. USA* **89,** 4452–4456.

31. Nakamura, Y., Nishisho, I., Kinzler, K. W., Vogelstein, B., Miyoshi, Y., Miki, Y., et al. (1992) Mutations of the *APC* (adenomatous polyposis coli) gene in FAP (familial polyposis coli) patients and in sporadic colorectal tumors. *Tohoku J. Exp. Med.* **168,** 141–147.

32. Nagase, H., Miyoshi, Y., Horii, A., Aoki, T., Petersen, G. M., Vogelstein, B., et al. (1992) Screening for germline mutations in familial adenomatous polyposis patients: 61 new patients and a summary of 150 unrelated patients. *Hum. Mutat.* **1,** 467–473.

33. Olschwang, S., Tiret, A., Laurent-Puig, P., Muleris, M., Parc, R., and Thomas, G. (1993) Restriction of ocular fundus lesions to a specific subgroup of *APC* mutations in adenomatous polyposis coli patients. *Cell* **75,** 959–968.

34. Smith-Ravin, J., Pack, K., Hodgson, S., Tay, S. K., Phillips, R., and Bodmer, W. (1994) *APC* mutation associated with late onset of familial adenomatous polyposis. *J. Med. Genet.* **31,** 888–890.

35. Spirio, L., Otterud, B., Stauffer, D., Lynch, H., Lynch, P., Watson, P., et al. (1992) Linkage of a variant or attenuated form of adenomatous polyposis coli to the adenomatous polyposis coli (*APC*) locus. *Am. J. Hum. Genet.* **51,** 92–100.

36. Spirio, L., Olschwang, S., Groden, J., Robertson, M., Samowitz, W., Joslyn, G., et al. (1993) Alleles of the *APC* gene: an attenuated form of familial polyposis. *Cell* **75,** 951–957.

37. Varesco, L., Gismondi, V., Presciuttini, S., Groden, J., Spirio, L., Sala, P., et al. (1994) Mutation in a splice-donor site of the *APC* gene in a family with polyposis and late age of colonic cancer death. *Hum. Genet.* **93,** 281–286.

38. Cross, I., Delhanty, J., Chapman, P., Bowles, L. V., Griffin, D., Wolstenholme, J., et al. (1992) An intrachromosomal insertion causing 5q22 deletion and familial adenomatous polyposis coli in two generations. *J. Med. Genet.* **29,** 175–179.

39. Tops, C. M., van-der-Klift, H. M., van-der-Luijt, R. B., Griffioen, G., Taal, B. G., Vasen, H. F., and Khan, P. M. (1993) Non-allelic heterogeneity of familial adenomatous polyposis. *Am. J. Med. Genet.* **47,** 563–567.

40. Stella, A., Resta, N., Gentile, M., Susca, F., Mareni, C., Montera, M. P., and Guanti, G. (1993) Exclusion of the *APC* gene as the cause of a variant form of familial adenomatous polyposis (FAP). *Am. J. Hum. Genet.* **53,** 1031–1037.

41. Burn, J. and Chapman, P. (1994) Familial adenomatous polyposis: heterogeneity? *Am. J. Hum. Genet.* **55**, 412,413.
42. Cotton, R. G., Rodrigues, N. R., and Campbell, R. D. (1988) Reactivity of cytosine and thymine in single-base-pair mismatches with hydroxylamine and osmium tetroxide and its application to the study of mutations. *Proc. Natl. Acad. Sci. USA* **85**, 4397–4401.
43. Grompe, M., Muzny, D. M., and Caskey, C. T. (1989) Scanning detection of mutations in human ornithine transcarbamylase by chemical mismatch cleavage. *Proc. Natl. Acad. Sci. USA* **86**, 5888–5892.
44. Dianzani, I., Camaschella, C., Saglio, G., Forrest, S. M., Ramus, S., and Cotton, R. G. (1991) Simultaneous screening for beta-thalassemia mutations by chemical cleavage of mismatch. *Genomics* **11**, 48–53.
45. Smooker, P. M. and Cotton, R. G. (1993) The use of chemical reagents in the detection of DNA mutations. *Mutat. Res.* **288**, 65–77.
46. Keen, J., Lester, D., Inglehearn, C., Curtis, A., and Bhattacharya, S. (1991) Rapid detection of single base mismatches as heteroduplexes on Hydrolink gels. *Trends Genet.* **7**, 5.
47. White, M. B., Carvalho, M., Derse, D., O'Brien, S. J., and Dean, M. (1992) Detecting single base substitutions as heteroduplex polymorphisms. *Genomics* **12**, 301–306.
48. van-der-Luijt, R., Khan, P. M., Vasen, H., van-Leeuwen, C., Tops, C., Roest, P., et al. (1994) Rapid detection of translation-terminating mutations at the adenomatous polyposis coli (*APC*) gene by direct protein truncation test. *Genomics* **20**, 1–4.
49. Naylor, J. A., Green, P. M., Rizza, C. R., and Giannelli, F. (1993) Analysis of factor VIII mRNA reveals defects in every one of 28 haemophilia A patients. *Hum. Mol. Genet.* **2**, 11–17.
50. Morton, D. G., Macdonald, F., Cachon-Gonzales, M. B., Rindl, P. M., Neoptolemos, J. P., Keighley, M. R., et al. (1992) The use of DNA from paraffin wax preserved tissue for predictive diagnosis in familial adenomatous polyposis. *J. Med. Genet.* **29**, 571–573.
51. Chomczynski, P. and Sacchi, N. (1987) Single-step method of RNA isolation by acid guanidinium thiocyanate-phenol-chloroform extraction. *Anal. Biochem.* **162**, 156–159.
52. Groden, J., Gelbert, L., Thliveris, A., Nelson, L., Robertson, M., Joslyn, G., et al. (1993) Mutational analysis of patients with adenomatous polyposis: identical inactivating mutations in unrelated individuals. *Am. J. Hum. Genet.* **52**, 263–272.
53. Soto, D. and Sukumar, S. (1992) Improved detection of mutations in the p53 gene in human tumors as single-stranded conformation polymorphs and double-stranded hetroduplex DNA. *PCR Methods Applic.* **2**, 96–98.
54. Tassabehji, M., Read, A. P., Newton, V. E., Patton, M., Gruss, P., Harris, R., and Strachan, T. (1993) Mutations in the *PAX3* gene causing Waardenburg syndrome type 1 and type 2. *Nature Genetics* **3**, 26–30.
55. Bhattacharyya, A. and Lilley, D. M. (1989) The contrasting structures of mismatched DNA sequences containing looped-out bases (bulges) and multiple mismatches (bubbles). *Nucleic Acids Res.* **17**, 6821–6840.

56. Maxam, A. and Gilbert, W. (1980) Sequencing end-labeled DNA with base-specific chemical cleavages. *Methods Enzymol.* **65,** 499–560.

57. Haris, I. I., Green, P. M., Bentley, D. R., and Giannelli, F. (1994) Mutation detection by fluorescent chemical cleavage: application to hemophilia B. *PCR Methods Applic.* **3,** 268–271.

58. Roest, P. A., Roberts, R. G., van-der-Tuijn, A. C., Heikoop, J. C., van-Ommen, G. J., and den-Dunnen, J. T. (1993) Protein truncation test (PTT) to rapidly screen the *DMD* gene for translation terminating mutations. *Neuromuscular Disord.* **3,** 391–394.

59. Spirio, L., Nelson, L., Ward, K., Burt, R., White, R., and Leppert, M. (1993) A CA-repeat polymorphism close to the adenomatous polyposis coli (*APC*) gene offers improved diagnostic testing for familial APC. *Am. J. Hum. Genet.* **52,** 286–296.

60. van-Leeuwen, C., Tops, C., Breukel, C., van-der-Klift, H., Fodde, R., and Khan, P. M. (1991) CA repeat polymorphism at the *D5S299* locus linked to adenomatous polyposis coli (*APC*). *Nucleic Acids Res.* **19,** 5805.

61. Breukel, C., Tops, C., van-Leeuwen, C., van-der-Klift, H., Fodde, R., and Khan, P. M. (1991) AT repeat polymorphism at the *D5S122* locus tightly linked to adenomatous polyposis coli (*APC*). *Nucleic Acids Res.* **19,** 6665.

62. Allan, G. J., Cottrell, S., Trowsdale, J., and Foulkes, W. D. (1994) Loss of heterozygosity on chromosome 5 in sporadic ovarian carcinoma is a late event and is not associated with mutations in *APC* at 5q21-22. *Hum. Mutat.* **3,** 283–291.

63. Heighway, J., Hoban, P. R., and Wyllie, A. H. (1991) *Ssp* I polymorphism in sequence encoding 3' untranslated region of the *APC* gene. *Nucleic Acids Res.* **19,** 6966.

64. Kraus, C. and Ballhausen, W. G. (1992) Two intragenic polymorphisms of the *APC* gene detected by PCR and enzymatic digestion. *Hum. Genet.* **88,** 705,706.

65. Olschwang, S., Laurent-Puig, P., Thuille, B., and Thomas, G. (1992) Frequent polymorphism in the 13th exon of the adenomatous polyposis coli gene. *Hum. Genet.* **90,** 161–163.

66. Chung, M. H., Kiyosawa, H., Ohtsuka, E., Nishimura, S., and Kasai, H. (1992) DNA strand cleavage at 8-hydroxyguanine residues by hot piperidine treatment. *Biochem. Biophys. Res. Commun.* **188,** 1–7.

67. Sambrook, J., Fritsch, E. F., and Maniatis, T. (1989) Appendix D: codons and amino acids, in *Molecular Cloning: A Laboratory Manual* (Nolan, C., Ford, N., and Ferguson, M., eds.), Cold Spring Harbor Laboratory Press, Cold Spring Harbor, NY, pp. D.2–D.5.

68. Xia, L., St. Denis, K. A., and Bapat, B. (1995) Evidence for a novel exon in the coding region of the adenomatous polyposis coli *(APC)* gene. *Genomics* **28,** 589–591.

69. Sulekova, Z., Reina-Sanchez, J., and Ballhausen, W. G. (1995) Multiple *APC* messenger RNA isoforms encoding exon 15 short open reading frames are expressed in the context of a novel exon 10A-derived sequence. *Int. J. Cancer* **63,** 435–441.

5

Methods for Screening in Cystic Fibrosis

Martin Schwarz and Geraldine Malone

1. Introduction
1.1. Cystic Fibrosis Mutation Analysis

Cystic fibrosis (CF) is the most common lethal autosomal recessive disorder in Whites, with an incidence of approx 1 in 2500 live births and a carrier frequency of approx 1 in 25. Since the discovery of the cystic fibrosis transmembrane conductance regulator (CFTR) gene in 1989 (1–3), molecular genetics laboratories throughout the world have endeavored to identify the mutations present in their population of CF-bearing chromosomes. Since the entire CFTR gene and its intron–exon boundaries have been sequenced, mutation analysis in CF has become relatively simple, although time consuming. Generally, a number of different methods are applied to mutation analysis, but all involve an initial step of amplification of part of the gene by polymerase chain reaction (PCR) (4), or a derivative of it, such as amplification refractory mutation system (ARMS) (5).

Since there are over 500 different mutations of the CFTR gene so far described (Cystic Fibrosis Genetic Analysis Consortium), one must be aware of the relative frequencies of the common mutations. Some of these (for the United Kingdom [6], with comparative figures for North America and North and South Europe [7]) are given in Table 1. The large number of mutations makes population screening problematical, since a negative result will only reduce carrier risk and cannot exclude CF carrier status. A number of approaches to CF screening have been taken (e.g., couple screening in pregnancy and preconceptual [20]; cascade screening [21]; and population screening), although general population screening has largely been ruled out (22).

From: *Methods in Molecular Medicine: Molecular Diagnosis of Genetic Diseases*
Edited by: R. Elles Humana Press Inc., Totowa, NJ

Table 1
Relative Frequencies of the Common CF Mutations in the United Kingdom (6), North America, and Northern and Southern Europe (7)[a]

Mutation	Exon	UK No.	UK %	North America No.	North America %	Northern Europe No.	Northern Europe %	Southern Europe No.	Southern Europe %	References
ΔF508	10	7387	75.32	6900	66.1	14,866	70.28	4007	55.03	3
G551D	11	302	3.08	206	1.97	356	1.68	37	0.51	8
G542X	11	165	1.68	234	2.24	439	2.08	259	3.56	9
621 + 1(G > T)	intron 4	91	0.93	154	1.48	97	0.46	37	0.51	10
1717 − 1(G > A)	intron 10	56	0.57	44	0.42	160	0.76	65	0.89	9
R117H	4	45	0.46	61	0.58	62	0.29	3	0.04	11
R553X	11	45	0.46	96	0.92	165	0.78	44	0.6	8
1898 + 1(G > A)	intron 12	45	0.46	2	0.02	41	0.19	10	0.14	12
N1303K	21	45	0.46	130	1.25	209	0.99	179	2.46	13
R560T	11	41	0.42	24	0.23	40	0.19	0	0	9
ΔI507	10	30	0.31	20	0.19	57	0.27	5	0.07	9,14
G85E	3	21	0.21	16	0.15	30	0.14	14	0.19	11
1154insTC	7	19	0.19	n/a	n/a	n/a	n/a	n/a	n/a	15
V520F	10	17	0.17	n/a	n/a	n/a	n/a	n/a	n/a	16
W1282X	20	17	0.17	245	2.35	120	0.57	43	0.59	17
E60X	3	16	0.16	n/a	n/a	n/a	n/a	n/a	n/a	Malone[b]
3659delC	19	14	0.14	14	0.13	39	0.18	1	0.01	9
1078delT	7	9	0.09	1	0.01	53	0.25	2	0.3	18

S549N	11	8	0.08	5	0.05	18	0.09	2	0.03	*8*
Q493X	10	7	0.07	n/a	n/a	n/a	n/a	n/a	n/a	*9*
R347P	7	6	0.06	26	0.25	55	0.26	24	0.33	*11*
3849 + 10 kb(C > T) intron	19	5	0.05	57	0.55	23	0.11	8	0.11	*19*
A455E	9	3	0.03	27	0.26	35	0.17	0	0	*9*

[a]n/a, Data not available.
[b]Personal communication.

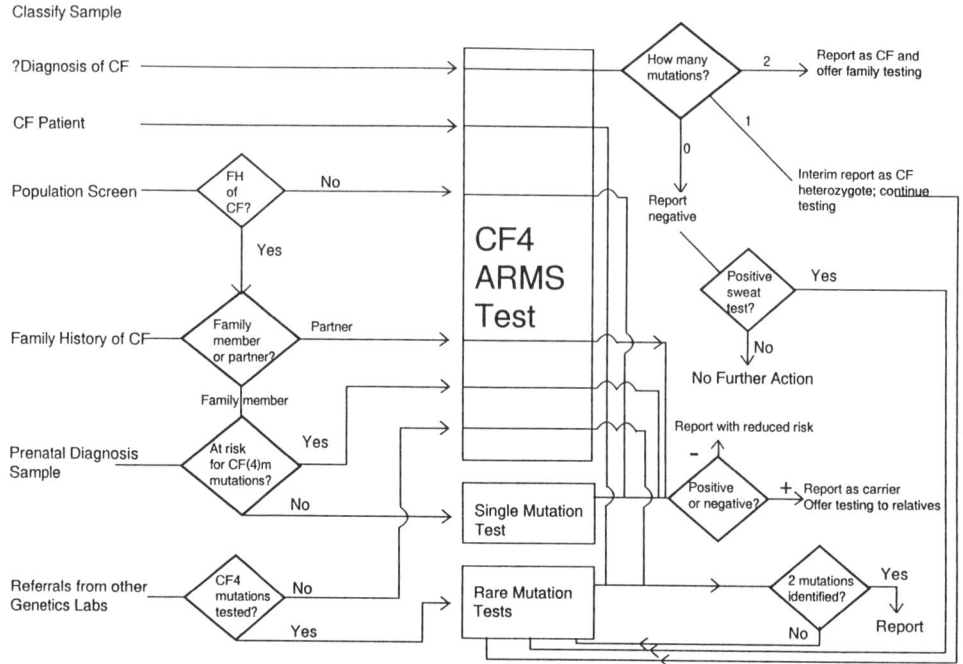

Fig. 1. Strategy for molecular analysis in CF.

1.2. Testing Strategy

In order to carry out the appropriate tests on a sample, a number of questions should be answered:

1. Is there a family history of CF?
2. If there is a family history of CF, is the genotype of the affected person known?
3. What is the ethnic origin of the person to be tested?

The extent and type of analysis performed on a sample depends on the family history of the individual to be tested; for example, to confirm CF in a patient, it is necessary to identify two mutant alleles, whereas someone with no family history of CF requires less comprehensive testing in order to reduce his or her risk of being a carrier of CF (Fig. 1). In addition, there are a number of "subsets" of patients, showing atypical CF phenotypes, in whom mutations of the CFTR gene can be found (e.g., congenital bilateral absence of the vas deferens [CBAVD] and chronic pancreatitis; *see* Section 1.2.8.). In this chapter a comprehensive strategy for detecting CF mutations is given, but the methods described in full detail are restricted to ARMS and allele-specific oligonucleotide (ASO) techniques.

1.2.1. CF Patients—Common Mutations

In all cases, the samples may be tested in the first instance either with the CF(4)m–PCR kit (Johnson & Johnson Clinical Diagnostics, Amersham, UK) *(23)*, which tests for the four most common CF mutations in the United Kingdom, or for just ΔF508 and ΔI507 by polyacrylamide gel electrophoresis (PAGE). In many populations more than half of all CF patients are homozygous for ΔF508 and it is therefore usually more efficient to test first for ΔF508 alone. If this is carried out using the PCR primers C16B and C16D (Table 2), it must be remembered that ΔF508 and ΔI507 can only be distinguished in heterozygous form (there being no heteroduplexes formed in ΔI507 and ΔF508 homozygotes, nor in ΔF508/ΔI507 compound heterozygotes, which would otherwise enable the two mutations to be differentiated). It is therefore preferable to test both the parents of a CF patient; since they are almost certain to be heterozygous for the relevant mutation, this strategy has the combined benefit of distinguishing between ΔF508 and ΔI507, and also confirming that both parents are indeed heterozygotes. (If this is not the case, further investigation of the family is required.) Alternatively, the use of the CF(4)m kit allows specific testing of ΔF508, together with the next three most common UK mutations.

1.2.2. CF Patients—Rare Mutations

If, after ΔF508/ΔI507 and ARMS CF(4)m testing, two mutations have not been identified, and CF has either been confirmed by sweat testing or there is a strong clinical suspicion of CF, the next tranche of mutations must be investigated (according to Table 1 and to local population variations). This is commonly performed in a specialist laboratory that is capable of rare mutation analysis.

These next mutations are not necessarily tested in descending order of frequency (as they are all fairly rare), since batching of samples and the combination of a number of tests may dictate which mutation analyses are performed first. A number of different techniques may now be employed simultaneously. As an extreme example, a sample may be tested for R560T and R117H by ARMS duplex (primers are detailed in Table 3, p. 106), for exons 5, 8, and 18 by denaturing gradient gel electrophoresis (DGGE), for exons 3 and 7 by single-stranded conformational polymorphism (SSCP), for W1282X and N1303K by ASO hybridization to dot-blots (Table 4, p. 106), and for R553X by restriction endonuclease digestion of PCR products. Because of the simplicity of detection of changes which alter restriction endonuclease recognition sequences (Table 5, p. 107), a number of diagnostic laboratories choose to test for these mutations (e.g., R553X, R560T) at an early stage. This may be followed by further SSCP and DGGE analysis, and ultimately DNA sequencing exon by exon. With the great spread of mutations within the gene, there is really no "correct" order.

Table 2
Sequences, Product Sizes, and Annealing Temperatures of PCR Primers Used in CF Analysis (*see* Note 10)[a]

Exon	Primer sequence 5' to 3'	Name	Product size, bp	Annealing temperature, °C
3	CTTGGGTTAATCTCCTTGGA	3i5	309	54
	ATTCACCAGATTTCGTAGTC	3i3		
4	TCACATATGGTATGACCCTC	4i5	438	54
	TTGTACCAGCTCACTACCTA	4i3		
7	AGACCATGCTCAGATCTTCCAT	7i5	410	54
	GCAAAGTTCATTAGAACTGATC	7i3		
9	TAATGGATCATGGGCCATGT	9i5	561	54
	ACAGTGTTGAATGTGGTGCA	9i3		
10 (part)	GTTTTCCTGGATTATGCCTGGGCAC	C16B	98	54
	GTTGGCATGCTTTGATGACGCTTC	C16D		
10	GCAGAGTACCTGAAACAGGA	10i5	491	54
	CATTCACAGTAGCTTACCCA	10i3		
11	CAACTGTGGTTAAAGCAATAGTGT	11i5	425	54
	GCACAGATTCTGAGTAACCATAAT	11i3		
12	GTGAATCGATGTGGTGACCA	12i5	426	57
	CTGGTTTAGCATGAGGCGGT	12i3		
13	TGCTAAAATACGAGACATATTGCA	13i5	528	58
	ATCTGGTACTAAGGACAG	C1-1M		
14a	AAAAGGTATGCCACTGTTAAG	14ai5	511	57
	GTATACATCCCCAAACTATCT	14ai3		
17b	TTCAAAGAATGGCACCAGTGT	17bi5	463	56
	ATAACCTATAGAATGCAGCA	17bi3		
19	GCCCGACAAATAACCAAGTGA	19i5	454	54
	GCTAACACATTGCTTCAGGCT	19i3		

104

	Sequence	Primer	Product size	Temp.
20	GGTCAGGATTGAAAGTGTGCA	20i5	473	59
	CTATGAGAAAACTGCACTGGA	20i3		
21	AATGTTCACAAGGACTCCA	21i5	476	54
	CAAAGTACCTGTTGCTCCA	21i3		
intron 6a	CAAGTCTTTCACTGATCTTC	FCO9	106/110	57
	TGAGCAGTTGTTAATAGATAA	6iRPT		
intron 8	TCTATCTCATGTTAATGCTG	NUR1	220	50
	GTTTCTAGAGGACATGATC	NUR2		
intron 17b	GACAATCTGTGTGCATCG	AT17R1.2	201–301	50
	GCTGCATTCTATAGGTTATC	AT17D1.2		
intron 17b	AAACTTACCGACAAGAGGA	AC17R2	140	50
	TGTCACCTCTTCATACTCAT	AC17D2		
intron 19	AGGCTTCTCAGTGATCTGTTG	i19F	437	50
	GAATCATTCAGTGGGTATAAGCAG	i19R		

[a]Sequences are provided courtesy of the Cystic Fibrosis Genetic Analysis Consortium.

Table 3
Sequences and Product Sizes for ARMS Primers *(23)* Used to Detect the CF Mutations R560T and R117H in a Duplex Reaction[a]

Mutation	Primer	Sequence 5' to 3'	Product size, bp
R560T	Common	AAAATTTCAGCAATGTTGTTTTTGACCAAC	
	Normal	GCTTGCTAGACCAATAATTAGTTATTCAAC	316
	Mutant	GCTTGCTAGACCAATAATTAGTTATTCAAG	
R117H	Common	CACATATGGTATGACCCTCTATATAAACTC	
	Normal	CCTATGCCTAGATAAATCGCGATAGAACC	237
	Mutant	CCTATGCCTAGATAAATCGCGATAGAAT	

[a]As for the CF(4)m test, a pair of tubes (A and B) is required for each DNA sample. Tube A contains R560T and R117H common, R560T normal, and R117H mutant primers; tube B contains R560T and R117H common, R560T mutant and R117H normal, primers. Thermal cycler and electrophoresis conditions are as for CF(4)m.

Table 4
Sequences of Normal (N) and Mutant (M) ASOs Used in the Detection of CF Mutations[a]

Mutation	ASO	Sequence 5' to 3'	Posthybridization wash temperature, C°
ΔF508	N	CACCAAAGATGATATTTC	42–44
	M	AACACCAATGATATTTCTT	
1717 – 1(G > A)	N	TGGTAATAGGACATCTC	42–44
	M	TGGTAATAAGACATCTC	
1898 + 1(G > A)	N	CAAAGAACATACCTTTCAA	42–44
	M	TGAAAGATATGTTCTTTG	
W1282X	N	CAACAGTGGAGGAAAGCCTT	42–44
	M	CAACAGTGAAGGAAAGCCTT	
N1303K	N	TAGAAAAAACTTGGATCC	42, 44, 46
	M	TAGAAAAAAGTTGGATCC	
PolyT(intron8)	5T	TGTGTGTGTTTTTAACAG	36, 40, 42
	7T	TGTGTGTTTTTTTAACAG	36
	9T	GTGTGTTTTTTTTTAACAG	36, 40, 42

[a]Posthybridization washes are carried out in 2X SSC, 0.1% SDS solution at incremental temperatures as shown (*see* Notes 9 and 10).

Table 5
CF Mutations Detectable by Restriction Endonuclease (RE) Digestion of PCR Products

| Mutation | PCR primers[a] | RE | RE digestion product sizes, bp[b,c] | |
			Normal	Mutant
G85E	3i5 and 3i3	*Hin*fI	105 + 204	309
621 + 1 (G > T)	4i5 and 4i3	*Mse*I	33, 35, 71, 118, 181	33, 35, 54, 71, 118, 127
1154insTC	7i5 and 7i3	*Msp*I, *Rsa*I	50, 68, 74 + 218[c]	50, 68, 76 + 218[c]
R334W	7i5 and 7i3	*Msp*I	192 + 218	410
R347P	7i5 and 7i3	*Cfo*I	151 + 259	410
G551D	11i5 and 11i3	*Mbo*I	425	182 + 243
R553X	11i5 and 11i3	*Hinc*II	186 + 239	425
R560T	11i5 and 11i3	*Mae*II	425	215 + 210
S549N	11i5 and 11i3	*Dde*I	13, 174 + 238	13 + 412
3849 + 10 kb (C > T)	i19F and i19R	*Hph*I	88 + 349	88, 127 + 222
W1282X	20i5 and 20i3	*Mnl*I	185 + 288	473

[a]*See* Table 2.
[b]The expected digestion product sizes for both normal and mutant sequences are shown.
[c]These products may be distinguished by PAGE.

1.2.3. Carrier Testing and Prenatal Diagnosis When Two Mutations Have Not Been Identified

If, after this quite extensive testing, two mutations have not been identified in a CF patient, it may be necessary to resort to using intragenic markers to make the family "informative" if prenatal diagnosis is required. This is the procedure to identify the parents' CF-bearing chromosomes so that their inheritance can be followed by linkage; the search for the second mutation, or rarely both mutations, of course, continues.

The large battery of highly polymorphic intragenic markers makes it highly likely that a family will be informative (Table 6). Although the dinucleotide repeats are by far the most polymorphic, it may not always be necessary to use them. For example, if exon 10 PCR products are available from a CF patient and his or her parents, it is quite straightforward to perform a restriction enzyme digest (*Hph*I) to look for the M470V polymorphism. Although only a dimorphism (A or G at nucleotide position 1540), this marker demonstrates quite a high degree of heterozygosity (0.24).

Table 6
Intragenic Polymorphisms Used to Determine Carrier Status in CF Family Studies[a]

Polymorphism			Analysis Method[c]	Allele/product sizes, bp	Refs.
Name	Type	Primers[b]			
IVS6bTTGA	TTGA repeat	FCO9, 6iRPT	PAGE	106 and 110	24
IVS8CA	CA repeat	NUR1, NUR2	PAGE	~220	25
IVS17bTA	TA repeat	AT17R1.2, AT17D1.2	PAGE	~201–299	26
IVS17bCA	CA repeat	AC17R2, AC17D2	PAGE	~140	26,27
M470V	A or G @ 1540	10i5, 10i3	RE (*Hph*I)	A (Met):492	9
				G (Val):191 + 301	
T854T	G or T @ 2694	14ai5, 14ai3	RE (*Cfr*13I)	G:511	28
				A:125 + 286	

[a]Mutations have not been characterized in the CF Index Case.
[b]See Table 2.
[c]PAGE, Separation of alleles by polyacrylamide gel electrophoresis; RE (enzyme), restriction endonuclease digestion and agarose gel electrophoresis.

It is here that one should consider the problem posed by consanguinity. Asian CF patients (or others from populations in which consanguinity is common) are frequently homozygous for a CF mutation and occasionally this may be a "private" mutation. It is therefore important to identify the mutation if possible and, if not, to find a marker for which the family is informative. This is usually possible, for even though the patient may be homozygous, the parents must be heterozygous for the mutation and are therefore likely to be heterozygous for a linked marker. Although a linked marker haplotype can be useful for prenatal diagnosis, it is unlikely to be of much use in carrier testing in a large extended family (but should be useful in a small family until the marker ceases to be informative), and for this purpose the mutation should be identified.

1.2.4. Testing Individuals with No Family History of CF

It may be sufficient to test an individual who has no family history of CF (for example, the partner of a relative of a CF patient) for enough mutations to enable a suitable reduction in their risk of carrying CF. The number and type of mutations tested will depend on the ethnic and geographical origin of that person (*see* Section 1.2.7.). If one assumes a carrier risk of 1 in 25 for the United Kingdom, and the ARMS CF(4)m kit detects 81% of mutations in the United Kingdom (Table 1), a person who is negative will have a risk of 1 in 166 of carrying CF. This figure can of course be reduced further by testing more mutations, but the reduction in risk becomes smaller with each mutation tested.

1.2.5. Testing Relatives of a CF Patient

In order to provide the most accurate information on carrier risks it is necessary to determine the genotype of the CF patient. This usually will have been achieved before relatives come forward for testing, but in certain cases the genotype will be unknown. For example, the CF patient may have died, moved overseas, or simply may not have been tested. If the patient has died, the parents (who are of course obligate carriers) may be available and willing to be tested. If the patient has moved away, it is usually possible to find out who the patient's physician is and then find out the genotype or obtain a sample. Occasionally, there may have been a CF patient who died 20 or 30 yr ago. One can only do so much to determine the strength of the diagnosis and in the end it is probably enough to test the relative for the common mutations in order to give a sufficiently reduced carrier risk.

1.2.6. Assistance with the Diagnosis of CF

A knowledge of the distribution of mutations in a given population is invaluable in the testing of individuals suspected of having CF. Table 1 shows the 20 most frequent mutations in the United Kingdom and their respective frequencies. It can be seen that testing for the four most common mutations covers 81% of all CF chromosomes in the United Kingdom and a negative result goes some way to reduce the possibility of CF, but of course does not exclude it altogether. Indeed, molecular analysis cannot exclude CF while the number of mutations continues to grow, and the best that can be attained is either the confirmation of CF by identifying two mutations, or a reduction in the likelihood of CF by testing for a number of mutations. It is not possible, after getting a negative result for several mutations, to provide a numerical risk of CF, since the clinical possibility of CF already has been raised and has consequently altered the prior risk of CF. When testing for the four most common CF mutations has yielded only one mutation in a person, a sweat test should be performed and further testing for rare mutations will then only take place after an abnormal sweat test result.

1.2.7. Testing CF Patients from Other Ethnic Origins and Their Relatives

The distribution of CF mutations varies from country to country *(7)*, even within the United Kingdom *(6)*, and it is therefore extremely important to ascertain an individual's ethnic origin before testing is undertaken. For example, there are particular mutations which should be tested in patients (and relatives and their partners) from particular ethnic backgrounds (e.g., W1282X in Ashkenazi Jews, 394delTT in Scandinavians, etc.). Pakistani mutations have been seen predominantly in exons 4, 10, and 12, and SSCP analysis of these exons covers most known mutations of this origin.

1.2.8. Clinical Presentation of CF Patients

The nature of the clinical presentation of the patient also should be determined before any extensive investigation is carried out, as this too may have a bearing on which mutations to test for. Although genotype:phenotype correlation in CF is not well defined, there are mutations which may be associated with particular presentations. For example, mild lung disease, pancreatic sufficiency and normal sweat chloride levels have been reported in individuals who have the 3849 + 10 kb (C > T) mutation. Consequently, ascertainment of the clinical features may give an indication of the mutations to test for.

In addition, there are a number of clinical subgroups in which particular mutations of the CFTR gene have been observed. For example the mutations ΔE115 and K1060T, as well as ΔF508, G542X, and R117H have been seen in CBAVD *(29)*. An increased frequency of CF heterozygotes has been observed among patients with chronic pancreatitis (Haworth, personal communication, February 1996).

The phenotypic effect of the R117H mutation has been seen to be dependent on the length of the intron 8 polythymidine tract immediately preceding exon 9 *(30)*. Three variants have been described (5T, 7T, and 9T) which give rise to varying degrees of exon 9 splicing. The R117H mutation is associated with the 5T variant in the majority of CF patients, but with the 7T variant in CBAVD patients. The 5T, 7T, and 9T variants may be determined by ASO hybridization (ASO sequences are detailed in Table 4).

2. Materials

2.1. Samples

Any sample which contains nucleated cells may be used as a source of DNA for molecular genetic analysis. Samples are usually blood (1–5 mL in K/EDTA) or mouthwash/ buccal swabs (taken in 10 mL of 4% sucrose solution). Since only small amounts of DNA are required when molecular analysis is performed by PCR, mouthwash and buccal swab samples provide sufficient material for testing. This technique is becoming increasingly popular with patients, since it is noninvasive and can be collected by the patient at home and sent to the laboratory by mail.

2.2. Reagents

1. CF(4)m PCR kit (product code PCR1012; Johnson & Johnson Clinical Diagnostics); includes *Taq* DNA polymerase.
2. T4 Polynucleotide kinase (product code 70031; United States Biochemical, Cleveland, OH/Amersham International plc, Little Chalfont, UK).
3. *Taq* DNA polymerase (product code 1146 173; Boehringer Mannheim, Lewes, UK).
4. Hybond N+ blotting membrane (product code RPN203B; Amersham International).
5. Proteinase K (product code 1092 766; Boehringer Mannheim).
6. 20X Saline sodium citrate (SSC): $3M$ NaCl, $0.3M$ trisodium citrate, pH 7.0.
7. Hybridization solution: 5X SSC, 0.1% sodium dodecyl sulphate (SDS), 0.1% Ficoll, 0.1% polyvinylpyrollidone (product code P-5288; Sigma, Poole, UK), 0.1% bovine serum albumin (product code A-9647; Sigma), 1% of a 10 mg/mL solution of sheared denatured herring sperm DNA (product code 223 646; Boehringer Mannheim) (*see* Note 1).
8. Blood lysis buffer: $0.32M$ sucrose, 10 mM Tris-HCl, pH 7.5, 5 mM $MgCl_2$, 1% Triton X-100 (product code X-100, Sigma). Store at 4°C.
9. Virkon detergent (product code 222/154; Merck, Lutterworth, UK). Prepare a 2% solution as required.
10. TE Buffer: 1 mM Tris-HCl, 10 mM EDTA, pH 7.5.
11. TBE Buffer: $0.089M$ Tris, $0.089M$ boric acid, $0.002M$ EDTA, pH 8.0.
12. Mineral oil (product code M-3516; Sigma).

2.3. Equipment

In addition to standard laboratory equipment, the following are required:

1. Thermal cycler (DNA Thermal Cycler, Perkin Elmer, Beaconsfield, UK).
2. Hybridization oven (HB1D, Techne, Cambridge, UK).
3. Vertical PAGE apparatus (9 × 8 cm AE6400, Genetic Research Instrumentation, Dunmow, UK; 40 × 20 cm V3, Anachem, Luton, UK).
4. Horizontal gel electrophoresis apparatus (HE series, Pharmacia Biotech, St. Albans, UK).
5. Heating block (Dri-Block DB-2A, Techne), useful but not essential.

3. Methods

3.1. Extraction of DNA from Mouthwash Samples

Mouthwash samples (in 10 mL of 4% sucrose solution) are collected by the patients themselves and returned to the laboratory by mail (*see* Note 2).

1. Centrifuge the samples at 1200g for 15 min (4°C) to pellet the buccal cells.
2. Discard the supernatant into a suitable detergent (e.g., 2% Virkon solution) and resuspend the pellet in 500 µL of 10 mM NaCl, 10 mM EDTA, pH 7.5 solution in a 1.5 mL screw-topped microcentrifuge tube.
3. Spin briefly (15 s) in a microcentrifuge to pellet the cellular material again.
4. Discard the supernatant, resuspend the pellet in 500 µL of 50 mM NaOH solution, and heat to 100°C for 10 min in a heating block (or a boiling water bath).
5. After the suspension has cooled, add to each tube 100 µL of 1M Tris-HCl, pH 7.5 solution to neutralize the NaOH, and mix by inversion.
6. Spin briefly in a microcentrifuge and transfer the supernatant to a fresh tube.
7. A 5-µL aliquot of DNA prepared in this way is sufficient for a single PCR reaction. DNA should be stored at –20°C until use.

3.2. Extraction of DNA from Blood Samples

Two methods are used to extract DNA from whole blood. The first requires only a small amount (~200 µL) of blood and is similar to the method described for extraction of DNA from mouthwash samples and produces sufficient DNA for PCR-based analysis. The second method requires 1–10 mL of blood and employs a proteinase K digestion followed by phenol and chloroform extraction. This latter method may yield ~200 µg of DNA from a 5-mL blood sample (*see* Note 3).

3.2.1. Small-Scale Extraction of DNA from Blood Samples

1. To 200 µL of blood (in EDTA), add 800 µL of cold 170 mM NH$_4$Cl solution in a screw-topped microcentrifuge tube and mix by rotating for 20 min.
2. Spin the tube in a microcentrifuge for 2 min to obtain a white-cell pellet. Discard the supernatant into a suitable detergent (e.g., 2% Virkon solution).

3. Resuspend the cell pellet in 300 μL of 10 mM NaCl, 10 mM EDTA, pH 7.5 solution, and then spin briefly. Collect the pellet. Gently rinse the surface of the pellet with an additional 300 μL of this solution to remove any visible hemoglobin residue.
4. Resuspend the resultant white-cell pellet in 500 μL of 50 mM NaOH solution.
5. Incubate the suspension in a heating block/water bath at 100°C for 10 min, then neutralize by adding 100 μL of Tris-HCl, pH 7.5 solution and vortex for 5 s.
6. Finally, centrifuge the suspension to pellet the cell debris and transfer the supernatant to a fresh tube.
7. A 5-μL aliquot of DNA prepared in this way is sufficient for a single PCR reaction. DNA should be stored at –20°C until use.

3.2.2. Large-Scale Extraction of DNA from Blood Samples

1. Transfer 1–10 mL of whole blood (in EDTA) into a 30-mL centrifuge tube. Add blood lysis buffer to a final vol of 30 mL (10 mL for blood vol <2 mL). Mix by inverting several times.
2. Centrifuge for 30 min at 1200g (4°C) to pellet the white cells.
3. Discard the supernatant into a suitable detergent (e.g., 2% Virkon solution), taking care not to dislodge the pellet. Keep the tube inverted and drain the pellet.
4. Resuspend the pellet in 2 mL of 0.075M NaCl, 0.024M EDTA, pH 8.0 solution and transfer to a 14-mL tube.
5. Add 200 μL of 10% SDS solution and 10 μL of proteinase K solution (20 mg/mL, *see* Note 4), and mix by inverting the tube.
6. Incubate overnight at 37°C.
7. Add 2 mL of phenol (saturated with 100 mM Tris-HCl, pH 8.0) (*see* Note 5).
8. Mix on a rotator for 10 min.
9. Separate the aqueous and organic phases by centrifugation at 1200g for 2 min.
10. Transfer the (upper) aqueous phase by pipet into a fresh tube containing 2 mL of phenol. Take care not to carry over any of the phenolic layer. Repeat steps 8 and 9.
11. Transfer the (upper) aqueous phase by pipet to a fresh tube containing 2 mL of chloroform:isoamyl alcohol (25:1). Repeat steps 8 and 9.
12. Transfer the (upper) aqueous phase by pipet into a fresh tube containing 4 mL of absolute ethanol. Allow the DNA to begin to precipitate at the interface, then mix gently to complete the precipitation.
13. Remove the DNA precipitate from the ethanol with a disposable plastic tip. Drain off the excess ethanol from the DNA by pressing against the side of the tube, and transfer to a 2-mL cryotube containing 100–500 μL of sterile distilled water.
14. Dissolve the DNA at room temperature by mixing on a rotator for 2–3 h.
15. Measure the DNA concentration and purity using a UV spectrophotometer, and adjust the concentration to 500 μg/mL.
16. A 0.5-μL aliquot of DNA prepared in this way is sufficient for a single PCR reaction. DNA should be stored at –20°C until use.

3.3. ARMS Multiplex

1. Prepare genomic DNA using one of the methods described in Sections 3.1–3.2.2.
2. Each Johnson & Johnson CF(4)m PCR test comprises one "A" reaction (yellow tube) and one "B" reaction (blue tube). These are stored at –20°C. Allow the required number of tubes to thaw before use, including an extra test to contain water in place of DNA as a control. Positive controls containing particular mutations may be included. Spin the tubes briefly in a microcentrifuge.
3. Add test DNA (5 or 0.5 µL depending on the extraction method) to each tube of an A and B pair at ambient temperature (*see* Note 6).
4. Add 1 drop (30–50 µL) of sterile mineral oil to each reaction tube; then re-cap the tubes firmly.
5. Prepare the *Taq* DNA polymerase (supplied in the kit) dilution by mixing 80 µL water, 10 µL ARMS buffer (10X), and 10 µL *Taq* DNA polymerase (45–60 U). This is sufficient for 20 tests (40 tubes).
6. Place the reaction tubes in the thermal cycler block which is set to run at 94°C. After the tubes have been at 94°C for 5 min, remove each tube in turn and add 2 µL of the diluted *Taq* DNA polymerase to the lower aqueous phase through the mineral oil layer. Ensure that the enzyme is not added to the oil layer. Replace each tube in the block at 94°C until enzyme has been added to each tube.
7. Stop the 94°C soak program and immediately run the amplification program for 35 cycles of: 94°C denaturation for 45 s, 60°C annealing for 45 s, and 72°C extension for 45 s, followed by a final extension of 10 min at 72°C and an indefinite soak at 4°C.
8. Take a 20-µL aliquot from each reaction tube and to each aliquot add 10 µL of gel loading buffer. Load 25 µL of each A and B pair next to each other on a horizontal 3% agarose gel (containing ethidium bromide at 0.5 µg/mL) (*see* Note 7).
9. Electrophorese the samples at 100V for 45 min (for a 20 × 25-cm gel) in 0.5X TBE buffer.
10. Visualize using a UV transilluminator and photograph the gel for a permanent record (*see* Fig. 2)

3.4. ASO Hybridization

In addition to the ARMS multiplex test, a number of mutations are tested for by ASO hybridization to dot-blots of PCR products. In the first instance, PCR products of the relevant CFTR exon are prepared according to standard procedures. These are fixed onto duplicate nylon membranes in the form of dot-blots, which are then hybridized to one of two ASOs, which are homologous to either the normal sequence or the mutant sequence at any given point.

3.4.1. Preparation of Dot-Blots

1. For each sample, label a 0.5-mL microcentrifuge tube. To each tube, add 6 µL of denaturing solution (0.4*M* NaOH, 25 m*M* EDTA). Carefully (from beneath the oil layer) take up 16 µL of PCR product from each sample and add to the denaturant.

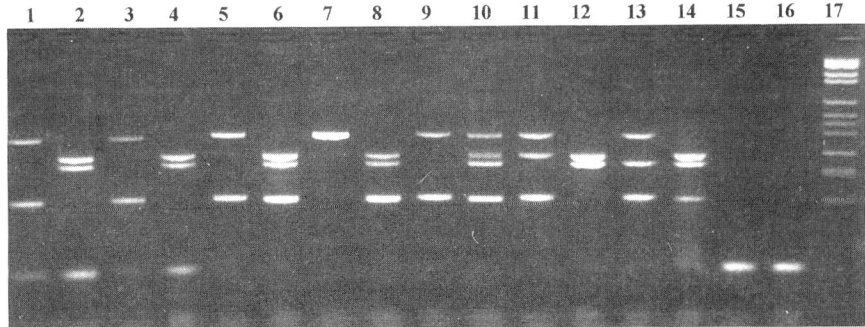

Fig. 2. Detection of four CF mutations by the CF(4)m PCR kit. Odd-numbered tracks contain the ARMS products for the normal alleles of 621 + 1(G > T) and ΔF508, plus the mutant alleles of G551D and G542X. Even-numbered tracks contain products for the normal alleles of G551D and G542X and the mutant alleles of 621 + 1(G > T) and ΔF508. Tracks 1 and 2 are from an individual who is negative for all four mutations, as are tracks 3 and 4. Tracks 5 and 6 are from a ΔF508 heterozygote (the extra band in track 6 represents the ΔF508 mutant allele). Tracks 7 and 8 are from a ΔF508 homozygote (the extra band in track 8 represents the ΔF508 mutant allele and the band representing the normal allele for ΔF508 is absent from track 7). Tracks 9 and 10 are from a compound heterozygote of 621 + 1(G > T) and ΔF508. Tracks 11 and 12 are from a G551D heterozygote. Tracks 13 and 14 are from a compound heterozygote of G542X and ΔF508. Tracks 15 and 16 are a negative (no DNA) control and track 17 is DNA molecular weight marker VI (Boehringer Mannheim).

2. Incubate the tubes at 94°C for 10 min in a heating block and then cool. Centrifuge the tubes briefly.
3. Cut a piece of charged nylon membrane (e.g., Hybond N+) sufficient for preparing duplicate membranes. In pencil, mark out a grid of squares 1.25 × 1.25 cm and number the membranes accordingly (*see* Note 8).
4. Transfer 8 μL of each sample onto duplicate squares of each membrane. Allow to dry.
5. Fix the DNA to the membrane by exposing to UV light at 312 nm (on a standard UV transilluminator) for 5 min.
6. Place the membrane between sheets of filter paper. Wrap in cling film, and store at 4°C until use.

3.4.2. ASO Labeling

Each ASO is 5' end-labeled with γ-^{33}P or ^{32}P using polynucleotide kinase (PNK) which catalyzes the transfer of the γ-phosphate of ATP to a 5'-OH terminus of DNA.

1. To a 0.5-mL tube add the following: 5 μL sterile distilled water, 1 μL PNK buffer (10X), 1 μL ASO (10–20 ng/μL), 1 μL ^{33}P-ATP or ^{32}P-ATP, 2 μL PNK (10–20 U).

2. Incubate the reaction mixture at 37°C for 1 h, then heat to 70°C for 2 min to denature the enzyme.
3. Dilute each reaction to 100 μL with distilled water for ease of dispensing.

3.4.3. Hybridization of ASOs to Dot-Blots

1. Place each of the duplicate membranes (A and B) in a clean, dry hybridization vessel. To each vessel add 10 mL of hybridization solution, taking care to avoid trapping air bubbles between the membrane and the vessel.
2. Prehybridize the membranes in the hybridization oven at 42°C for 1 h.
3. To the A vessel, add the ^{33}P- or ^{32}P-labeled "mutant" ASO (from Section 3.4.2.), ensuring that the ASO is mixed throughout the vessel. Likewise, add the labeled "normal" ASO to the B vessel.
4. Incubate the two vessels overnight at 42°C in the hybridization oven.
5. Discard the hybridization solution, replace with 30 mL of wash solution (2X SSC, 0.1% SDS), and return to the hybridization oven for 45 min.
6. Repeat step 5, adjusting the oven temperature according to the ASO used (Table 4) (see Note 9).
7. After the final wash, remove the membrane from the vessel, blot dry, and place between polythene sheets in an X-ray cassette. Place a sheet of X-ray film against the membrane and expose at −70°C for 1–4 d before developing if using ^{33}P, or at room temperature for 2–3 h if using ^{32}P.

4. Notes

1. Prepare a solution of herring sperm DNA (10 mg/mL) preferably leaving it to dissolve overnight. The DNA may be sheared either by passing the solution several times through a narrow gage (G21) needle, or by using a sonicating water bath (60 min, full power for 100 mL of DNA solution). The DNA solution may then be stored in 10-mL aliquots at −20°C until required. The DNA solution should be placed in a boiling water bath for 5–10 min to denature the DNA immediately prior to its use in the preparation of hybridization solution.
2. It has been reported that if patients eat apples or chocolate before performing a mouthwash sample there may be some inhibition of PCR when using those samples (Cellmark Diagnostics, personal communication, March 1994). We recommend that patients do not perform mouthwash sampling immediately after eating. Patients are also advised not to brush their teeth immediately before sampling. For babies/children who are too young to perform a mouthwash, sufficient cellular material may be collected by gently wiping inside each cheek using a swab/cotton bud and rinsing this into the sucrose solution.
3. DNA prepared from mouthwash samples or from blood using the small-scale (NaOH) method could probably be stored for several years (not investigated), but the phenol/chloroform extraction method from blood is recommended for preparation of DNA destined for long-term storage. DNA for storage should be dissolved in TE buffer pH 7.5 rather than in water.
4. Prepare an aqueous solution of proteinase K (20 mg/mL) and store at −20°C in 500-μL aliquots.

5. Phenol is highly corrosive, can cause severe burns, and should be handled with care.
6. Multiplex ARMS CF(4)m is a very sensitive test and the use of filter pipet-tips throughout is recommended to avoid problems with contamination.
7. Ethidium bromide is a powerful mutagen and should be handled with care. A stock solution (10 mg/mL) should be prepared and stored at 4°C in a lightproof bottle.
8. Hybond membrane should be handled as little as possible, always using clean, dry gloves.
9. Posthybridization wash temperatures are given, but since different ovens will have different specifications, these conditions should be used as a guide and monitoring of the membranes after each wash, using a Geiger-Muller detector, is advised.
10. Working solutions of primer pairs are made at a concentration of 20 μM of each primer. Stock solutions of each primer are stored at 10X working concentration. Working solutions of ASOs are made at 10 ng/μL, and stock solutions at 100X working concentration. All primer and ASO solutions are stored at –20°C.

References

1. Rommens, J. M., Ianuzzi, M. C., Kerem, B., Drumm, M. L., Melmer, G., Dean, M., et al. (1989) Identification of the cystic fibrosis gene: chromosome walking and jumping. *Science* **245,** 1059–1065.
2. Riordan, J. R., Rommens, J. M., Kerem, B., Alon, N., Rozmahel, R., Grzelczak, Z., et al. (1989) Identification of the cystic fibrosis gene: cloning and characterization of complementary DNA. *Science* **245,** 1066–1073.
3. Kerem, B., Rommens, J. M., Buchanan, J. A., Markiewicz, D., Cox, T. K., Chakravarti, A., et al. (1989) Identification of the cystic fibrosis gene: genetic analysis. *Science* **245,** 1073–1080.
4. Mullis, K. and Faloona, F. (1987) Specific synthesis of DNA in vitro via a polymerase catalyzed chain reation, in *Methods in Enzymology,* vol. 155 (Wu, R., ed.), Academic, New York, pp. 335–350.
5. Newton, C. R., Graham, A., Heptinstall, L. E., Powell, S. J., Summers, C., Kalsheker, N., and Smith, J. C. (1989) Analysis of any point mutation in DNA: the amplification refractory mutation system. *Nucleic Acids Res.* **17,** 2503–2516.
6. Schwarz, M. J., Malone, G. M., Haworth, A., Cheadle, J. P., Meredith, A. L., Gardner, A., et al. (1995) Cystic fibrosis mutation analysis: report from 22 UK regional genetics laboratories. *Hum. Mut.* **6,** 326–333.
7. Kazazian, H. H., Jr. and The Cystic Fibrosis Genetic Analysis Consortium (1994) Population variation of common cystic fibrosis mutations. *Hum. Mut.* **4,** 167–177.
8. Cutting, G. R., Kasch, L. M., Rosenstein, B. J., Tsui, L-C., Antonarakis, S. E., and Kazazian, H. H., Jr. (1990) A cluster of cystic fibrosis mutations in the first nucleotide-binding fold of the cystic fibrosis conductance regulator protein. *Nature* **346,** 366–369.
9. Kerem, B., Zielenski, J., Markiewicz, D., Bozon, D., Gazit, E., Yahaf, J., et al. (1990) Identification of mutations in regions corresponding to the 2 putative nucleotide (ATP)-binding folds of the cystic fibrosis gene. *Proc. Natl. Acad. Sci. USA* **87,** 8447–8451.

10. Zielenski, J., Bozon, D., Kerem, B., Markiewicz, D., Rommens, J. M., and Tsui, L.-C. (1991) Identification of mutations in exons 1 through 8 of the cystic fibrosis transmembrane conductance regulator (CFTR) gene. *Genomics* **10**, 229–235.

11. Dean, M., White, M., Amos, J., Gerrard, B., Stewart, C., Khaw, K.-T., and Leppert, M. (1990) Multiple mutations in highly conserved residues are found in mildly affected cystic fibrosis patients. *Cell* **61**, 863–870.

12. Strong, T. V., Smit, L. S., Nasr, S., Wood, D., Cole, J. L., Ianuzzi, M., Stern, R., and Collins, F. S. (1992) Characterisation of an intron 12 splice donor mutation in the cystic fibrosis transmembrane conductance regulator (CFTR) gene. *Hum. Mut.* **1**, 380–387.

13. Osborne, L., Knight, R. A., Santis, G., and Hodson, M. (1991) A mutation in the second nucleotide binding fold of the cystic fibrosis gene. *Am. J. Hum. Genet.* **48**, 608–612.

14. Schwarz, M. J., Summers, C., Heptinstall, L. E., Newton, C., Markham, A., and Super, M. (1991) A deletion mutation of the cystic fibrosis transmembrane conductance regulator (CFTR) locus: ΔI507. *Adv. Exp. Med. Biol.* **290**, 393–398.

15. Iannuzzi, M. C., Stern, R. C., Collins, F. S., Hon, C. T., Hidaka, N., Strong, T., et al. (1991) Two frameshift mutations in the cystic fibrosis gene. *Am. J. Hum. Genet.* **48(2)**, 227–231.

16. Jones, C. T., McIntosh, I., Keston, M., Ferguson, A., and Brock, D. J. H. (1992) Three novel mutations in the cystic fibrosis gene detected by chemical cleavage: analysis of variant splicing and a nonsense mutation. *Hum. Mol. Genet.* **1(1)**, 11–17.

17. Vidaud, M., Fanen, P., Martin, J., Ghanem, N., Nicolas, S., and Goossens, M. (1990) Three mutations in the CFTR gene in French cystic fibrosis patients: identification by denaturing gradient gel electrophoresis. *Hum. Genet.* **85**, 446–449.

18. Claustres, M., Gerrard, B., White, M. B., Desgeorges, M., Kjellberg, P., Rollin, B., and Dean, M. (1992) A rare mutation (1078delT) in exon 7 of the CFTR gene in a Southern French adult with cystic fibrosis. *Genomics* **13**, 907,908.

19. Highsmith, W. E., Burch, L. H., Zhou, Z., Olsen, J. C., Boat, T. E., Spock, A., et al. (1994) A novel mutation in the cystic fibrosis gene with pulmonary disease but normal sweat chloride concentration. *N. Engl. J. Med.* **331**, 974–980.

20. Livingstone, J., Axton, R. A., Gilfillan, A., Mennie, M., Compton, M., Liston, W. A., et al. (1994) Antenatal screening for cystic fibrosis: a trial of the couple model. *Br. Med. J.* **308**, 1459–1462.

21. Super, M., Schwarz, M. J., Malone, G., Roberts, T., Haworth, A., and Dermody, G. (1994) Active cascade testing for carriers of cystic fibrosis gene. *Br. Med. J.* **308**, 1462–1468.

22. American Society of Human Genetics Board of Directors (1992) Statement of the American Society of Human Genetics on Cystic Fibrosis Carrier Screening. *Am. J. Hum. Genet.* **51(6)**, 1443,1444.

23. Ferrie, R. M., Schwarz, M. J., Robertson, N. H., Vaudin, S., Super, M., Malone, G., and Little, S. (1992) Development, multiplexing, and application of ARMS tests for common mutations in the CFTR gene. *Am. J. Hum. Genet.* **51(2)**, 251–262.

24. Gasparini, P., Dognini, M., Bonnizzato, A., Pignatti, P. F., Morral, N., and Estivill, X. (1991) A tetranucleotide repeat polymorphism in the cystic fibrosis gene. *Hum. Genet.* **86,** 625.

25. Morral, N., Nunes, V., Casals, T., and Estivill, X. (1991) CA/GT microsatellite allele within the cystic fibrosis transmembrane conductance regulator (CFTR) gene are not generated by unequal crossing over. *Genomics* **10,** 692–698.

26. Zielenski, J., Markiewicz, D., Rininsland, F., Rommens, J. M., and Tsui, L.-C. (1991) A cluster of highly polymorphic dinucleotide repeats in intron 17B of the CFTR gene. *Am. J. Hum. Genet.* **49,** 1256–1262.

27. Morral, N., Girbau, E., Zielenski, J., Nunes, V., Casals, T., Tsui, L.-C., and Estivill, X. (1992) Dinucleotide (CA/GT) repeat polymorphism in intron 17B of the cystic fibrosis conductance transmembrane regulator (CFTR) gene. *Hum. Genet.* **88,** 356.

28. Zielenski, J., Rozmahel, R., Bozon, D., Kerem, B., Grzelczak, Z., Riordan, J. R., et al. (1991) Genomic DNA sequence of the cystic fibrosis conductance regulator (CFTR) gene. *Genomics* **10,** 214–228.

29. Casals, T., Bassas, L., Ruiz-Romero, J., Chillon, M., Giminez, J., Ramos, M. D., et al. (1995) Extensive analysis of 40 infertile patients with congenital absence of the vas deferens: in 50% of cases only one CFTR allele could be detected. *Hum. Genet.* **95,** 205–211.

30. Kiesewetter, S., Macek, M., Jr., Davis, C., Curristin, S. M., Chu, C.-S., Graham, C., et al. (1993) A mutation in CFTR produces different phenotypes depending on chromosomal background. *Nature Genet.* **5,** 274–278.

6

Characterization of Gene Rearrangements and Gene Conversion Events in the 21-Hydroxylase Gene

Simon C. Ramsden and Paul J. Sinnott

1. Introduction

Congenital adrenal hyperplasia (CAH) is an inherited disorder of steroidogenesis with a wide spectrum of expression. In about 95% of cases, the disease is the result of 21-hydroxylase deficiency, an autosomal recessive condition that maps to the major histocompatibility complex (MHC) on 6p21.3 *(1)*.

Classical CAH results in excessive androgen production. Females with this disorder are frequently diagnosed at birth because of ambiguous development of external genitalia, whereas males may not present until age 4–7 when they begin to manifest inappropriate virilization. Approximately 30% of individuals with classical CAH have this simple virilizing form of the disease. The remaining 70% in addition manifest the potentially life-threatening salt-wasting form of classical CAH characterized by an inability to retain dietary sodium.

Pang and coworkers *(2)* estimated the incidence of classical CAH based on biochemical criteria as 1 in 14,000 with a carrier frequency of 1 in 60. Nonclassical CAH is likely to be equally as common, and although accurate estimates are not available, the prevalence of all clinical forms of the disease is likely to vary from one population to the next *(3)*. When an individual at population risk requests carrier testing, we estimate a prior carrier risk of 1 in 50. This cannot account for racial differences and, in addition, will be an underestimate, not accounting for the mildest mutations.

1.1. The Genetics of 21-Hydroxylase Deficiency

There are two 21-hydroxylase loci at 6p21.3, a functional gene (termed P450c21B, CYP21, or 21B) and a nonfunctional pseudogene (termed P450c21A,

From: *Methods in Molecular Medicine: Molecular Diagnosis of Genetic Diseases*
Edited by: R. Elles Humana Press Inc., Totowa, NJ

CYP21P, or 21A). These loci are duplicated in tandem with the C4A and C4B loci, respectively, which encode the fourth component of the serum complement *(4)*. What we see today is assumed to be the consequence of an ancestral duplication of approx 30 kb of DNA encoding the 21-hydroxylase and C4 genes *(see* Fig. 1). Sequencing studies have confirmed the presence of a number of mutations within the 21A pseudogene incompatible with gene function *(5,6)*. The tandem duplication involving the 21-hydroxylase gene results in high levels of mutation owing to gene deletions and gene conversion.

1.1.1. Gene Deletions

Gross deletions of the entire 21B gene account for approximately one-third of 21-hydroxylase-deficient chromosomes. The high degree of sequence homology between the A and B units means that unequal pairing may occur across this region during meiosis. If this is accompanied by a recombination event within the mispaired region, then a triplication and a deletion of a complete unit will result in the meiotic products. The position of the recombination event will dictate the exact composition of the resultant recombinant chromosomes. Figure 2 shows a range of theoretical possibilities given different recombination events. Recombination events at position A, for example, will result in a chromosome lacking the entire 21B gene. Clearly, this is not the full picture since a recombination event between A and B will result in a 21B/21A fusion gene, nonfunctional by virtue of the 21A sequences.

Figure 2 also demonstrates the generation of deletions and triplications that will have no consequence on 21-hydroxylase activity. Indeed, these rearrangements can be demonstrated in the normal population. It has been estimated, for example, that 14% of normal chromosomes in the French population carry a 21A unit deletion *(7)*. These nonpathogenic deletions and triplication haplotypes may be used as extremely close polymorphisms for 21-hydroxylase deficiency gene tracking.

1.1.2. Gene Conversion

Approximately two-thirds of 21-hydroxylase-deficient chromosomes show no evidence of gross 21B deletions. In these instances, sequencing has identified point mutations, and small insertions and deletions. Closer examination reveals that these mutations are usually already present in the 21A pseudogene, and they appear to pass into the 21B gene by the process of gene conversion, a process first described in ascomycete fungi *(8)*. Gene conversion in this system relies on the heteroduplex formed by the nonhomologous pairing between the 21A and B genes. Mispaired bases, corresponding to the sites of mutation in the 21A gene, are subject to mismatch repair. Consequently, the strands may be correctly or incorrectly repaired, the latter case resulting in the transfer of pseudogene sequence into the active 21-hydroxylase gene.

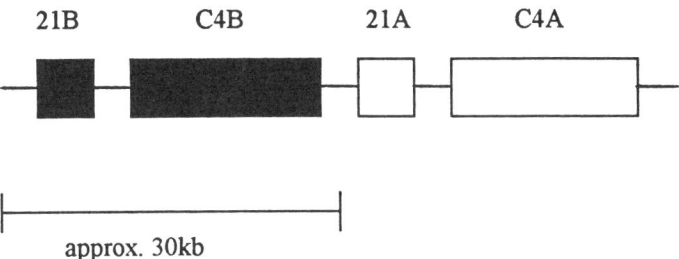

Fig. 1. Schematic representation of the genomic organization around the 21-hydroxylase locus.

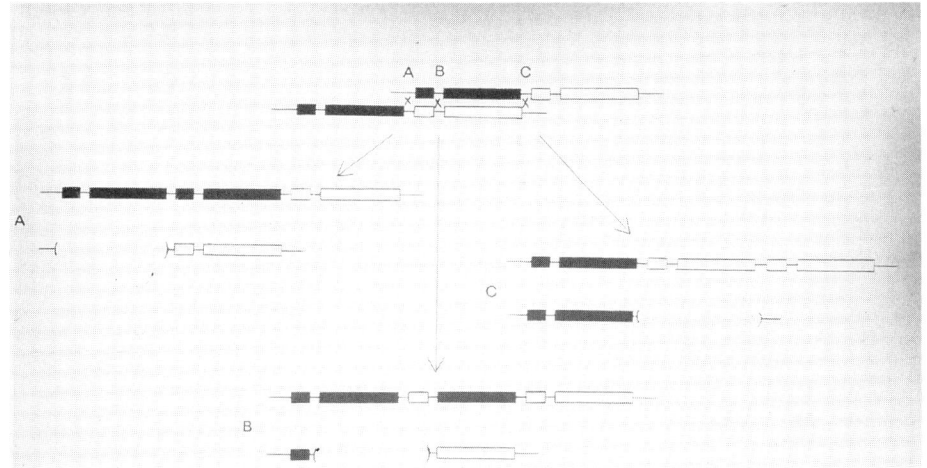

Fig. 2. Possible outcomes of nonhomologous recombination events around the 21-hydroxylase gene.

1.2. Referrals

Individuals will be referred for the molecular diagnosis of 21-hydroxylase deficiency for a variety of reasons:

1. An early and accurate prenatal diagnosis in a family with a previous history of 21-hydroxylase deficiency will identify affected female fetuses *in utero*. In these cases, dexamethasone treatment will assist normal genital development in the fetus.
2. For individuals with either a mild or atypical manifestation of the disease, molecular techniques may identify mutations in the 21-hydroxylase gene that will confirm the diagnosis. Unfortunately, since no routine screening strategy would be likely to identify all possible mutations, the inability to identify a mutation can never exclude the diagnosis.

3. Individuals will often present to clinic requesting carrier screening. These may be individuals at an elevated prior risk owing to an affected relative or individuals at population risk with a partner who is affected or a known carrier.

Haplotype analysis incorporating markers closely flanking the disease locus is the most useful technique in the prenatal diagnosis of CAH where affected members of a family have been previously diagnosed. These requests are often at short notice, and gene tracking will always offer quick, accurate risks. For diagnostic purposes and carrier detection, however, direct mutation analysis is usually necessary.

2. Materials

The polymerase chain reaction (PCR) procedures used throughout this chapter are standard techniques, and the materials and equipment required have been described in detail elsewhere (*see* particularly Chapter 2). Southern analysis for major gene rearrangements will be highlighted as the key technique in this chapter.

2.1. PCR

1. The materials required for the PCR amplification are detailed in Chapter 2.
2. The oligonucleotides required are given in Tables 1 and 2.
3. For the visualization of microsatellites, one will require apparatus suitable for running 8% native polyacrylamide (19:1 ratio of crosslinking) gels and silver staining is required (*see* Chapter 2).
4. For the visualization of amplification refractory mutation system (ARMS) products, one will require apparatus suitable for running 1–3% horizontal agarose gels and ethidium bromide staining (*see* Chapter 2).

2.2. Southern Analysis

Analytical-grade reagents should be used at all times.

1. A 20 × 20 cm submarine gel electrophoresis tank suitable for running agarose gels is essential, i.e., Horizon 20.25 system (Life Technologies, Gaithersburg, MD).
2. An electrophoresis power pack.
3. A temperature-controlled hybridization oven, capable of maintaining 65°C.
4. Electrophoresis-grade agarose.
5. *Taq*I restriction enzyme: This is available from numerous manufacturers at a concentration of approx 10 U/µL and will be supplied with a suitable reaction buffer. Store at –20°C.
6. Probes 21A1.8 *(11)* and C4B550 *(12)*.
7. TBE electrophoresis buffer: Make as a 10X stock solution, 0.89M Tris, 0.89M boric acid, 0.02M EDTA (pH 8.0), and store at room temperature.
8. 5X TBE gel loading buffer, to make 10 mL: 4.9 mL glycerol, 100 µL of 10% SDS, 3 mg bromophenol blue, and 15 mg xylene cyanole. Store at room temperature.
9. Phosphate prehybridization/hybridization solution (PPH): Prepare prehybridization solution as a 2X stock (i.e., 0.5M NaH$_2$PO$_4$, 0.5M NaCl, 1 mM EDTA, adjust to pH 7.5 with 5M NaOH), and store at room temperature. When ready to

Table 1
Microsatellite Primers[a]

Oligonucleotide	Sequence, 5'–3'
IR2	GCCTCTAGATTTCATCCAGCCACA
IR4	CCTCTCTCCCCTGCAACACACA

[a] Primer sequences taken from ref. *9*.

Table 2
ARMS Primers[a]

Oligonucleotide	Sequence, 5'–3'
P1	TTC AGG CGA TTC AGG AAG GC
P4	TCT CGC ACC CCA GTA TGA CT
P5	GGT GCT GAA CTC CAA GAG G
P11	GGA GCA ATA AAG GAG AAA CTG A
P19	TTG AGC AAG GGC AGC CGT G
P48	CAG AGC AGG GAG TAG TCT C
P55	CCT GTC CTT GGG AGA CTA CT
P659A	ACC CTC CAG CCC CCA A
P659C	ACC CTC CAG CCC CCA C
P659G	ACC CTC CAG CCC CCA G
P1004T	CCG AAG GTG AGG TAA CAG A
P1004A	CGA AGG TGA GGT AAC AGT
P1688G	ACT GCA GCC ATG TGC AC
P1688T	CAC TGC AGC CAT GTG CAA
P2113C	GGG CAC AAC GGG CCG
P2113T	AAG GGC ACA ACG GGC CA

[a] Primer sequences taken from ref. *10*.

use the prehybridization buffer, dilute with water and add SDS to a final concentration of 1X PPH, 0.5% SDS. To make the hybridization buffer, remove 20 mL into a screw-capped plastic tube, and add PEG 6000 to a final concentration of 6%. No further blocking is required for these probes.

10. Probe-labeling reagents: In a laboratory not already routinely labeling probes, a commercial random priming labeling kit (e.g., The Random Primed DNA Labeling Kit, Boehringer Mannheim [East Sussex, UK], product number 1004 760) is the easiest option.

11. α^{32}PdCTP radioisotope label: Can be purchased at 10 µCi/µL from Amersham International (Buckinghamshire, UK). Note that storage and use of radioactive materials are governed by national and local safety regulations.

12. Denaturing solution: 1.5M NaCl, 0.5M NaOH. Store at room temperature.
13. 20X SSC: 3M NaCl, 0.3M Na-citrate. Store at room temperature.
14. Positively charged nylon membrane for DNA transfer, i.e., Hybond N+ (Amersham International).
15. 250- and 500-μ gage polythene layflat tubing (P & B Plastics, Stockport, UK).
16. Glass plates.
17. Autoradiograph cassettes fitted with blue emitting intensifying screens, i.e., High Speed X (X-Ograph, Wiltshire, UK).
18. X-Ray film: Fuji RX (Fuji Photo Film Co., Japan).
19. −70°C Freezer.
20. A slow orbital shaker.
21. A short-wave UV transilluminator.

3. Methods

3.1. Gene Tracking

The 21-hydroxylase locus resides within the class III region of the MHC, and typing for the linked human leucocyte antigen (HLA) loci have been widely used in tracking this gene. Although associations are well established between CAH and certain HLA types *(13–16)*, they are rarely of much practical use in routine diagnosis. DNA-based markers have proven most useful for the molecular diagnosis of 21-hydroxylase deficiency. These can be divided into two broad types, namely markers derived from DNA-based HLA typing and microsatellite markers representing anonymous polymorphisms.

3.1.1. DNA-Based HLA Typing

Although it is outside the scope of this chapter to describe the practical details behind HLA typing, they are worth a brief note since they do offer a rich source of highly polymorphic markers for 21-hydroxylase gene tracking if HLA typing facilities are available. A complete system of HLA-DR and DQ typing devised by Bidwell and Jarrold *(17)* relying on Southern analysis has now been adopted by many typing laboratories.

More recently, an alternative to restriction fragment length polymorphism (RFLP) typing has been developed, the use of PCR amplification followed by hybridization with allele-specific oligonucleotide probes *(18)*. The principle of so-called oligotyping is the determination of nucleotide sequences that occur in the polymorphic exons of the HLA genes. In the HLA class II genes, for example, most of this variation occurs in the second exon.

One of the most elegant strategies for HLA typing at the molecular level involves the design of specific oligonucleotide primers for PCR amplification, which will amplify, exclusively, the desired allele. This sequence-specific amplification (or ARMS—*see* Section 3.2.2.) technique is now available for the rapid nonradioactive typing of HLA-A, -B, -C, -DR, and -DQ loci *(19–21)*.

Table 3
Conditions for Amplifying a Microsatellite Repeat at the TNF Locus

Microsatellite	Primers	Product sizes, bp	Cycling[a]	Number of cycles
TNFα	IR2 + 4	80–110	93°C, 1 min 65°C, 1 min 72°C, 1 min	27

[a]Cycling is preceeded by 93°C for 3 min and followed by 72°C for 5 min.

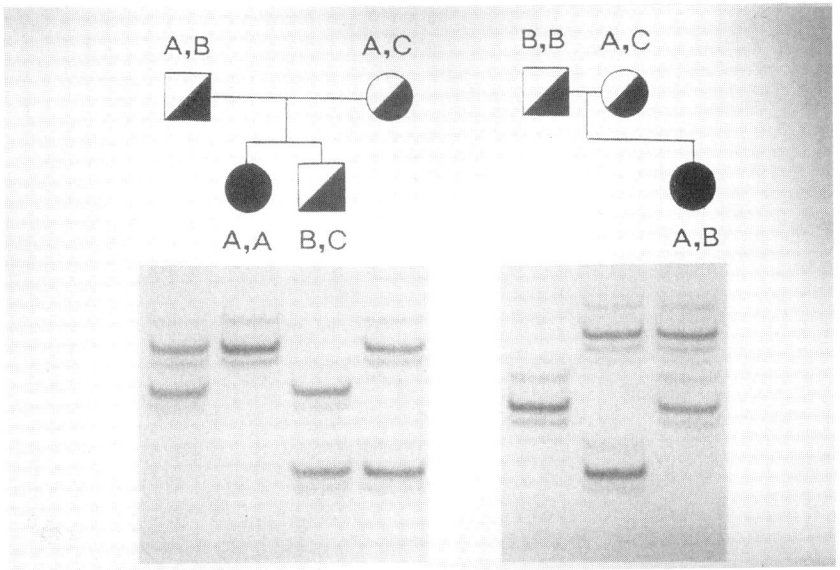

Fig. 3. Microsatellite TNFα. This marker shows approx 0.5% recombination with the 21-hydroxylase locus.

3.1.2. Microsatellite Markers

These offer a rapid nonradioactive alternative to HLA typing. Microsatellites have been described at the TNF locus approx 0.5 cM distal to the disease gene (9). These have proven particularly useful in the diagnosis of this disease. Table 3 shows the amplification conditions used for a particularly useful microsatellite. Fragments are resolved on 8% native polyacrylamide gels and visualized using ethidium bromide or silver staining (*see* Chapter 2). Figure 3 shows this marker segregating through two families.

It is envisaged that as the HLA region becomes better characterized, further microsatellites will become available offering flanking markers that might be amplified in a multiplex reaction making gene tracking for this disease more efficient.

3.2. Mutation Analysis

3.2.1. Short Range Mapping

Rearrangements involving the 21-hydroxylase gene are best determined by a short-range mapping strategy using Southern analysis (adapted from ref. *22*). Although a number of restriction digests can provide information regarding genomic organization around this locus, we use a simple *Taq*I digest with a mixed radiolabeled probe representing the p450c21 cDNA, 21A1.8 *(11)*, and a 5' C4 cDNA, C4B550 *(12)*. For the purposes of this chapter, the technical details of the process of Southern analysis are given in full. However, it is the interpretation of the resulting autoradiographs that makes this particular application most interesting.

3.2.1.1. RESTRICTION DIGESTION AND GEL ELECTROPHORESIS

1. The genomic DNA is cut with *Taq*I prior to electrophoresis. Prepare restriction digests of all the samples to be analyzed in either 0.6- or 1.6-mL microcentrifuge tubes as follows: 5 μg of genomic DNA, 3 μL of 10X restriction enzyme buffer (supplied by the manufacturer), 10 U of restriction enzyme (typically 1 μL). Add sterile dH$_2$O to 30 μL and incubate in a water bath at 65°C for at least 4 h, preferably overnight.
2. While the samples are digesting, prepare a 0.8% agarose gel for electrophoresis of the samples. For a typical 20 × 20 cm format, the following amounts should be sufficient:, 35 mL of 10X TBE, 315 mL of dH$_2$O, 2.8 g of agarose. The gel should be heated gently to dissolve the agarose either in a microwave oven or on a hotplate with a magnetic stirrer bar. Once the agarose has completely dissolved, add 17.5 μL of a 10 mg/mL solution of ethidium bromide, swirl gently to mix, and allow the gel solution to cool to 65°C.
3. Place an appropriate comb in the gel former, and seal the open ends with plastic tape. When the gel has cooled down, pour carefully into the former. Check for air bubbles, especially around the comb. These can be removed using a Pasteur pipet. Allow the gel to set for at least 1 h before running. If the gel is not required immediately, it may be wrapped in cling film and stored in a refrigerator at 4°C for up to 48 h. When ready to run, remove the tape and immerse in 1X TBE buffer to a depth over the gel surface of about 1.5 mm. Only remove the comb once the gel is fully submerged in the running buffer.
4. The samples should be monitored for complete digestion before running. Take 3 μL of each restriction digest, and mix with 1 μL of 5X TBE loading buffer, and run for 30 min at 60 mA on a 0.8–1.0% agarose monitor gel. The digested samples should then be visualized on a UV transilluminator. Undigested or partially digested samples have a characteristic streaky appearance. Add a further 10 U of restriction enzyme to any uncut samples and reincubate for at least 2 h.

5. Once the samples are completely digested, mix each with 9 μL of dH$_2$O and 9 μL of 5X TBE loading buffer. Load the whole sample onto the gel using a fresh micropipeter tip for each sample. A mol-wt standard, i.e., 1-kb ladder (Life Technologies), should also be loaded in one of the outer wells. Set the gel to run at 55 mA in constant current mode for at least 16 h. You will need to resolve fragments ranging from 3.2–7.0 kb.

3.2.1.2. SOUTHERN BLOTTING

1. When the gel has electrophoresed the correct distance, place the gel on a UV transilluminator. Cut off the mol-wt marker, the wells, and any waste agarose. Remember to slice off a corner of the gel to allow it to be oriented, and note the dimensions of the trimmed gel. Transfer the gel into a plastic tray, and submerge in denaturing solution. Denature on a slow orbital shaker for 1 h.

2. While the gel is denaturing, cut a piece of charged Nylon membrane and two pieces of Whatman 3MM filter paper to a size slightly larger than the gel. Mark or cut one corner of the membrane to correspond to the cut corner of the gel. Transfer the gel onto an inverted gel casting tray, and carefully place the nylon membrane onto the gel avoiding introducing air bubbles. Briefly wet the sheets of filter paper in denaturing solution, and place on top of the membrane. Complete the blot by adding a stack of paper towels to a depth of approx 6 cm and compress with a suitable weight (approx 500 g). Leave to blot for 12–16 h (*see* Note 1).

3. Dismantle the blot and discard any damp paper towels. Place the membrane into a tray containing 200 mL of 3X SSC, and shake gently for 2 min, pour off the 3X SSC, and repeat twice. The filter should now be of neutral pH, and may be probed immediately or sealed in plastic while still damp and stored at 4°C almost indefinitely.

3.2.1.3. PROBE LABELING AND HYBRIDIZATION

1. The instructions supplied with the labeling kit need to be followed with care for successful labeling. Remember you will be handling dangerous radioisotopes and need to use adequate protection in the form of perspex shields. Monitor both the working area and yourself adequately during and after handling radioisotopes. Between 50 and 100 ng of probe should be labeled for each Southern blot, and most kits recommend that 2.5–5 μCi of α^{32}PdCTP be used per labeling reaction. For this analysis, the two probes, 21A1.8 and C4B550, should be labeled in separate reactions. Remember that single-stranded DNA is needed as a template for the labeling reaction, so you must denature the probe by heating to 100°C in a dry block or boiling water bath before adding to the rest of the reaction. For safety reasons, labeling reactions should always be carried out in screw-capped Eppendorfs.

2. Make up 200 mL of prehybridization solution per filter by diluting down the 2X stock to 1X and adding SDS to a final concentration of 0.5%. Before use, remove 10 mL of this solution into a screw-capped 30-mL plastic tube, and add 0.6 g PEG 6000. This will make up the hybridization buffer, and should be placed at 65°C during the period of prehybridization to dissolve the PEG and assist in

degassing the solution. Place the filters in a sealable plastic box, add the prehybridization solution, and seal the lid tightly. Place in an oven at 65°C for at least 1 h to prehybridize (*see* Note 2).

3. After the required prehybridization and labeling, the hybridization can be set up in sealed plastic bags. First add 200 μL of prehybridization buffer (without SDS) to the probes, mix them together, and then boil them for 5 min, after which the probe mixture should be placed on ice. While the probes are being boiled, the filter should be placed in 500-gage plastic and double sealed on three sides. The hybridization buffer is then added followed by the denatured probes and the bag sealed, taking care to exclude bubbles. The filters should then be placed between two glass plates and incubated at 65°C overnight (Note 3).

3.2.1.4. FILTER WASHING AND AUTORADIOGRAPHY

1. Prepare 1 L of a stringent 0.2X SSC, 0.1% SDS wash solution and 1 L of a less stringent solution (i.e., 1X SSC, 0.1% SDS), and equilibrate at 65°C.
2. Cut the sealed plastic containing the hybridizing filter open with a scalpel, and remove the filter into 500 mL of the less stringent wash in a sealable plastic box. After a few minutes, replace this wash with the remaining 500 mL and place at 65°C for 30 min. Finally, replace this wash with the more stringent wash, and leave for a further 30 min at 65°C.

   All wash solutions and the hybridization solutions should be disposed of down a sink designated for the disposal of radioactive waste. The plastic and glass plates should be washed thoroughly in running water before handling and disposal of the plastic.
3. Remove the filter after the first stringent wash with a clean pair of forceps, and place on a clean surface. Monitor the radioactivity using a Geiger counter, if this is above 10 counts/s (cps) (with the plastic shield left over the Geiger detection window), wash in fresh solution for a further 30 min. Repeat this final wash until the activity is between 5 and 10 cps or until no drop in activity is observed between washes.
4. Either heat-seal the filter in 250-gage plastic or wrap in cling film. Place with a sheet of X-ray film inside an autoradiograph cassette fitted with intensifying screens in a darkroom.
5. Leave to expose at –70°C for 1–5 d before developing. The film is usually developed after an overnight exposure to judge the length of time needed for a good result.
6. Filters can be stripped ready for reprobing by soaking them in boiling 0.1% SDS for 10 min (*see* Note 4).

3.2.1.5. INTERPRETATION OF RESULTS

The C4B gene exists in two forms, long (22 kb) and short (16 kb), the difference being the result of the presence or absence of a 6.8-kb intron at the 5' end of the gene *(23)*. As a result of this polymorphism, the 5' end of the C4B gene is characterized by 6.0- or 5.4-kb *Taq*I fragments corresponding to the long and short forms, respectively. The 5' end of the C4A gene can be distinguished

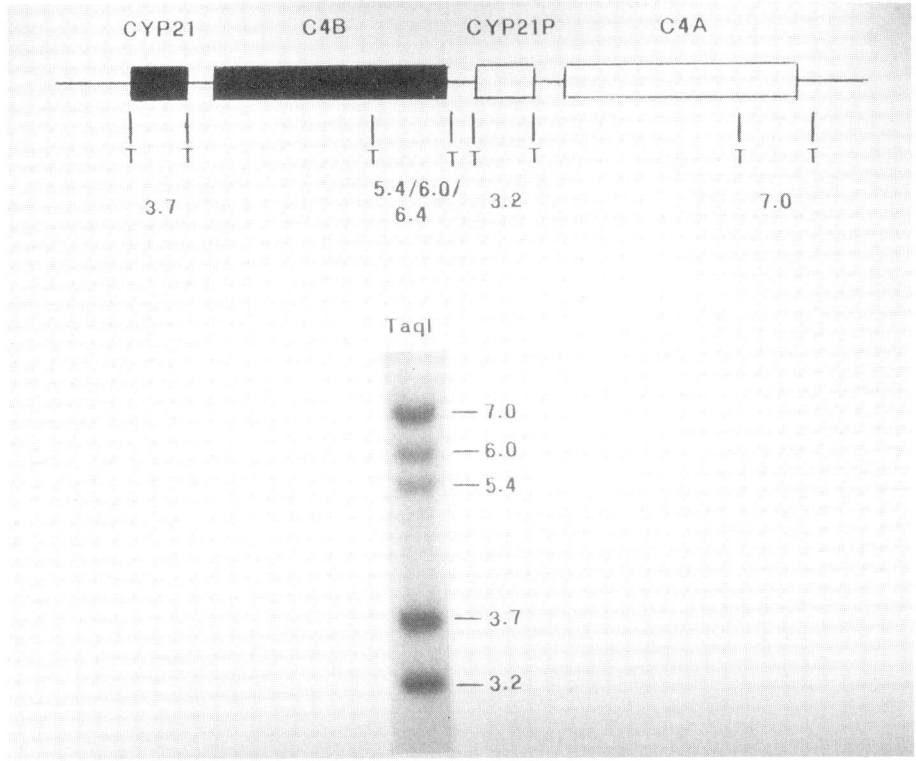

Fig. 4. Key to characterizing the genomic organization around the 21-hydroxylase gene (CYP21) using Southern analysis as described in the text. A *Taq*I (T) digest and a mixed probing with 21A1.8 and C4B550 reveal an individual with no deletions and heterozygous for the 5.4- and 6.0-kb C4B alleles. Note the C4B signals are half the intensity of the C4A signal.

from C4B alleles since it lies on a 7.0-kb fragment *(20)*. The 21B gene lies largely on a 3.7-kb *Taq*I fragment and the 21A gene lies largely on a 3.2-kb *Taq*I fragment by virtue of an additional *Taq*I site at its 5' end *(see* Fig. 4).

A 21A1.8 and C4B550 mixed probe hybridized against a *Taq*I genomic digest will usually be sufficient to elucidate the genomic organization around this locus. By comparing band intensities within gel lanes, one can identify deleted and duplicated genes. In this system, the C4 alleles act as internal lane controls for interpreting the dosage of the 21A and B alleles *(see* Fig. 5).

In a few rare cases, the short-range mapping strategy described will not be sufficient to elucidate the genomic organization fully around the 21-hydroxylase locus. When this situation occurs, pulsed-field gel electrophoresis must be used *(24)*.

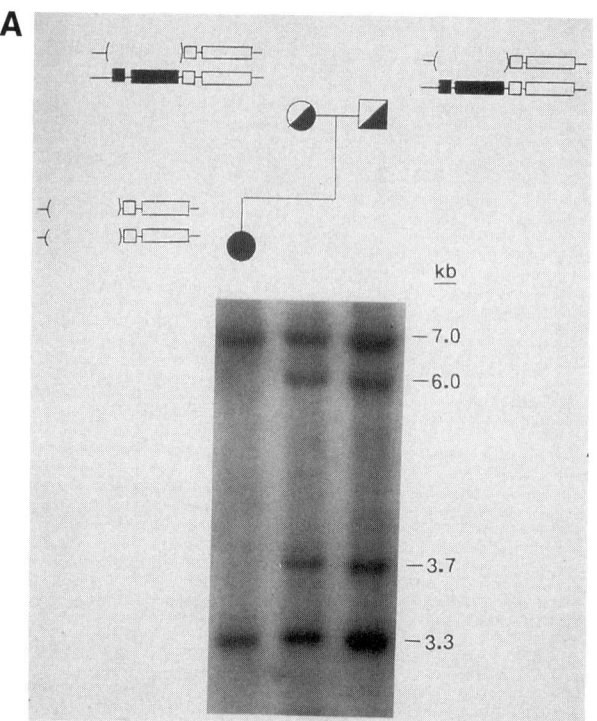

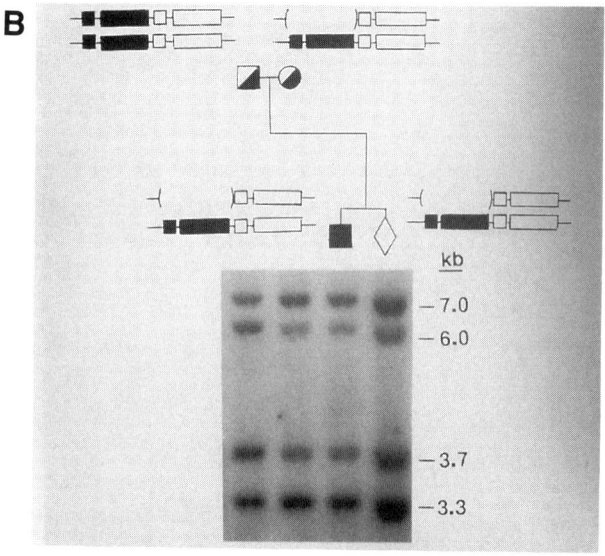

Fig. 5. (A,B) *(Caption on page 134)*

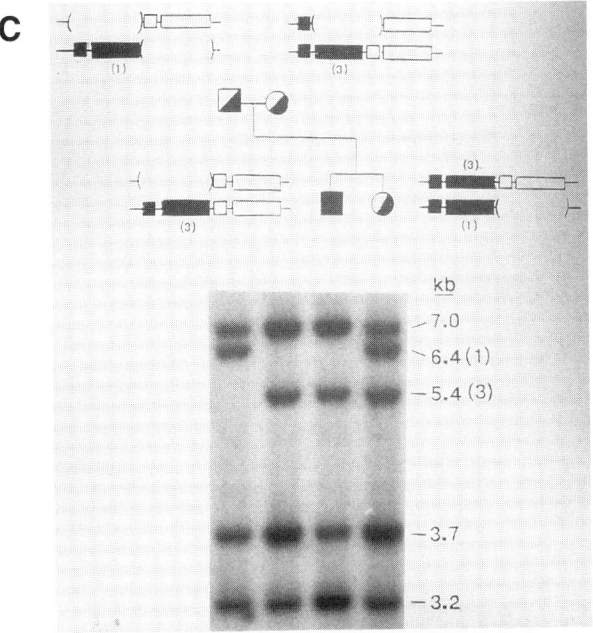

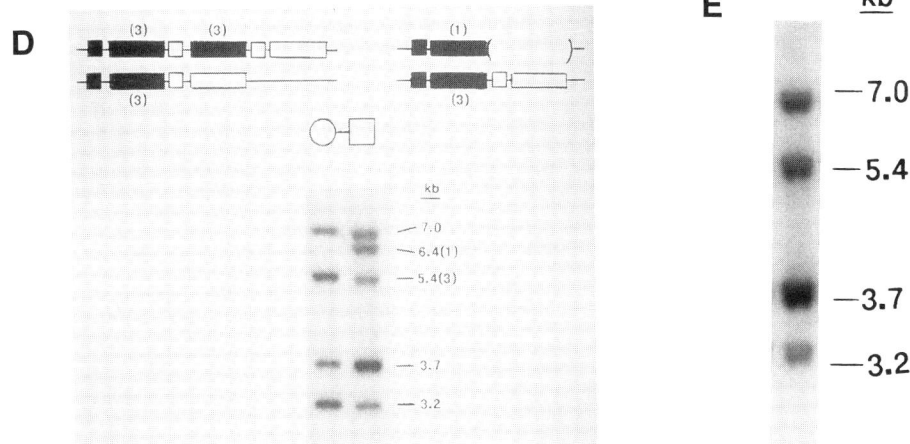

Fig. 5. (C,D,E) *(Caption on page 134)*

3.2.2. Detection of Point Mutations

Only a minority of gene conversion events will involve the *Taq*I sites diagnostic of the 21B gene (*see* Fig. 5C). The remainder will not be detected using Southern analysis as described. As most pathogenic mutations within the 21B gene will have derived from the 21A pseudogene, we know what mutations to look for. However, any mutation detection method must be able to distinguish those mutant sequences within the 21B gene from the same sequences present within the pseudogene.

Fig. 5. (A) A severe salt-wasting female has 21-hydroxylase deficiency by virtue of being homozygously deleted for her 21B genes. Note she has no signal at 3.7 kb. This gene would only normally be expected to be deleted as a part of a larger 30-kb deletion, and consistent with this, we see no C4B alleles either. The parents are both carriers of this deletion as evidenced by reduced 21B and C4B band intensities. (B) A male has 21-hydroxylase deficiency. Allele dosage on Southern analysis reveals 21B and C4B alleles of reduced intensity, indicating that he is a carrier of a B unit deletion, which he has inherited from his mother. The father's short-range mapping results show a pattern consistent with no deletion, and he is most likely to carry a point mutation within one of his 21B genes. (C) This family has three deletions segregating. The father has both an A unit and a B unit deletion. He therefore has a single copy of each of the four genes in the region, and as expected, all four bands on the Southern analysis are of equal intensity. Note that an A unit deletion is always accompanied by a 6.4-kb C4B allele (allele 1) owing to the unique *Taq*I fragment created by this deletion. The mother has an interstitial deletion (note the relative band intensities 21B:C4B:21A:C4A [2:1:1:2]). The affected son has inherited the 21B unit deletion and presumably a point mutation from his mother. The daughter has inherited the 21A unit deletion (note the C4B 1 allele). (D) This demonstrates some of the nonpathogenic variation around this locus in two individuals, neither of whom have (or are carriers of) the disease. The man's A unit deletion is indicated by the 6.4-kb C4B allele. The woman, however, carries a triplication. This can often be hard to spot, especially if one cannot observe the chromosomes segregating through at least two generations. In this case, one must use the relative allele dosages 21B:C4B:21A:C4A (2:3:3:2). (E) In all the above examples, the variation around the 21-hydroxylase locus has resulted from unequal recombination as discussed in Section 1.1.1. Gene conversion events that involve the *Taq*I sites relevant to this diagnostic technique also will be identified. This figure shows the results from an individual who appears to have an imbalance of 21B and 21A genes without an accompanying imbalance between the C4B and C4A alleles resulting from gene conversion. In this case, 21A sequence has been converted into 21B sequence, and so this would not be expected to have pathogenic consequences (given all other things being equal, there will still be two functional 21B genes). This interpretation has been confirmed in this individual by observing the segregation of the converted 21-hydroxylase gene. Clearly, the reverse situation, conversion of 21B sequence into 21A, could have serious implications.

Table 4
Common Point Mutations in the 21-Hydroxylase Gene

Nucleotide position[a]	Position gene	Sequence change	Protein change	Clinical phenotype
659	Intron 2	A or C → G	Splice mutation	Salt wasting
1004	Exon 4	ATC → AAC	Ile 173 → Asn	Simple virilizing
1688	Exon 7	GTG → TTG	Val 282 → Leu	Nonclassical
2113	Exon 8	CGG → TGG	Arg 357 → Trp	Salt wasting

[a]Nucleotide positions have been taken from ref. *10*.

Table 5
First-Round ARMS-PCR Amplification of the 21B Gene

Region amplified	Exons 1–3, fragment A	Exons 3–10, fragment B
Primers	P1 + P48	P4 + P55
Final primer concentrations	0.5 μ*M*	0.5 μ*M*
Cycling conditions[a]	93°C, 1 min	93°C, 1 min
	54°C, 1 min	54°C, 1 min
	72°C, 1 min	72°C, 1 min
Number of cycles	20	20

[a]Cycling is preceded by 93°C for 3 min and followed by 72°C for 5 min.

A strategy has been described based on the use of sequence-specific PCR or ARMS *(10)*. In this technique, a preamplification step is employed to amplify specifically the 21B sequence in preference to the 21A. This is achieved by designing primers to amplify only in the absence of an 8-bp deletion present within the 21A pseudogene. A second round of ARMS is then used to identify mutations using the amplified 21B sequence as a template. The following describes a method for identifying a number of the more common mutations summarized in Table 4.

3.2.2.1. PROTOCOL FOR DETECTION OF POINT MUTATIONS

1. Amplify the 21B gene in two halves using 20-μL standard PCR reactions (*see* Table 5 and Note 5).
2. Dilute the reactions with 20 μL water and use 2 μL of product to seed the second round of mutation-specific PCR.
3. For the second round, prepare 20 μL PCR reactions to amplify a mutation-specific fragment as well as a larger control fragment. The two fragments share a common primer. In this duplex reaction, working primer concentrations are 0.5 μ*M* for the common primer and the ARMS primers (specific to the variant you wish to amplify), and 0.15 μ*M* for the control primer (*see* Note 5 and Table 6).

Table 6
Second-Round ARMS-Mutation Detection in the 21B Gene

Mutation	659	1004	1688	2113
Template fragment (*see* Table 4)	A	B	B	B
Control primer	P5	P19	P11	P11
Common primer	P48	P55	P55	P55
ARMS primers	P659A, P659C, P659G	P1004T P1004A	P1688G P1688T	P2113C, P2113T
Cycling[a]	93°C, 1 min 60°C, 1 min 72°C, 3 min	93°C, 1 min 54°C, 1 min 72°C, 3 min	93°C, 1 min 54°C, 1 min 72°C, 3 min	93°C, 1 min 54°C, 1 min 72°C, 3 min
Number of cycles	30	30	30	30
Control fragment size, bp	423	1385	2064	2064
ARMS fragment size, bp	86	323	1005	1428

[a]Cycling is followed by 72°C for 5 min.

4. Resolve the products of the second round of amplification on agarose gels (3% for the 659 mutation and 1% for the others) and visualize using ethidium bromide (*see* Table 6 and Fig. 6).

3.3. Quoting Risks

For carrier detection, mutation analysis will offer a means of modifying the prior risk of 1 in 50. Accurate estimates of frequencies for mutations within the 21-hydroxylase gene are not yet available. However, experience has led us to estimate that approximately one-third of deficient genes carry a gross deletion detected by the short-range mapping.

At least 16 mutations have been described within the 21B gene. Most have derived originally from the 21A pseudogene. However, novel mutations will always be a possibility. Consequently, it will not be feasible to screen exhaustively for all mutations within a service environment. We find that by screening for the common point mutations at positions 659, 1004, 1688, and 2113 (*see* Table 4) in addition to the short-range mapping strategy described for identifying deletions and gene conversion events, we are able to identify the majority of pathogenic mutations (Note 6). In a pilot study (unpublished results), this system identified a causative mutation in 69 of 81 21-hydroxylase-deficient chromosomes.

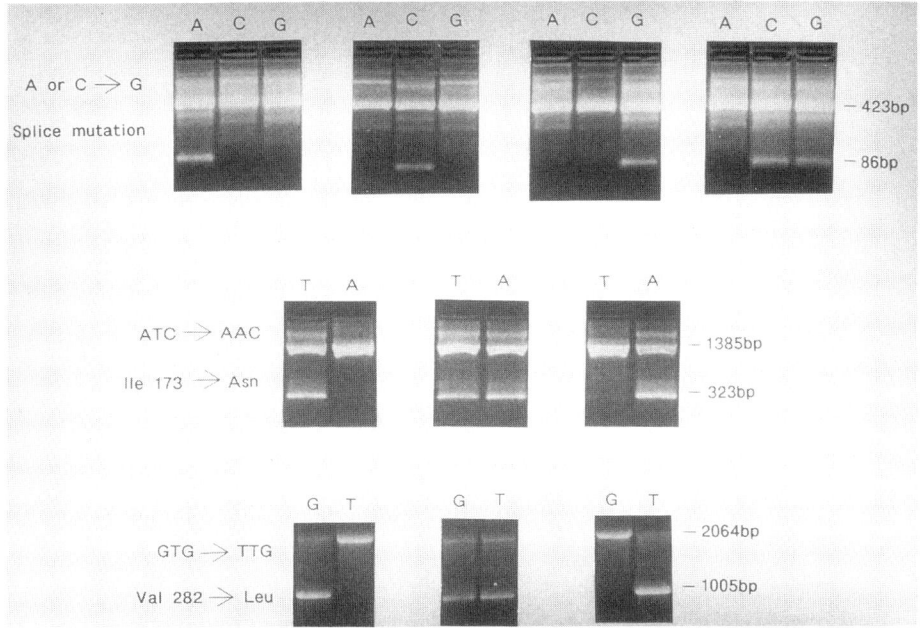

Fig. 6. Genotyping the common point mutations using the ARMS technique. Genotypes for the mutations are as follows (left to right): Splice mutation 659 A/C→G, AA, CC, GG, CG. Ile173→Asn ATC/ATC, ATC/AAC, AAC/AAC. Val282→Leu GTG/GTG, GTG/TTG, TTG/TTG. All these genotypes assume that a single ARMS product signifies homozygosity and not hemizygosity. This would have to be verified using the short-range mapping strategy described.

4. Notes

1. There are almost as many variations on Southern analysis methodologies as there are labs doing the technique. Described here is our preferred approach to the technique. It is probably the simplest we have tried, but by no means the most rapid. Depurination of gels to nick the DNA is not usually necessary unless one is looking at particularly large target fragments (>10 kb), and by using charged membrane in conjunction with an alkali blot, we avoid the need for crosslinking of the genomic DNA onto the filter. We find that with capillary blotting there is generally no need to set up a reservoir. The "dry blotting" method described here will generally suffice. Clearly much more rapid blotting procedures, such as vacuum blotting, are available to speed up the procedure. Different membranes may require different blotting protocols. For best results, refer to the manufacturer's instructions.

2. The prehybridization and hybridization buffers described here are ideal for the probes outlined in this chapter. However, they are not suitable for all probes. If more blocking is required, alternative buffers are available (*see* Chapter 3).

3. Described here is a simple (some might say archaic) method of setting up a hybridization. Nowadays a range of commercially available purpose-built hybridization ovens are available to simplify the procedure and minimize radiation exposures.

4. If the alkali blotting technique is used in conjunction with a charged membrane, then filters must not be stripped using sodium hydroxide as often recommended for nylon filters.

5. Standard PCR conditions will usually suffice. However, with the products being so large, conditions may need to be optimized. Particularly we find that the following 20X buffer has given the most consistent results—1.0M Tris-HCl (pH 9.0 at 25°C), 400 mM ammonium sulfate, 30 mM MgCl$_2$. This buffer has a relatively low magnesium chloride concentration, and the concentration of dNTPs will have to be calculated to give a free magnesium concentration of 0.7 mM (*see* Chapter 2). Hot start (adding the enzyme after the initial denaturing step, while the reaction is still hot) will often improve the quality of results.

6. If two point mutations are identified in an affected individual, one cannot assume that they are on different chromosomes since gene conversion can transfer more than one mutation as a single event. To establish phase, their independent segregation must be observed.

References

1. Aston, C. E., Sherman, S. L., Morton, N. E., Spieser, P. W., and New, M. I. (1988) Genetic mapping of the 21-hydroxylase locus: estimation of small recombination frequencies. *Am. J. Hum. Genet.* **43**, 304–310.
2. Pang, S., Wallace, M. A., Hofman, L., Thuline, H. C., Dorche, C., Lyon, I. C. T., et al. (1988) Worldwide experience in newborn screening for classical congenital adrenal hyperplasia due to 21-hydroxylase deficiency. *Paediatrics* **81**, 866–874.
3. Spiezer, P. W., Dupont, B., Rubenstein, P., Piazza, A., Kastelan, A., and New, M. I. (1985) High frequency of non-classical steroid 21-hydroxylase deficiency. *Am. J. Hum. Genet.* **37**, 650–667.
4. Carroll, M. C., Campbell, R. D., and Porter, R. R. (1985) Mapping of steroid 21-hydroxylase genes to complement component C4 genes in HLA, the major histoincompatability locus in man. *Proc. Natl. Acad. Sci. USA* **83**, 521–525.
5. White, P. C., New, M. I., and Dupont, B. (1986) Structure of the human 21-hydroxylase genes. *Proc. Natl. Acad. Sci. USA* **83**, 5111–5115.
6. Higashi, Y., Yoshioka, H., Yamane, M., Gotoh, O., and Fujii-Kuriyama, Y. (1986) Complete nucleotide sequence of two steroid 21-hydroxylase genes tandemly arranged in human chromosome: a pseudogene and a genuine gene. *Proc. Natl. Acad. Sci. USA* **83**, 2841–2845.
7. Morel, Y., Andre, J., Uring-Lambert, B., Hauptman, G., Bétuel, H., Tosi, M., et al. (1989) Rearrangements and point mutations of the p450c21 genes are distinguished by five restriction endonuclease haplotypes identified by a new probing strategy in 57 families with congenital adrenal hyperplasia. *J. Clin. Invest.* **83**, 527–536.

8. Holliday, R. (1964) A mechanism for gene conversion in fungi. *Genetic Res.* **5,** 282–304.
9. Udalova, I. A., Nedospasov, S. A., Webb, G. C., Chaplin, D. D., and Turetskaya, R. L. (1993) Highly informative typing of the human TNF locus using six adjacent polymorphic markers. *Genomics* **16,** 180–186.
10. Wedell, A. and Luthman, H. (1993) Steroid 21-hydroxylase deficiency: two additional mutations in salt wasting disease and rapid screening of disease causing mutations. *Hum. Mol. Genet.* **2,** 4499–4504.
11. Sinnott, P. J., Dyer, P. A., Price, D. A., and Strachan, T. (1989) 21-Hydroxylase deficiency patients with HLA identical affected and unaffected siblings. *J. Med. Genet.* **26,** 10–17.
12. Schneideer, P. M., Carroll, M. C., Alper, C. A., Rittner, C., Whitehead, A. S., Yunis, E. J., and Colten, H. R. (1986) Polymorphism of the human complement C4 and steroid 21-hydroxylase genes. *J. Clin. Invest.* **78,** 650–657.
13. Partenan, J., Koskimies, S., Sipilia, I., and Lipsanen, V. (1989) Major histocompatibility—complex gene markers and restriction fragment analysis of steroid 21-hydroxylase (CYP21) and complement C4 genes in classical congenital adrenal hyperplasia patients in a single population. *Am. J. Hum. Genet.* **44,** 660–670.
14. Fleischnick, E., Awdeh, Z. L., Raum, D., Granados, J., Alosco, S. M., Crigler, J. R., Jr., et al. (1983) Extended MHC haplotypes in 21-hydroxylase deficiency congenital adrenal hyperplasia: shared genotypes in unrelated patients. *Lancet* **I,** 152–156.
15. Holler, W., Scholtz, S., Knorr, D., Bidlingmaier, F., Keller, E., and Ekkehard, D. A. (1985) Genetic differences between the salt-wasting simple virilising and nonclassical types of congenital adrenal hyperplasia. *J. Clin. Endocrinol. Metab.* **60,** 757–763.
16. Pollack, M. S., Levine, L. S., and O'Neill, G. L. (1981) HLA linkage and B14, DR1, BfS haplotype association with the genes for late onset and cryptic 21-hydroxylase deficiency. *Am. J. Hum. Genet.* **33,** 540–550.
17. Bidwell, J. L. and Jarrold, E. A. (1986) HLA-DR allogenotyping using exon specific cDNA probes and application of minigel methods. *Mol. Immunol.* **23,** 1111–1115.
18. Dyer, P. A., Jawaheer, D., Ollier, B., Poulton, K., Sinnott, P. J., and Thomson, W. (1993) HLA allele detection using molecular techniques. *Disease Markers* **1,** 145–160.
19. Browning, M. J., Krausa, P., Rowan, A., Bicknell, D. C., Bodmer, J. G., and Bodmer, W. F. (1993) Tissue typing the HLA-A locus from genomic DNA by sequence specific PCR: comparison of HLA genotype and surface expression on colorectal tumour lines. *Proc. Natl. Acad. Sci. USA* **90,** 2842–2845.
20. Olerup, O. and Zetterquist, H. (1992) HLA-DR typing by PCR amplification with sequence specific primers (PCR-SSP) in 2 hours: an alternative to serological DR typing in clinical practice including donor recipient matching in cadaveric transplantation. *Tissue Antigens* **39,** 225–235.
21. Bunce, M. and Welsh, K. I. (1994) Rapid DNA typing for HLA-C using sequence-specific primers (PCR-SSP): identification of serological and non-serologically defined HLA-C alleles including several new alleles. *Tissue Antigens* **43,** 7–17.

22. Morel, Y. and Miller, W. L. (1991) Clinical and molecular genetics of congenital adrenal hyperplasia due to 21-hydroxylase deficiency, in *Advances in Human Genetics*, vol. 20 (Harris, H. and Hirschorn, K., eds.), Plenum, New York, pp. 1–88.
23. Yu, Y. C., Belt, K. T., Giles, C. M., Campbell, R. D., and Porter, R. R. (1986) Structural basis of the polymorphism of the human complement components C4A and C4B: gene size, reactivity and antigenicity. *EMBO J.* **5,** 2873–2881.
24. Collier, S., Sinnott, P. J., Dyer, P. A., Price, D. A., Harris, R., and Strachan, T. (1989) Pulsed field gel electrophoresis identifies a high degree of variability in the number of tandem 21-hydroxylase and complement C4 repeats in 21-hydroxylase deficiency haplotypes. *EMBO J.* **8,** 1393–1402.

7

Molecular Analysis of X-Chromosome Inactivation

David O. Robinson and John F. Harvey

1. Introduction

Analysis of X-chromosome inactivation patterns can be a useful tool in the identification of carriers of certain X-linked diseases and also for other investigations, such as gene mapping and clonality analysis. X inactivation is the process in females whereby one of the two X chromosomes of a cell is maintained in an inactive state with most genes remaining untranscribed. It occurs early in embryogenesis at the late blastocyst stage and normally is random such that for each cell there is an equal chance of either X chromosome being inactive. Once a cell has undergone X inactivation, all cells originating from it maintain the same chromosome inactive throughout life. Adult tissues therefore are normally a mosaic of groups of cells with the same X chromosome inactive.

1.1. The Applications of X-Inactivation Analysis

1.1.1. Female Carriers of X-Linked Diseases

Sometimes it is difficult to determine by direct mutation analysis the carrier status of asymptomatic female relatives of individuals with X-linked diseases because of the presence of the normal X. However, in certain cases X inactivation status can be used as an indicator of carrier status. In females where one X chromosome carries a mutation that is incompatible with cell viability, only those cells with the mutation on the inactive X survive, thus generating a unilateral pattern of X inactivation (*see* Notes 1 and 2). Examples of this include carriers of Bruton-type agammaglobulinemia *(1)*, Wiskott–Aldrich syndrome *(2)*, X-linked severe combined immunodeficiency *(3)*, and X-linked immunodeficiency with hyper IgM *(4)* (*see* Note 3). In some cases non-random X inactivation is restricted to certain cell lineages (*see* Note 4).

From: *Methods in Molecular Medicine: Molecular Diagnosis of Genetic Diseases*
Edited by: R. Elles Humana Press Inc., Totowa, NJ

1.1.2. Females with Symptoms of X-Linked Diseases

X-linked diseases, which are normally recessive, occasionally manifest themselves in females, for example, Duchenne muscular dystrophy *(5)*, adrenoleucodystrophy *(6)*, and X-linked retinitis pigmentosa *(7)*. This is sometimes caused by non-random X inactivation, but there are other possible causes including X-chromosome monosomy with the single X carrying a mutation, homozygosity for a mutation, an X-autosome translocation, or the presence of an autosomal phenocopy. X-inactivation analysis therefore can be of use in identifying the causative mechanism of disease and thus facilitate risk calculation for other family members. In the case of X-linked retinitis pigmentosa type 2, X-inactivation analysis also can be of prognostic value, those females with a less severe skew in X inactivation developing less severe symptoms *(8)*.

1.1.3. The Mapping of Diseases to the X Chromosome

Some X-linked diseases, such as agammaglobulinemia and focal dermal hypoplasia, have or may have autosomal phenocopies. In sporadic cases of these diseases the X-inactivation status of female relatives has been used to determine the mode of inheritance of the disease *(9,10)*, thus facilitating recurrence risk and carrier risk calculations within the pedigree.

1.1.4. Carriers of Structural Abnormalities of the X Chromosome

In pedigrees in which a structural abnormality of the X chromosome, such as a partial deletion or an inversion, is segregating, molecular analysis of X inactivation can be used to identify asymptomatic female carriers *(11)*. Carriers usually exhibit nonrandom X inactivation such that the normal X is exclusively active. A random pattern of X inactivation can be the cause of an abnormal phenotype *(12)*.

1.1.5. Females with Small Ring X Chromosomes

In some cases of females with a 46,Xr(X) karyotype the severity of the phenotype is thought to be influenced by the inactivation status of the marker chromosome. In those cases where not only the normal chromosome but also the marker chromosome is active, the phenotype is more severe because of functional disomy for genes on the marker *(13)*. If the marker chromosome contains a site amenable to molecular analysis, then X inactivation can be ascertained without the need for cell culture and late replication analysis.

1.1.6. The Origin of X-Autosome Translocations

Females with balanced X-autosome translocations exhibit nonrandom X inactivation such that the derived X is exclusively active. In cases where the translocation has arisen *de novo*, X-inactivation studies using molecular probes have superseded more lengthy procedures in determining the parental origin of the aberration *(14)*.

1.1.7. Clonality in Tumor Cell Lines

X-inactivation analysis has been used as an indicator of clonal composition in lymphoproliferative diseases and other human cancers in order to study tumor progression and evolution *(15,16)*.

1.2. Strategies for Molecular Analysis of X Inactivation

X inactivation is associated with the methylation of specific CpG sites on the X chromosome. The majority of such sites found so far are associated with genes, and usually the inactive X is methylated. However, there are at least two sites, M27β *(17)* and DX74 *(18)*, at which the reverse is the case with the active X being methylated. A number of methylation sites have been found that are close to DNA polymorphisms and can be used to determine X-inactivation patterns in informative females *(17,19–23)*. Two strategies are available, one using Southern blotting and the other using the polymerase chain reaction (PCR).

1.2.1. The Use of Methylation-Sensitive Restriction Enzymes and Southern Blotting

This approach uses DNA probes to analyze polymorphic sites that are differentially methylated on active and inactive X chromosomes. The example used here is the probe M27β which recognizes a VNTR polymorphism (too large for routine PCR amplification) in Xp11.22 and which is informative in 90% of females *(24)*. The internal cytosine residue of a CCGG sequence lying 5' to the VNTR is methylated on all active X chromosomes and unmethylated only on inactive X chromosomes, although in blood cells a variable proportion of inactive X chromosomes are methylated at this site *(25)*. Methylation status can be determined by Southern blotting using the restriction enzyme *Hpa*II and its isoschizomer *Msp*I (as a control) that recognize the sequence CCGG. *Msp*I cleaves this sequence whether or not it is methylated, whereas *Hpa*II only cleaves CCGG sites that are unmethylated on the internal cytosine. A comparison is made of the Southern blot banding patterns of a DNA sample cleaved with *Msp*I and independently cleaved with *Hpa*II. All samples are also cleaved simultaneously with *Ava*II in order to separate a variably methylated CCGG site lying 3' to the VNTR from the VNTR and its associated 5' CCGG sequence *(25)* (*see* Note 5). This also generates fragments of a size resolvable by standard agarose gel electrophoresis. After hybridization with the probe M27β, the *Msp*I track will show two allelic bands in informative females. In the *Hpa*II track, inactive X chromosomes that are unmethylated will be represented by a band of the same size as that in the *Msp*I digest. Bands larger than those in the *Msp*I track will represent active (methylated) X chromosomes and also, in DNA extracted from blood, a proportion of inactive X chromosomes that are methylated at this site. (This proportion differs from female to female and ranges from 0–60% *[25]*.)

In cases with random X inactivation the *Hpa*II track will contain both bands present in the *Msp*I track and also their larger methylated counterparts. However, in the case of unilateral X inactivation when the CCGG site is unmethylated exclusively on one allele, then only one of the two bands present in the *Msp*I track will be present in the *Hpa*II track. This fragment is that derived from the exclusively inactive X chromosome. Similar analysis can also be carried out using other probes such as phosphoglycerate kinase (PGK) *(19)* and hypoxanthine-guanine phosphoribosyltransferase (HPRT) *(20)*, but they are considerably less polymorphic than M27β (*see* Note 6).

1.2.2. PCR Amplification of DNA
Cleaved with Methylation-Sensitive Restriction Enzymes

This technique relies on the availability of PCR primers that can amplify a length of DNA containing both a repeat sequence polymorphism and a site that is differentially methylated on active and inactive X chromosomes. A comparison is made of the PCR amplification products of DNA with and without prior cleavage with a methylation-sensitive restriction enzyme, such as *Hpa*II or *Hha*I, which only cleaves its recognition site if it is unmethylated. Females with unilateral X inactivation who are informative for the polymorphism will show two allelic PCR bands when the DNA sample is undigested prior to PCR, but only one band when the sample is digested prior to PCR.

In this chapter primers that bracket the polymorphic repeat sequence within the human androgen receptor gene (HUMAR) are described *(22,26)*. They also amplify a CCGG site that is methylated only on inactive X chromosomes. If DNA from a female with unilateral X inactivation is digested with *Hpa*II, then the unmethylated CCGG site on the active X will be cleaved, thus amplification of only the allele on the inactive X is possible. Subsequent PCR amplification products (approx 280 bases long depending on the size of the repeat sequence) are compared with the two bands produced from undigested DNA. A polymorphism within the monoamine oxidase A (MAOA) gene can be employed in a similar fashion *(21)*. Such PCR methods are more rapid than blotting and require much less DNA, however, not all females are informative. The HUMAR polymorphism is heterozygous in 90% *(22)* and the MAOA polymorphism in 75% *(27)* of females (*see* Note 6).

2. Materials

2.1. X-Inactivation Analysis
Using M27β and Southern Blotting

1. Sample DNA.
2. Restriction enzymes *Hpa*II, *Ava*II, and *Msp*I at 10 U/μL.
3. 10X Concentrated restriction enzyme buffer: 10 mM Tris-HCl, 10 mM magnesium chloride and 1 mM dithiothreitol (DTT), pH 7.5.
4. Incubator or water bath at 37°C.
5. Gel loading buffer consisting of 40% sucrose, 0.25% bromophenol blue, and 1 mM EDTA.
6. M27β probe (ATCC cat no. 61516/61517).
7. 0.25M HCl solution.
8. Denaturing solution: 0.5M sodium hydroxide, 1M sodium chloride.
9. Neutralizing solution: 1M Tris-HCl, 1.5M sodium chloride, pH 8.0.
10. Horizontal gel electrophoresis apparatus with 20 × 20 cm gel formers, combs, and 3000-V power supply.
11. Agarose.
12. 5 mg/mL Ethidium bromide solution.
13. UV transilluminator, UV protective visor, and goggles (Ultra-Violet Products Inc., San Gabriel, CA).
14. CU-5 Polaroid camera and hood with Kodak Wratten 22A or 23A red filter and black and white 667 Polaroid film.
15. Blotting membrane, e.g., Zeta-Probe GT (Bio-Rad Labs, Ltd., Hemel Hempstead, UK).
16. Oven at 80°C.
17. 25 × 35-mm Plastic "radiation bags" (Jencons Scientific Ltd., Leighton Buzzard, UK).
18. Bag sealer.
19. Trays for gel and filter washings.
20. Prehybridization and hybridization buffer: 7% SDS, 0.25M Na$_2$HPO$_4$, pH 7.2.
21. Shaking water bath or incubator.
22. Redivue [α^{32}P]dCTP at 3000 Ci/mmol (Amersham International, Amersham, UK).
23. DNA labeling kit, e.g., "High Prime" (Boehringer Mannheim, Lewes, UK).
24. Wash buffer 1: 20 mM Na$_2$HPO$_4$, pH 7.2, 5% SDS.
25. Wash buffer 2: 20 mM Na$_2$HPO$_4$, pH 7.2, 1% SDS.
26. Sephadex G50-150 equilibrated in 10 mM Tris-HCl, 1 mM EDTA, pH 7.5 (TE), and a 0.7 × 20-cm glass column.
27. Autoradiography cassettes, intensifying screens, and X-ray film (e.g., Kodak Xomat AR5).

2.2. X-Inactivation Analysis
Using the HUMAR Primers and PCR

1. Sample DNA.
2. 10 U/μL *Hpa*II restriction enzyme.
3. 10X *Hpa*II buffer: 10 mM Tris-HCl, 10 mM magnesium chloride, and 1 mM DTT, pH 7.5.

4. Water bath or incubator at 37°C.
5. PCR primers as follows *(26)*: HUMAR Primer 1 5' GCTGTGAAGGTTGCTGTT-CCTCAT 3' and HUMAR Primer 2 5' TCCAGAATCTGTTCCAGAGCGTGC 3'.
6. T4 Polynucleotide kinase (PNK) at 10 U/μL.
7. 10X PNK buffer: 330 mM Tris-acetate pH 7.8, 660 mM potassium acetate, 100 mM magnesium acetate, and 5 mM DTT.
8. γ^{32}P[dATP] at 3000 Ci/mmol (Amersham International).
9. 5 U/μL *Taq* polymerase.
10. 10X concentrated PCR buffer: 100 mM Tris-HCl and 500 mM potassium chloride, pH 8.3.
11. 25 mM magnesium chloride solution.
12. 100 mM solutions of dATP, dGTP, dCTP, and dTTP.
13. Mineral oil for PCR.
14. Gel loading buffer: 45% formamide, 20 mM EDTA, 0.05% bromophenol blue, and 0.05% xylene cyanol.
15. Vertical "sequencing" gel electrophoresis apparatus with 3000-V power supply.
16. Thermal cycler and thin-walled PCR reaction tubes.
17. Electrophoresis buffer (1X TBE): 10.8 g Tris base, 5.5 g boric acid, and 4 mL 0.5M EDTA, pH 8.0, in 1 L distilled water.
18. 6% (w/v) acrylamide/bisacrylamide (19:1), 7M urea in 1X TBE (Severn Biotech Ltd., Kidderminster, UK).
19. N,N,N',N',-Tetramethylene-ethylenediamine (TEMED).
20. Ammonium persulfate: 1% aqueous solution (store at –20°C in 1-mL aliquots).
21. Autoradiography cassettes with intensifying screens.
22. X-ray film (e.g., Kodak X-Omat AR5).

3. Methods

3.1. X-Inactivation Analysis
Using M27β and Southern Blotting

1. For restriction enzyme digestions, prepare three tubes each containing 6 μL of 10X restriction enzyme buffer and 10 μg of sample DNA and make up to a volume of 58 μL with distilled water.
2. To each tube add 1 μL (10 U) of *Ava*II.
3. To tube 2 add 1 μL (10 U) of *Msp*I.
4. To tube 3 add 1 μL (10 U) of *Hpa*II.
5. Incubate for 16 h at 37°C.
6. For gel electrophoresis add 12 μL of loading buffer to each tube and load all the sample on to a 0.8% 20 × 20 × 1 cm horizontal agarose gel in 1X TBE containing 5 μg/mL ethidium bromide.
7. Run at 50 mA for 40 h.
8. Visualize the DNA in the gel by transilluminating with long wavelength UV light (302 nm) to ensure that the DNA is fully digested and has run evenly. Record by photographing.

9. Immerse the gel in 500 mL of 0.25M HCl at room temperature for 25 min with gentle shaking.
10. Pour off the HCl solution, rinse in denaturing solution, and gently shake the gel in 500 mL of denaturing solution for 70 min at room temperature.
11. Pour off the denaturing solution, rinse in neutralizing solution, and gently shake the gel in 500 mL of neutralizing solution for 70 min at room temperature.
12. Transfer the DNA from the gel onto a blotting membrane (e.g., Zeta-Probe GT) using the standard Southern blotting capillary transfer procedure. (For details of Southern blotting procedure, *see*, for example, Chapter 12, Section 3.4.).
13. Label 50 ng of M27β probe with 50 μCi of [α^{32}P]dCTP [3000 Ci/mmol] using the labeling kit according to the manufacturer's instructions. After a 30-min incubation at 37°C, run the labeled probe through a column of approx 12 cm of Sephadex G50–150 in TE to remove free nucleotides. Monitor the separation of free nucleotides from labeled probe on the column with a hand-held Geiger counter. Collect the labeled probe peak (the first peak of activity to come off the column) in a screwcap Eppendorf tube held with a pair of forceps. Replace the tube cap, denature the probe in a boiling water bath for 10 min, and cool rapidly on ice.
14. Prehybridize the blotted membrane in a plastic "radiation" bag for 5–30 min with 20 mL of hybridization buffer at 65°C. Add the labeled probe, seal the bag, and incubate overnight with gentle shaking at 65°C. Wash the membrane at 65°C for 2 × 30 min in wash buffer 1, and 2 × 30 min in wash buffer 2. Enclose the filter in clear plastic wrap and expose to X-ray film at –80°C overnight, or longer depending on the efficiency of the hybridization, and develop.
15. Banding patterns are shown in Fig. 1 (*see* Note 7).

3.2. X-Inactivation Analysis
Using the HUMAR Primers and PCR

1. For restriction enzyme digestion prepare two tubes for each DNA sample containing 1 μg of DNA in 20 μL of 1X *Hpa*II buffer.
2. Add 1 μL (10 U) *Hpa*II to tube 1 (tube 2 serves as the undigested control).
3. Incubate at 37°C for 16 h.
4. To end label add 7 μL of 500 μg/mL primer 1 (enough for 10 reactions) to 2 μL 10X T4PNK buffer, 1 μL T4PNK (10 U), 9 μL H$_2$O, and 1 μL γ^{32}P[dATP] 3000 Ci/mmol (*see* Note 8).
5. Incubate at 37°C for 30 min.
6. Place on ice.
7. For 10 reactions prepare a mix containing 501 μL of 10X PCR buffer, 30 μL 25 mM MgCl$_2$, 7 μL unlabeled HUMAR primer 2 at 500 μg/mL, 1.2 μL of each dNTP at 100 mM, 387 μL H$_2$O, and 1 μL (5 U) of *Taq* polymerase. Keep on ice.
8. Pipet 2 μL of each DNA sample (*Hpa*II digested or undigested control DNA) and 3 μL H$_2$O into a PCR tube and add 1 drop of mineral oil.
9. Place the tubes in the thermal cycler and incubate for 6 min at 96°C to denature the DNA prior to PCR and to inactivate the restriction enzyme.

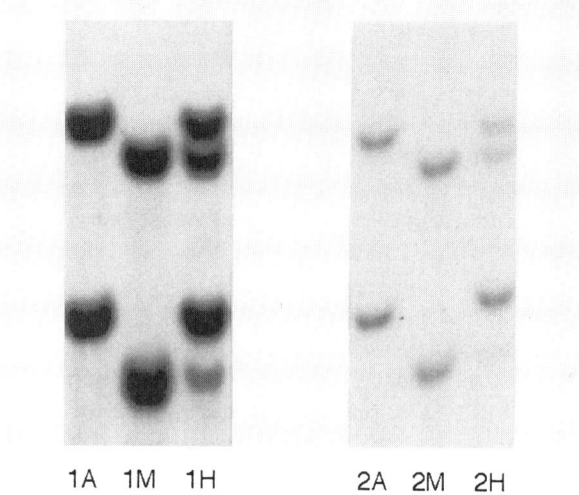

1A   1M   1H   2A   2M   2H

Fig. 1. Autoradiograph of Southern blot analysis of X-inactivation status using M27β. Tracks 1A, 1M, 1H represent an individual with random X inactivation and tracks 2A, 2M, and 2H represent an individual with unilateral X inactivation. Tracks A: DNA digested with *Ava*II only. Tracks M: DNA digested with *Ava*II and *Msp*I. Tracks H: DNA digested with *Ava*II and *Hpa*II.

10. Add the 20 μL of labeled HUMAR primer 1 to the PCR mix on ice and add 45 μL of this to the denatured DNA in the thermocycler.
11. Cycle at 96°C for 1 min, 60°C for 1 min, and 72°C for 2 min for 25 cycles, with a final elongation time of 7 min at 72°C.
12. Add an equal volume of formamide loading buffer, heat at 100°C for 5 min, and place on ice.
13. Load 5 μL onto a 6% PAGE/urea sequencing gel and run at 100 W for 3–4 h.
14. Expose to phosphoimaging screen or X-ray film for 2–24 h, depending on the efficiency of the labeling.
15. Banding patterns are shown in Fig. 2.

4. Notes

1. A proportion of apparently normal females with no family history of X-linked disease have a unilateral or a severely skewed pattern of X inactivation, either owing to an unidentified rare mutation on the X chromosome or to chance variation. Also, the X-inactivation pattern can vary in different tissues *(27)*. The proportion of normal females with severely skewed X inactivation has been variously estimated as 4 *(15)*, 7 *(28)*, and 9.5% *(29)*. This can lead to the misinterpretation of X-inactivation data. Also, the results of biochemical tests for carrier status can be influenced by X inactivation, for example, in pyruvate dehydrogenase deficiency *(30)* and Lesch-Nyhan syndrome *(31)*. Therefore it is prudent to determine the X-inactivation status of samples used for such assays.

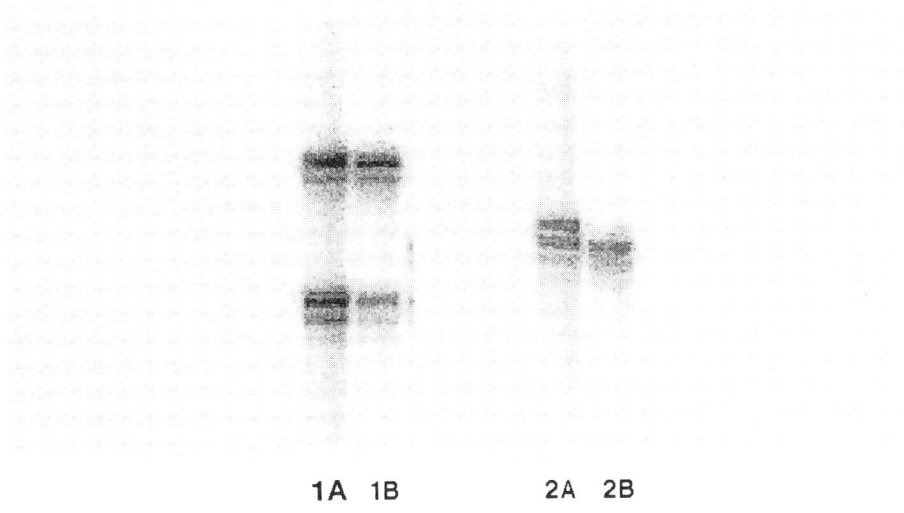

1A 1B   2A 2B

Fig. 2. Phosphoimage of PCR analysis of X-inactivation status using the HUMAR primers. Tracks 1A and 1B represent an individual with random X inactivation and tracks 2A and 2B represent an individual with unilateral X inactivation. Tracks A: PCR without predigestion of DNA with *Hpa*II. Tracks B: PCR after digestion of DNA with *Hpa*II.

2. In chorionic villus biopsies the level of skewing of X inactivation may be fairly high in normal individuals and is potentially misleading *(30)*.
3. Some mothers of isolated cases of disease may be mosaic carriers of a mutation and, although still at risk of having a second affected child, may not exhibit a unilateral pattern of X inactivation in the cells available for testing.
4. The tissue of origin of the cells analyzed can be important for the ascertainment of carrier status. Carriers of some diseases exhibit a unilateral pattern of X inactivation only in one or a limited number of cell types. For Wiskott–Aldrich syndrome, DNA from whole blood lymphocytes is sufficient to identify nonrandom X inactivation in female carriers, however, in X-linked agammaglobulinemia only B-lymphocytes manifest unilateral X inactivation in carriers and must first be isolated to the appropriate level of purity (95%) *(32)* before analysis. X-linked severe combined immunodeficiency carriers have unilateral X inactivation in T- and B-lymphocytes, but not in monocytes and neutrophils *(3,33)*. Carriers of X-linked immunodeficiency with hyper IgM exhibit nonrandom X inactivation in T-cells, B-cells, and neutrophils, but not in fibroblasts *(4)*. In all such cases, cells in which X inactivation is unaffected by the disease also should be analyzed to ensure that the X-inactivation pattern is not skewed for reasons other than carrier status.
5. For M27β analysis, *Pst*I can be used in place of *Ava*II. We use *Ava*II because it functions optimally in the same buffer as *Hpa*II and *Msp*I, whereas *Pst*I requires a higher salt concentration. Both *Ava*II and *Pst*I serve to exclude another *Hpa*II site on the 3' side of the VNTR that does not correlate well with X-inactivation

status. Some of the earlier publications on this method describe the use of restriction enzymes that do not exclude the 3' site and give a less clear picture of X-inactivation status.

6. Although PCR-based analysis of X inactivation is more rapid than blotting, there are cases where Southern blotting is still the method of choice. For example, the M27β locus is closely linked to the gene responsible for Wiscott–Aldrich syndrome and female carriers of the mutation exhibit nonrandom X inactivation *(2)*, therefore, both linkage and X-inactivation analysis can be performed at the same time. Also a small proportion of females are uninformative for the available PCR-based polymorphisms and it is then necessary to try M27β and Southern blotting.

7. Occasionally the difference in size between the two M27β alleles is the same as that between the methylated and unmethylated bands such that the lower methylated band is the same size as the upper unmethylated band. This can be misinterpreted as unilateral X inactivation. In such cases X-inactivation analysis should be repeated using another methylation site.

8. When using the HUMAR PCR method in principle either primer can be end labeled, however, in our laboratory we get better results labeling primer 1. It is also possible to visualize PCR products, without radiolabeling, by staining with ethidium bromide, although more than 25 rounds of thermocycling are necessary. Radiolabeling and restricting the cycle number to within the linear range facilitates a more accurate determination of the degree of bias of X inactivation by measuring the relative band intensities using densitometry or a phosphoimager.

References

1. Fearon, E. R., Winkelstein, J. A., Civin, C. I., Pardoll, D. M., and Vogelstein, B. (1987) Carrier detection in X-linked agammaglobulinaemia by analysis of X chromosome inactivation. *N. Engl. J. Med.* **316,** 427–431.
2. Fearon, E. R., Kohn, D. B., Winkelstein, J. A., Vogelstein, B., and Blaese, R. M. (1988) Carrier detection in the Wiskott–Aldrich syndrome. *Blood* **72,** 1735–1739.
3. Puck, J. M., Nussbaum, R., and Conley, M. E. (1987) Carrier detection in X-linked severe combined immunodeficiency based on patterns of X chromosome inactivation. *J. Clin. Invest.* **79,** 1395–1400.
4. Notarangelo, L. D., Parolini, O., Albertini, A., Duse, M., Mazolari, E., Plebani, A., et al. (1991) Analysis of X-chromosome inactivation in X-linked immunodeficiency with hyper-IgM (HIGM1): evidence for the involvement of different hematopoietic cell lineages. *Hum. Genet.* **88,** 130–134.
5. Moser, H. and Emery, A. E. H. (1974) The manifesting carrier in Duchenne muscular dystrophy. *Clin. Genet.* **5,** 271–284.
6. Moser, A. B., Naidu, S., Kumar, A. J., and Rosenbaum, A. E. (1987). The adrenoleucodystrophies. *CRC Clin. Rev. Neurobiol.* **3,** 29–88.
7. Warburg, M. (1971) Random inactivities of the X chromosome in intermediate X-linked retinitis pigmentosa. Two hypotheses. *Trans. Ophthalmol. Soc. UK* **91,** 553–560.

8. Friedrich, U., Warburg, M., and Jorgensen, A. L. (1993) X-inactivation pattern in carriers of X-linked retinisis pigmentosa: a valuable means of prognostic evaluation? *Hum. Genet.* **92**, 359–363.

9. Tsuge, I., Matsuoka, H., Abe, T., Kamachi, Y., and Torii, S. (1993) X chromosome inactivation analysis to distinguish sporadic cases of X-linked agammaglobulinaemia from common variable immunodeficiency. *Eur. J. Pediat.* **152(11)**, 900–904.

10. Gorski, J. L. (1991) Father-to-daughter transmission of focal dermal hypoplasia associated with non-random X inactivation: support for X-linked inheritance and paternal X chromosome mosaicism. *Am. J. Med. Genet.* **40(3)**, 332–337.

11. Wells, S., Mould, S., Robins, D., Robinson, D., and Jacobs, P. (1991) Molecular and cytogenetic analysis of a familial microdeletion of Xq. *J. Med. Genet.* **28**, 163–166.

12. Francke, U. (1984) Random X inactivation resulting in mosaic nullisomy of region Xp21→1p21.3 associated with heterozygosity for ornithine transcarbamylase deficiency and for chronic granulomatous disease. *Cytogenet. Cell Genet.* **38**, 298–307.

13. Migeon, B. R., Luo, S., Stasiowski, B., Jani, M., Axelman, Y., Van Dyke, D. L., et al. (1993) Deficient transcription of MST from tiny ring chromosomes in females with severe phenotypes. *Proc. Natl. Acad. Sci. USA* **80**, 19,920–19,924.

14. Robinson, D. O., Boyd, Y., Cockburn, D., Collinson, M. N., Craig, I., and Jacobs, P. A. (1990) The parental origin of de novo X-autosome translocations in females with Duchenne muscular dystrophy revealed by M27β methylation analysis. *Genet. Res. Camb.* **56**, 135–140.

15. Vogelstein, B., Fearon, E. R., Hamilton, S. R., Preisinger, A. C., Willard, H. F., Michelson, A. M., et al. (1987) Clonal analysis using recombinant DNA probes from the X chromosome. *Cancer Res.* **47**, 4806–4813.

16. Abrahamson, G., Fraser, N. J., Boyd, Y., Craig, I., and Wainscoat, J. S. (1990) A highly informative X chromosome probe, M27β, can be used for the determination of tumour clonality. *Br. J. Haematol.* **74**, 371,372.

17. Boyd, Y. and Fraser, N. J. (1990) Methylation patterns at the hypervariable X chromosome locus DXS255 (M27β) correlate with X inactivation status. *Genomics* **7**, 182–187.

18. Giacalone, J., Friedes, J., and Francke, U. (1992) A novel GC rich human microsatellite VNTR in Xq24 is differentially methylated on active and inactive X chromosomes. *Nature Genet.* **1**, 137–143.

19. Keith, D. H., Singer-Sam, J., and Riggs, A. D. (1986) Active X chromosome DNA is unmethylated at eight CCGG sites clustered in a guanine -plus-rich island at the 5' end of the gene for phosphoglycerate kinase. *Mol. Cell. Biol.* **6**, 4122–4125.

20. Yen, P. H., Patel, P., Chinault, A. C., Mohandas, T., and Shapiro, L. J. (1984) Differential methylation of hypoxanthine phosphoribosyltransferase genes on active and inactive X chromosomes. *Proc. Natl. Acad. Sci. USA* **81**, 1759–1763.

21. Hendricks, R. W., Chen, Z. Y., Hinds, H., Schuurman, R. K. B., and Craig I. W. (1992) An X chromosome inactivation assay based on differential methylation of a CpG island coupled to a VNTR polymorphism at the 5' end of the monoamine oxidase A gene. *Hum. Mol. Genet.* **1(3)**, 187–194.

22. Allen, R. C., Zoghbi, H. Y., Moseley, A. B., Rosenblatt, H. M., and Belmont, J. W. (1992) Methylation of the *Hpa*II and *Hha*I sites near the polymorphic CAG repeat in the human androgen-receptor gene correlates with X chromosome inactivation. *Am. J. Hum. Genet.* **51,** 1229–1239.

23. Tonioli, D., D'Urso, M., Martini, G., Persico, M. G., Tufano, V., Battistuzzi, G., et al. (1984) Specific methylation pattern at the 3' end of the human housekeeping gene for glucose-6-phosphate dehydrogenase. *EMBO J.* **3,** 1987–1995.

24. Fraser, N. J., Boyd, Y., and Craig, I. (1989) Isolation and characterisation of a human variable copy number tandem repeat at Xcen-p 1.22. *Genomics* **5,** 146–148.

25. Hendricks, R. W., Kraakman, M. E. M., Mensink, R. G. J., and Schuurman, R. K. B. (1991) Differential methylation at the 5' and the 3' CCGG sites flanking the X chromosomal hypervariable DXS255 locus. *Hum. Genet.* **88,** 105–111.

26. Tilley, W. D., Marcelli, M., Wilson, J. D., and McPhaul, M. J. (1989) Characterisation and expression of a cDNA encoding the human androgen receptor. *Proc. Natl. Acad. Sci. USA* **86,** 327–331.

27. Gale, R. E., Wheadon, H., Boulos, P., and Linch, D. C. (1994) Tissue specificity of X chromosome inactivation patterns. *Blood* **83(10),** 2899–2905.

28. Vetrie, D., Flinter, F., Bobrow, M., and Harris, A. (1992) X inactivation patterns in females with Alport's syndrome: a means of selecting against a deleterious gene? *J. Med. Genet.* **29(9),** 663–666.

29. Harris, A., Collins, J., Vetrie, D., Cole, C., and Bobrow, M. (1992) X inactivation as a mechanism of selection against lethal alleles: further investigation of incontinentia pigmenti and X linked proliferative disease. *J. Med. Genet.* **29,** 608–614.

30. Brown, R. M. and Brown, G. K. (1993) X chromosome inactivation and the diagnosis of X linked disease in females. *J. Med. Genet.* **30,** 177–184.

31. Marcus, S., Steen, A.-M., Andersson, B., Larnbert, B., Kristoffersson, U., and Francke, U. (1992) Mutation analysis and prenatal diagnosis in a Lesch-Nyhan family showing non-random X-inactivation interfering with carrier detection tests. *Hum. Genet.* **89,** 395–400.

32. Alterman, L. A., de Alwis, M., Genet, S., Lovering, R., Middleton-Price, H., Morgan, G., et al. (1993) Carrier determination for X linked agammaglobulinaemia using X inactivation analysis of purified B cells. *J. Immunol. Methods* **166,** 111–116.

33. Conley, M. E., Lavoie, A., Briggs, C., Brown, P., Guerra, C., and Puck, J. M. (1988) Non-random X chromosome inactivation in B cells from carriers of X chromosome linked severe combined immunodeficiency. *Proc. Natl. Acad. Sci. USA* **85,** 3090–3094.

8

Risk Analysis

Andrew P. Read

1. Introduction

Every genetic laboratory diagnosis carries some degree of uncertainty, even if only the risk of laboratory error. Increasingly, diagnosis is based on direct tests that tell us whether or not the patient carries a given mutation. In these cases formal risk analysis is scarcely necessary—although it is important to remember that the patient wants to know the risk of disease, not the probability of possessing a certain genotype. Variable expression, nonpenetrance, or late onset may mean that carrying the mutation is not the same thing as having the disease. Unfortunately, there are still many situations where direct mutation tests are not available as part of a routine diagnostic service. Some disease genes have not yet been cloned; for others, although the gene is known, mutations are hard to find (e.g., in neurofibromatosis 1 and adult polycystic kidney disease type 1); sometimes direct tests easily reveal a proportion of all mutations, but the remainder are too diverse to be hunted down in a busy diagnostic laboratory (as happens in cystic fibrosis families). In all these cases family studies require the use of linked markers to track the disease gene through the family. Gene tracking always requires a risk calculation. A further complication arises when the same clinical disease can be caused by mutations at more than one locus, as with polycystic kidney disease or tuberous sclerosis.

Some aspects of risk analysis involve no more than common sense arithmetic or standard calculations of false-positive and false-negative rates. These calculations are covered in any standard text on elementary statistics (e.g., ref. *1*), and are not considered further here, although it is important that genetic laboratory workers should feel comfortable with simple statistics. This chapter concentrates on the two specialized techniques that are widely used in genetics

From: *Methods in Molecular Medicine: Molecular Diagnosis of Genetic Diseases*
Edited by: R. Elles Humana Press Inc., Totowa, NJ

laboratories for risk estimation, Bayesian analysis and pedigree analysis using linkage programs.

Genetic risk analysis usually involves calculating the probability of each of a small number of mutually exclusive outcomes: The person either carries the gene or does not; the fetus is either affected, a carrier, or homozygous normal. This type of problem lends itself well to analysis by Bayesian methods. Bayes' theory gives a formula for combining the probabilities of diverse pieces of evidence in order to get an overall probability, and allows simple hand calculations, at least in straightforward situations. Typically, Bayesian methods are used to combine pedigree risks with results of marker studies. Advantages of Bayesian methods are their generality—any risk factors can be incorporated into the calculation—and their simple logical structure. The main drawback is that the calculation can get excessively complicated for large pedigrees. A few people develop a great aptitude for reducing almost any problem to a Bayesian calculation, done by hand on a suitably large piece of paper, but for most of us, Bayesian methods are best kept for simple pedigrees. A recent book *(2)* gives examples of almost every conceivable application of Bayesian methods to genetic laboratory diagnosis.

The main alternative to Bayes is to use a linkage program on the computer (*see* Note 1). At first sight it may seem surprising that programs written for calculating lod scores should be useful for estimating risks. Actually the problems are not so very different. Each problem involves three interrelated sets of information: the segregation of the disease, the segregation of the marker(s), and the linkage relationship between the disease and the marker. Any two can be used to calculate the third. The core of linkage analysis programs, such as Liped and Mlink is a formula (the Elston–Stewart algorithm) *(3)* for calculating the overall likelihood of a pedigree, including disease and marker types. For linkage analysis, the overall likelihood is calculated twice, once on the assumption that the disease and marker loci are unlinked, and again on the assumption that they are linked with recombination fraction θ. The ratio of these two likelihoods is the odds for or against linkage with recombination fraction θ. The logarithm of these odds is the lod score $z(\theta)$ at that recombination value.

For risk estimation the odds of two alternative genotypes must be worked out for the proband. The likelihood of the pedigree is calculated twice. Both times the same, known, recombination fraction for the marker is specified; but for the two calculations the two alternative genotypes for the proband are used. Again, the ratio of the likelihoods gives the relative probabilities of the two genotypes. The advantages of using a linkage program are that very complicated pedigrees can be handled just as easily as simple ones, and the computer does not make arithmetical mistakes. The main disadvantage is that the calculation requires a very specific genetic model to be provided, including precise values for gene frequencies, genetic distances, and so on, which in reality are rarely known precisely. Additionally, none of the available programs is totally simple to run, still less to run correctly. Courses are available through various organizations (e.g., in the United Kingdom, through the Human Genome Project Resource Centre, *see* Note 2), and it is strongly recommended that at least one person in each center using these programs should have taken such a course. Most people need some help to get started, and plenty of guided practice before they feel confident. Two excellent books describe the principles of human linkage analysis *(3)* and some more practical details of using linkage programs *(4)*.

2. Materials

The main linkage analysis program is Mlink. This is part of a package called Linkage, currently in version 5.2, which includes several programs necessary for using Mlink, and some handy utility programs. All the Linkage programs run on a PC under DOS or OS/2, and are available free of charge to noncommercial users from various sources, including Professor Jurg Ott (*see* Note 1). Computation times can be quite lengthy, and it is best to use at least a 486 machine. The programs are supplied in both compiled and Pascal source code forms. If you want to alter any of the adjustable parameters (to allow larger families, more alleles at a locus, and so on) you will need an appropriate Pascal compiler, such as Borland's Turbo Pascal. This is a commercial package that must be bought from a software supplier. Alternatives to Mlink include Liped, again running on a PC and obtainable free from Professor Ott.

The other "material" necessary for risk analysis is the most accurate and up-to-date information on map distances and other properties of markers. For this reason, everybody doing risk analysis should have access over a computer network to the Genome Database (GDB) and to the online Mendelian Inheritance in Man (OMIM). At the time of writing both GDB and OMIM are freely accessible over the Internet, in addition to access in the United Kingdom for registered users at the Human Genome Project Resource Centre (*see* Note 2).

3. Methods
3.1. Bayesian Calculations

1. Set up a table with one column for each of the alternative hypotheses. Cover all the alternatives.
2. Assign a *prior probability* to each alternative. The prior probabilities of all the hypotheses must sum to 1. It is not important at this stage to worry about exactly what information you should use to decide the prior probability, as long as it is consistent across the columns. You will not be using all the information (other-

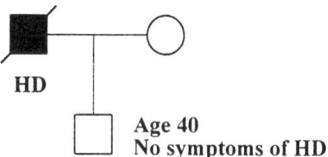

Fig. 1. Pedigree of HD.

wise there would be no point in doing the calculation because you would already have the answer), and any information not used in the prior probability can be used later.

3. Using one item of information not included in the prior probabilities, calculate a *conditional probability* for each hypothesis. The conditional probability is the probability of the information, given the hypothesis (*not* the probability of the hypothesis given the information!). The conditional probabilities for the different hypotheses do not necessarily sum to 1.

4. If there are further items of information not yet included, repeat step 3 as many times as necessary until all information has been used once and once only. The end result is a number of lines of conditional probabilities in each column.

5. Within each column, multiply together the prior and all the conditional probabilities. This gives a *joint probability*. The joint probabilities do not necessarily sum to 1 across the columns.

6. Scale the joint probabilities to give *final probabilities* that do sum to 1. This is done by dividing each joint probability by the sum of all the joint probabilities. The final probability is the desired answer (*see* Note 3).

3.1.1. Bayesian Calculation of the Risk of Carrying the Huntington's Disease (HD) Gene

Figure 1 illustrates a simple application. A man wishes to know the risk that he carries the HD gene. He is 40 yr old and on examination is free of symptoms.

1. Set up the calculation with two columns, for the two alternative hypotheses, that he has the HD gene or that he does not have it.

2. Use the mendelian probability, 1 in 2, as the prior risk.

3. For the "HD" column, the conditional probability is the chance that somebody age 40 shows no symptoms, given that they have a paternally inherited HD gene. Consulting an age-of-onset curve shows that this is 50%. For the "No HD" column, the probability that somebody age 40 shows no symptoms, given that they do not have the HD gene, is needed. Common sense suggests this figure is 1; the small possibility of a phenocopy could be allowed by setting the figure to, say, 0.999. Note that the conditionals do not sum to 1.

4. Calculate the joint and final probabilities (Table 1). The risk is 1 in 3 (Note 4).

Table 1
Bayesian Calculation of the Risk that II₁ (Fig. 1)
Has the HD Gene

Hypothesis: Man has	HD gene	No HD gene
Prior probability	1/2	1/2
Conditional		
Free of symptoms at age 40	0.5	1
Joint probability	0.25	0.5
Final probability	0.25/0.75 = 1/3	0.5/0.75 = 2/3

3.1.2. Bayesian Calculations for X-Linked Conditions

3.1.2.1. CARRIER RISK OF DUCHENNE'S MUSCULAR DYSTROPHY (DMD)

This example shows calculation of carrier risk of DMD, given an obligate carrier, with DNA and creatine kinase data. The proband is III_2 (Fig. 2).

1. There are two alternative hypotheses, and therefore two columns in the calculation.
2. II_2 is an obligate carrier, therefore, the prior risk is 1 in 2.
3. Put in the DNA information as a conditional probability. III_2 has inherited the low-risk allele of a marker that shows 5% recombination with DMD in a collection of family data. Given that she is a carrier, the probability of this is 0.05; given that she is not a carrier the probability is 0.95. (It happens that these conditional probabilities sum to 1.)
4. Put in the CK data as a second, independent conditional probability (*see* Note 5). III_2 has a CK level that gives 2.3:1 odds she is a carrier.
5. Work out the joint and final probabilities (Table 2). The final carrier risk is 10.8%.

3.1.2.2. DMD CARRIER RISK WITH NO OBLIGATE CARRIERS

What is the risk that II_4 (Fig. 3) is a carrier? The prior risk that a randomly selected woman is a carrier of DMD is 4 μ where μ is the mutation rate (Note 6). First the chance that her mother is a carrier is calculated (Table 3). The mother has a 1 in 3 chance of being a carrier (*see* Note 7). Therefore, ignoring the very small extra risk of a second new mutation, the daughter has a 1 in 6 risk. This could be modified by DNA marker studies and CK testing, as in previous examples.

3.1.2.3. PRIOR RISK FOR NONLETHAL X-LINKED CONDITIONS

For a nonlethal X-linked condition such as hemophilia, an important parameter is f, the biological fitness of affected males ($f = 0$ if none has children, $f = 1/3$ if they have on average only one third the number of children that unaffected men do, and so on). The prior risk that a female is a carrier is $x = 2 \mu(2 + f)/(1 - f)$ (*see* Note 8). For hemophilia A, the fitness of affected males is estimated to be 0.7, giving a prior risk of 18 μ.

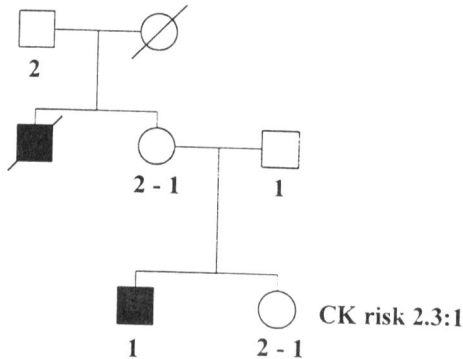

Fig. 2. Pedigree of DMD. II_2 is an obligate carrier.

Table 2
Bayesian Calculation of the Risk that III_2 (Fig. 2)
Carries the DMD Gene

Hypothesis: III_2 is	A carrier	Not a carrier
Prior probability	1/2	1/2
Conditional (1)		
DNA result	0.05	0.95
Conditional (2)		
CK data	2.3	1
Joint probability	0.0575	0.475
Final probability	0.0575/0.5325 = 0.108	0.475/0.5325 = 0.892

3.2. Risk Analysis Using Mlink

3.2.1. Prenatal Diagnosis
of Spinal Muscular Atrophy Using Linked Markers

1. Set up the pedigree file, setting out the pedigree structure and the disease and marker types in the standard format described in the program documentation (Fig. 4D, *see* pp. 160,161). Any word processor or text editor can be used, provided the result is an ASCII (plain text) file. Be careful not to leave any blank lines at the end. If the number of possible haplotypes exceeds 64, it must be reduced below this threshold by recoding alleles or eliminating markers (*see* Note 9). The pedigree in Fig. 4A has been simplified as shown in Fig. 4C.
2. Use the Makeped program that is part of the Linkage package to convert this to a processed pedigree file (Fig. 4E; *see* Note 10).

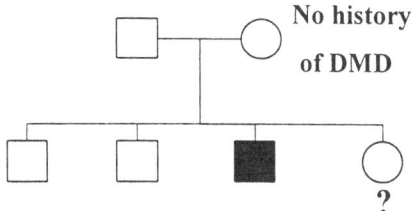

Fig. 3. Pedigree of DMD. A family that has no obligate carrier.

Table 3
Bayesian Calculation of the Risk that II$_4$ (Fig. 3)
Carries the DMD Gene

Hypothesis: Mother is a	Carrier	Noncarrier
Prior probability	4μ	$1-4\mu$
Conditional (1)		
She has an affected son	1/2	μ
Conditional (2)		
She has two unaffected sons	1/4	1
Joint probability	$\mu/2$	μ
Final probability	$\mu/2/(\mu/2+\mu)=1/3$	$\mu/(\mu/2+\mu)+2/3$

3. Use the Preplink program that is part of the Linkage package to create a file describing the genetics of the disease and markers (Fig. 4F). The map locations of all loci must be specified.
4. Use LCP, the Linkage Control Program in the Linkage package, to set up a DOS batch file to run the problem.
5. Run the batch file to calculate the risk. Figure 4G shows the output: The risk the fetus is affected is 98.9%.

3.2.2. Risk Analysis Using Mlink in DMD

1. Set up the pedigree file, with the disease and marker types, as before. Incorporate CK data by using liability classes (*see* Note 11).
2. Use the Makeped program to convert this to a processed pedigree file.
3. Use the Preplink program to create the file describing the genetics of the disease and markers. The mutation rate, 1×10^{-4}, is specified. The frequency of the disease allele is set at 2×10^{-4} (*see* Note 12). Figure 5 (*see* p. 162) shows a Preplink file that allows 10 different CK risk categories, and flanking markers, each with four alleles.
4. Use LCP, the Linkage Control Program, to set up a DOS batch file to run the problem.
5. Run the batch file to calculate the risk.

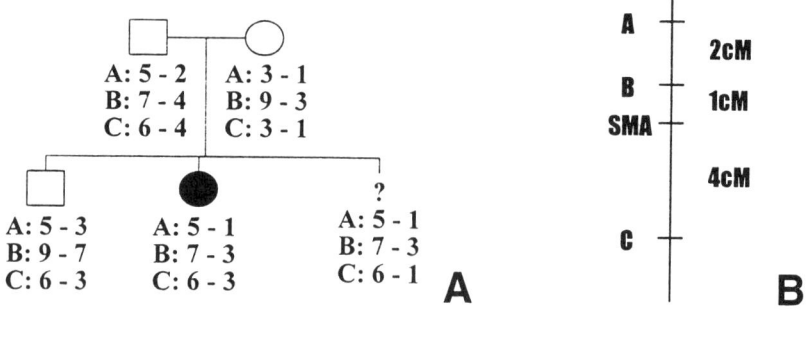

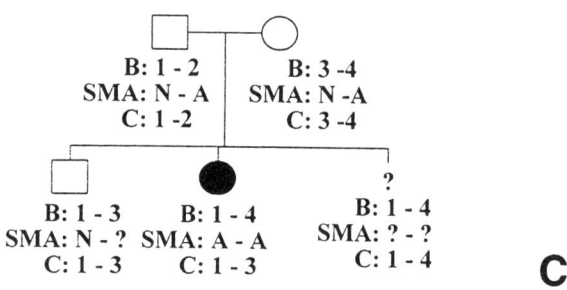

```
1 1 0 0 1 1 1 2 1 2    Father       1 1 0 0 3 0 0 1 0 1 1 2 1 2    Father Ped: 1 Per: 1
1 2 0 0 2 1 3 4 3 4    Mother       1 2 0 0 3 0 0 2 0 1 3 4 3 4    Mother Ped: 1 Per: 2
1 3 1 2 1 1 1 3 1 3    Son          1 3 1 2 0 4 4 1 0 1 1 3 1 3    Son Ped: 1 Per: 3
1 4 1 2 2 2 1 4 1 3    Daughter     1 4 1 2 0 5 5 2 0 2 1 4 1 3    Daughter Ped: 1 Per: 4
1 5 1 2 0 0 1 4 1 4    Fetus        1 5 1 2 0 0 0 1 1 0 1 4 1 4    Fetus Ped: 1 Per: 5
```

D   **E**

Fig. 4. Use of Mlink program to calculate risk in a prenatal diagnosis of spinal muscular atrophy using linked markers. (**A**) The pedigree, with types for three hypothetical markers, A, B, and C. No attempt has been made to draw out the haplotypes. (**B**) Genetic map. (**C**) Pedigree simplified for input to Mlink (*see* Note 9). Again, no attempt has been made to draw out the haplotypes; Mlink will do this. (**D**) Raw pedigree file for input to Mlink. (**E**) Pedigree file as processed by Makeped (*see* Note 10). (**F**) Preplink file describing the genetics. (**G**) Mlink output. The fetus has 98.9% risk of being affected.

```
3 1 0 5  << NO. OF LOCI, RISK LOCUS, SEXLINKED (IF 1) PROGRAM
0 0.0 0.0 0  << MUT LOCUS, MUT RATE, HAPLOTYPE FREQUENCIES (IF 1)
 2 1 3
1  2  << AFFECTION, NO. OF ALLELES
0.970000 0.030000  << GENE FREQUENCIES
1 << NO. OF LIABILITY CLASSES
0.0000 0.0000 1.0000 << PENETRANCES
 2 << ALLELE AT RISK
3  4  << ALLELE NUMBERS, NO. OF ALLELES
0.250000 0.250000 0.250000 0.250000  << GENE FREQUENCIES
3  4  << ALLELE NUMBERS, NO. OF ALLELES
0.250000 0.250000 0.250000 0.250000  << GENE FREQUENCIES
0 0  << SEX DIFFERENCE, INTERFERENCE (IF 1 OR 2)
0.01000 0.04000 << RECOMBINATION VALUES
1 0.10000 0.12000 << REC VARIED, INCREMENT, FINISHING VALUE
```

F

```
THETAS  0.010 0.040
-----------------------------------
PEDIGREE |  LN LIKE  | LOG 10 LIKE
-----------------------------------
RISK FOR PERSON     5 IN PEDIGREE     1
HOMOZYGOTE CARRIER      : 0.98882
HETEROZYGOTE CARRIER  : 0.01107
NORMAL                              : 0.00011
      1  -24.367676  -10.582725
-----------------------------------
TOTALS     -24.367676  -10.582725
-2 LN(LIKE) =  48.735351
```

G

Fig. 4. (F,G)

Special problems in DMD include possible ambiguity in the position of the DMD mutation relative to an intragenic marker (*see* Note 13) and germinal mosaicism (*see* Note 14). Sometimes it happens that a woman's carrier risk is negligible unless her father or grandfather is a germinal mosaic, in which case it is significant but hard to quantify. Risk estimation by any method is exceedingly difficult in such cases, and these are families where it is worth putting in extra efforts to define the mutation so that direct testing can be offered.

3.3. Risk Estimation in Cystic Fibrosis (CF)

As described in Chapter 5, most CF mutations are detected using direct mutation analysis. The necessity for risk calculations arises when no mutation is seen. A negative result on mutation screening does not exclude the presence of a rare mutation that is not included in the direct testing panel. For any particular geographical location and testing protocol, one can estimate the population frequency of these "invisible" CF mutations. It is a function of the overall CF frequency, of the distribution of mutations in that population, and of the proto-

```
3 1 1 5  << NO. OF LOCI, RISK LOCUS, SEXLINKED (IF 1) PROGRAM
1 1.00E-0004  1.00E-0004 0  << MUT LOCUS, MUT RATE, HAPLOTYPE FREQUENCIES (IF 1)
  2 1 3
1  2  << AFFECTION, NO. OF ALLELES        [DMD locus]
0.999800 0.000200   << GENE FREQUENCIES
11 << NO. OF LIABILITY CLASSES
0.0000 0.0000 1.0000                      [liability class for obligate carriers]
0.0000 1.0000
0.1000 0.9000 1.0000                      [liability class for CK C:NC odds 1:9]
0.0000 1.0000
0.2000 0.8000 1.0000                      [liability class for CK C:NC odds 2:8]
0.0000 1.0000
0.3000 0.7000 1.0000                      [liability class for CK C:NC odds 3:7]
0.0000 1.0000
0.4000 0.6000 1.0000                      [liability class for CK C:NC odds 4:6]
0.0000 1.0000
0.5000 0.5000 1.0000                      [liability class for CK C:NC odds 5:5]
0.0000 1.0000
0.6000 0.4000 1.0000                      [liability class for CK C:NC odds 6:4]
0.0000 1.0000
0.7000 0.3000 1.0000                      [liability class for CK C:NC odds 7:3]
0.0000 1.0000
0.8000 0.2000 1.0000                      [liability class for CK C:NC odds 8:2]
0.0000 1.0000
0.9000 0.1000 1.0000                      [liability class for CK C:NC odds 9:1]
0.0000 1.0000
0.9900 0.0100 1.0000                      [liability class for manifesting carriers]
0.0000 1.0000 << PENETRANCES
  2 << ALLELE AT RISK
3  4  << ALLELE NUMBERS, NO. OF ALLELES   [marker locus with 4 alleles]
0.2500000 0.2500000  0.2500000 0.2500000   << GENE FREQUENCIES
3  4  << ALLELE NUMBERS, NO. OF ALLELES   [2nd marker with 4 alleles]
0.2500000 0.2500000  0.2500000 0.2500000  << GENE FREQUENCIES
0 0  << SEX DIFFERENCE, INTERFERENCE (IF 1 OR 2)  [these next 3 lines are required, but
0.05000 0.05000 << RECOMBINATION VALUES          in fact not used by the program, if
1 0.10000 0.06000 << REC VARIED, INCREMENT, FINISHING VALUE    you use LCP].
```

Fig. 5. Preplink file for risk estimation in DMD using Mlink. The 11 liability classes allow creatine kinase data to be incorporated in the risk calculation (*see* Note 11).

col used for direct testing. Invisible mutations must then be considered in two contexts, population screening and family studies.

3.3.1. CF Population Screening

If the frequency of invisible mutations in a population is q, the risk of a CF child to a couple both of whom test negative is $q^2/4$. This is likely to be negligibly low, but the risk to couples one of whom tests positive and the other negative is much higher, at q/4. It has been suggested that a screening program does more harm than good unless q/4 is lower than the prescreening risk. For the United Kingdom this would require detection of 96% of all CF mutations. Most authors agree that this criterion is excessively stringent.

3.3.2. Diagnosis in CF Families

Chromosomes come in four classes:

1. Those carrying visible mutations;
2. Those known to carry invisible mutations (tracked from the parent of an affected child who has an invisible mutation);
3. Those with no visible mutation but the population risk q of carrying an invisible mutation; and
4. Those known not to carry any mutation (identified as the other chromosome of a known carrier, who would be affected if it carried any mutation).

When only one mutation can be detected in a CF-affected child, the parents can still be offered prenatal diagnosis in future pregnancies, using a combination of direct testing for the visible mutation and gene tracking for the invisible one. With multiallele microsatellite markers, no complicated calculation should be needed, because each parental chromosome usually can be distinguished. Giving carrier risks to a relative of the invisible mutation carrier is more tricky. Chromosomes must be tracked across the family. Unless all intervening relatives are available for study, the uncertainties mount rapidly because of the risk of recombination and because of possible failure to distinguish chromosomes identical by state but not by descent.

3.4. The Problem of Locus Heterogeneity

Extra uncertainty attends the interpretation of gene tracking results when the identical disease can be produced by mutations at more than one locus. In the occasional large family, linkage analysis can identify which locus is involved. Usually, however, one does not know. Adult polycystic kidney disease (APKD) is an example: 86% of families have a mutation mapping to the PKD1 locus on chromosome 16p13, while the rest mostly have a mutation at the currently unidentified PKD2 locus on chromosome 4q. Risk estimation is based on gene tracking, using the many polymorphic markers tightly linked to the PKD1 and PKD2 loci. Somebody who inherits a low-risk PKD1 marker from an affected parent has a risk of inheriting a disease allele given by: (the chance the disease is PKD1 and there is a recombinant) + (the chance the disease is not PKD1 × 1/2). The 1/2 is because if the disease is unlinked to the markers studied, there is the standard mendelian 1 in 2 risk.

Flanking markers are very much more powerful than single markers for pinpointing heterogeneity. Informative meioses can be classified into three types:

1. Nonrecombinants;
2. Single recombinants (with a marker—marker recombination); and
3. Apparent double recombinants, where somebody inherits a nonrecombinant haplotype of flanking markers in conjunction with the "wrong" disease status.

Single recombinants are uninformative: They merely show that a crossover has occurred somewhere between the flanking markers. Apparent double recombinants are likely to be the result of misdiagnosis or locus heterogeneity. The patient should be reevaluated to confirm the disease status. Two or more confirmed "double recombinants" in a family make it virtually certain that the disease locus is unlinked to the markers used.

The probabilities can be quantified by a Bayesian calculation, or more simply by using the Linkage programs. Suppose the markers M1 and M2 flank the normal disease locus D with recombination fractions $\theta 1$ and $\theta 2$. The likelihood of the data is calculated for two alternative maps:

$$M1—\theta 1—D—\theta 2—M2 \text{ and } D—0.5—M1—(\theta 1 + \theta 2)—M2$$

The ratio of the likelihoods is the odds of heterogeneity (*see* Note 15).

4. Notes

1. Noncommercial users can obtain the Linkage package by anonymous ftp from ftp york.ccc.columbia.edu (give login name ANONYMOUS; no password required; details in README.TXT file) or on disk from Professor Jurg Ott (Columbia University Unit 58, 722 West 168th St., New York, NY 10032). The standard version is for a PC using DOS, but other versions are available.

2. For UK users, the HGMP-RC is at Hinxton Hall (Cambridge CB10 1RQ). Consult your network supervisor about access to the Internet and World Wide Web (WWW). At the time of writing one of the easiest ways to access all biological databases is through the Baylor College of Medicine Genome Centre at Houston (WWW address http://gc.bcm.tmc.edu:8088). The Genome Database and OMIM are accessible at http://gdbWWW.gdb.org/, and the HGMP-RC at http://www.hgmp.mrc.ac.uk/.

3. A formal statement of Bayes' theorem is:

$$P(H_i|E) = P(H_i)P(E|H_i)/\Sigma P(H_i)P(E|H_i)$$

$P(H_i)$ means the probability of the ith hypothesis, and the vertical line means "given," so that $P(E|H_i)$ means the probability of the evidence (E) given hypothesis H_i (a conditional probability).

4. You might have expected the answer to be $1/2 \times 1/2 = 1/4$. This discrepancy illustrates an important general point about risk calculations. Both answers are correct, but they are answers to different questions. Of all 40-yr-olds whose father had HD, one in four will carry the HD gene but be free of symptoms. A second one of the four will have the gene and already be showing symptoms. Therefore, of all symptom-free 40-yr-olds whose father had HD, one in three carries the HD gene. It often happens that two logical and correct methods of calculating the same risk give different answers because they are answering subtly different questions. It is important to be sure that you are answering the question the patient asked.

5. If more than one conditional probability is used, it is essential that they should be logically independent of each other. If there were types for a second, flanking DNA marker, these could not be used as a separate conditional probability. The two markers are linked, and so the information they give is not independent. Assuming the flanking markers have not recombined with each other, a single conditional probability would be used, based on the likelihood of a double recombination.

6. Considering a lethal X-linked condition such as DMD, let the carrier risk of any randomly chosen woman be x. Then the risk that her daughter is a carrier is made of three components:
   a. A risk $x/2$ that she is a carrier by inheritance from her carrier mother.
   b. A risk μ that she has a new mutation on the maternal X chromosome (μ is the mutation rate in females).
   c. A risk ν that she has a new mutation on the paternal X chromosome (ν is the mutation rate in males).

   The daughter's overall risk is therefore $x/2 + \mu + \nu$. But since the daughter is equally a randomly chosen female, her risk must also be x. It follows that $x = 2(\mu + \nu)$. Usually one makes the assumption that the mutation rates are the same in both sexes, in which case the prior risk $x = 4\mu$.

7. Note that μ cancels out in the calculation, so it does not matter that its value is not known. The term in μ^2 in the noncarrier joint probability can be ignored, because for any realistic value of μ, μ^2 will be orders of magnitude smaller.

8. A woman can also be a carrier because her father was affected. The frequency of affected males will be $q = (x/2 + \mu)$, and the frequency of carrier females will be $x = (x/2 + 2\mu + qf)$, assuming equal male and female mutation rates. It follows that $x = x/2 + 2\mu + (x/2 + \mu)f$, which simplifies to $2\mu(2 + f)/(1 - f)$.

9. The number of possible haplotypes is the number of alleles at the disease locus, multiplied by the number of alleles at marker locus 1, multiplied by the number of alleles at marker locus 2, and so on. A disease with two alleles (affected, unaffected), tracked with microsatellites with 8 and 10 alleles, respectively, creates $2 \times 8 \times 10 = 160$ possible haplotypes. The time required to run the analysis rises exponentially with the number of haplotypes, and quickly becomes impossibly long; moreover, the standard versions of the Linkage package, run on a PC under DOS, cannot handle more than 64 haplotypes. One way around this problem is to redefine the markers to have fewer alleles (5). In a typical recessive family, at most, four different alleles of any marker are seen, even though the marker may have 10 different alleles in the wider population. Even with markers reduced to four alleles, only two ($4 \times 4 \times 2$ haplotypes including the disease) can be handled, plus maybe an extra 2-allele marker. It is important, therefore, to look carefully at the data and ask which markers actually are contributing useful information. In Fig. 4A, marker A gives no information that the more tightly linked marker B does not give. Markers B and C are recoded as having four alleles each, to give the pedigree in Fig. 4C.

10. The processed pedigree file contains added pointers to the pedigree structure, calculated automatically by the Makeped program.

11. The Linkage package allows a disease to have several liability classes with different penetrances. Each person in the pedigree is assigned to a liability class. This operates in an obvious way for age-dependent penetrances, as in HD. For DMD, the liability classes are used in a nonintuitive way to manipulate the penetrances so that the computer ends up putting in the appropriate CK odds ratio. The CK distribution is divided arbitrarily into n different classes, each giving odds carrier:noncarrier of R(n). In the Preplink file, n corresponding liability classes are defined for DMD with penetrances:

Genotype	1-1 (normal homozygote)	2-1 (carrier)	2-2 (affected homozygote)
Penetrance	$R(n)/[1 + R(n)]$	$1/[1 + R(n)]$	1

The penetrance assigned to the affected homozygote is immaterial—the computer demands a number, but in practice there will not be any such females. The other two penetrances work as follows. Suppose R(n) is 2, that is, the CK gives 2:1 odds a woman is a carrier. Mlink assigns penetrances 2/3 for homozygous normal and 1/3 for a carrier. The penetrance is the probability of being affected, given the genotype. Mlink calculates that an unaffected woman in this liability class is twice as likely to be a carrier as to be a normal homozygote, because the penetrances tell it that homozygous normal women are less likely to be unaffected. Thus the computer is tricked into including the CK data. The trickery matters only for unaffected women who may or may not be carriers. For obligate carrier females, a special liability class can be used, with the standard penetrances of 0, 0, and 1 for genotypes 1-1, 2-1, and 2-2, respectively. The pedigree must include the relevant affected males, so that the computer can work out that she is an obligate carrier. Males are either affected or unaffected, and every liability class has the male penetrances 0 and 1, as common sense requires. Thus males can be assigned to any liability class. An alternative to using liability classes is to define DMD as a quantitative phenotype instead of as a disease, but this seems even more counterintuitive.

12. Mlink uses the standard Hardy–Weinberg equation to calculate the frequency of carriers as $2pq$, where p and q are the frequencies of the normal and disease alleles. Thus the prior probability of a woman being a carrier is $2pq$. But the prior probability needs to be 4 μ (*see* Note 6). To get correct results, therefore, the frequency of the disease allele is given as 2×10^{-4}, regardless whether this is the true value in the population. A similar maneuver would be used for nonlethal diseases, where the prior carrier probability is a different function of μ, as explained (Note 8).

13. The unique size and complexity of the dystrophin gene means that in different DMD families the mutation might map to different sides of an intragenic marker. Linkage programs require a definite map. One has to use common sense in defin-

ing the locus order and recombination fractions. If the common strategy of having one intragenic and two flanking markers is used, it may be necessary to calculate the risk twice, once for mutations lying either side of the intragenic marker. The final risk is then an average, maybe weighted by a "guesstimate" of the prior probability that a mutation would map in either interval.

14. The linkage programs do not allow for germinal mosaicism (or the risk of nonpaternity, switched samples, maternal contamination of a chorion villus sample, and so on).

15. It is important in this calculation to use the actual likelihood of the pedigree at the correct recombination fractions, which is included on the Mlink output. Mlink also outputs the lod score, but this is contaminated by the known linkage of M1 and M2, and should not be used for estimating heterogeneity.

References

1. Mosteller, F., Rourke, R. E. K., and Thomas, G. B. (1970) *Probability with Statistical Applications,* 2nd ed., Addison-Wesley, London.
2. Bridge, P. (1993) *The Analysis of Genetic Risks.* Johns Hopkins University Press, Baltimore, MD.
3. Ott, J. (1991) *Analysis of Human Genetic Linkage.* Johns Hopkins University Press, Baltimore, MD.
4. Terwilliger, J. and Ott, J. (1994) *Handbook for Human Genetic Linkage.* Johns Hopkins University Press, Baltimore, MD.
5. Ott, J. (1978) A simple scheme for the analysis of HLA linkages in pedigrees. *Ann. Hum. Genet.* **42,** 255–257.

9

Hemoglobinopathies

Community Clues to Mutation Detection

John M. Old

1. Introduction

The hemoglobinopathies are a diverse group of inherited recessive disorders consisting of the structural hemoglobin variants and the thalassemias. They can occur at very high carrier frequencies in the malarious regions of the world and are regionally specific, with each population having a unique combination of structural variants and thalassemia mutations. Therefore, knowledge of the ethnic origin of a patient is usually essential for the quick identification of the underlying molecular defect(s) in the globin genes.

1.1. Regional Variation

Of the structural variants, the most important clinically is Hb S (β-globin codon 6, A $\rightarrow$ T), which reaches its highest frequencies in Africa, Saudi Arabia, and India. Sickle cell disease results from the homozygous state for the mutation, and also in varying degrees from the combination of a Hb S mutation coupled with either a Hb D Punjab, Hb O Arab, Hb C, or β-thalassemia mutation in the other β-gene. Hb D Punjab (codon 121, G $\rightarrow$ C) is found in India, Hb O Arab (codon 121, G $\rightarrow$ A) in the Middle East, and Hb C (codon 6, G $\rightarrow$ A) in West Africa. The second most important abnormal hemoglobin is Hb E (codon 26, G $\rightarrow$ A). The mutation causes a splicing defect resulting in a mild β^+ thalassemia phenotype and it can combine with β-thalassaemia trait to produce a severe hemoglobinopathy, depending on the type of β-thalassemia mutation. Hb E is extremely common in a region stretching from northern India to China, reaching frequencies of up to 50% in some populations.

From: *Methods in Molecular Medicine: Molecular Diagnosis of Genetic Diseases*
Edited by: R. Elles Humana Press Inc., Totowa, NJ

More than 120 different β-thalassemia mutations have been described world-wide *(1)*, and for most countries the spectrum of mutations has been determined *(2)*. The relative frequencies of the mutations in selected countries are listed in Table 1 (pp. 172,173). Although this information can be very useful for mutation screening in specific cases, for practical purposes the β-thalassemia mutations can be classified into four ethnic groups: Mediterranean, Asian Indian, Chinese, and Black African. For each group there are just a small number of common mutations that account for more than 90% of those found and therefore mutations can be identified for most couples at risk in one screening assay.

The α-thalassemia mutations are classed as either the α^+ types (one inactive α-globin gene per chromosome) or the α^0 types (two inactive α-globin genes per chromosome) *(3)*. The α^0 types all result from large DNA deletions and are found in Mediterranean countries, e.g., Italy, Greece, and Cyprus (the --^{MED} and $-[\alpha]^{20.5}$ alleles) or southeast Asia (--^{SEA}), Thailand (--^{THAI}), and the Philippines (--^{FIL}). It has also been found to occur at very low frequencies in nonmalarious regions, e.g., northern Europe (--^{BRIT} allele). The α^+ types can result from either gene deletions or point mutations. The most common alleles are the 3.7-kb deletion ($-\alpha^{3.7}$), found in African, Mediterranean, and Asian populations, and the 4.2-kb deletion ($-\alpha^{4.2}$), found in southeast Asian and Pacific populations. Of the nondeletion types, the most widespread is Hb Constant Spring, found throughout southeast Asia. In general, both nondeletion and α^0-thalassemia are rare in comparison to the α^+ thalassemia deletion-genes.

1.2. Methods of Detection

Three α^0-thalassemia deletions can be detected by PCR using primers to amplify across the breakpoints *(4)*. However, in my laboratory I have encountered much difficulty in getting reliable amplification with these primers because of the high G-C content of the α-globin gene region and continue to identify α-thalassemia deletions by Southern blot analysis. *Bam*HI digests are hybridized with an α-gene probe and *Bgl*II digests with a ζ-gene probe initially and then if required the filters can be stripped and rehybridized to the other probe. Table 2 (p. 174) lists the abnormal fragments (underscored) observed for all the common deletions *(4–7)*. The two alleles,--^{THAI} and --^{FIL}, cannot be identified with these probes because they involve deletions that remove the entire α-globin gene complex and require a probe from a region 4 kb upstream of the ζ-gene for their detection *(8)*.

The β-globin gene cluster DNA sequence is very easily amplified and nearly all the known mutations can be diagnosed by PCR. Four β^0-thalassemia deletion mutations *(9)*, five $(\delta\beta)^0$-thalassemia deletions, three deletions resulting in hereditary persistence of fetal hemoglobin, and the intergene deletion creating the abnormal Hb Lepore *(10)* can be diagnosed by amplification across the deletion breakpoints. Point mutations and insertions or deletions of just a few nucleotides in the β-globin gene are detected directly by the polymerase chain reaction (PCR) techniques of allele-specific oligonucleotide hybridization *(11)* or the allele-specific priming method *(12)*, the technique discussed in the next section and in Chapter 5. A few of the mutations create or abolish a restriction enzyme site *(see* Table 5) and can be screened for in a similar manner to restriction fragment length polymorphisms (RFLPs). This approach can be useful for the confirmation of a particular β-thalassemia mutation, but is of limited use for general screening of unknown samples. However, it is widely used for the molecular diagnosis of the β-globin variants giving rise to Hb S, Hb E, Hb D Punjab, and Hb O Arab. The primer sequences used in my laboratory for this purpose are listed in Table 3 (p. 175) *(see* Note 7). Finally, more than 17 RFLPs have been described in the β-globin gene cluster and a number of these are extremely useful for haplotype analysis and prenatal diagnosis *(13)*. The primer sequences for the investigation of 10 of these RFLPs by PCR are presented in Table 4 (p. 176).

1.3. Allele-Specific Priming Technique

This technique is illustrated in Fig. 1 (p. 177) and is known as the amplification refractory mutation system (ARMS). It was first described by Newton et al. *(14)*. For prenatal diagnosis two primers must be designed that will generate specific amplification products, one with the mutant allele and the other with the normal sequence. The nucleotide at the 3'-terminus of each primer is complementary to the base in the respective target sequence at the site of the mutation. In addition a deliberate mismatch to the target sequence is included at the third or fourth base from the 3' end. The deliberate mismatch enhances the specificity of the primer since all 3' terminal mismatches on their own except for C-C, G-A, and A-A mismatches will allow some extension of the primer and thus generate nonspecific amplification product *(15)*. The mutation-specific ARMS primers for the most common β-thalassemia mutations and β-globin variants are listed in Table 5 (p. 178,179) . All are the same length (30 mers) so that all can be used at one annealing temperature (65°C). Primers for the specific detection of the corresponding normal allele are listed in Table 6 (p. 180). These are required for prenatal diagnosis in cases where both partners of a couple at risk for β-thalassemia carry the same mutation. Each normal ARMS primer must be tested to check that it is working correctly using DNA from an individual homozygous for that particular mutation. The list of primers in Table 6 is shorter than Table 5 because of the lack of appropriate DNA controls in the laboratory.

Each ARMS primer requires a second primer to generate the allele-specific product and in addition, two control primers must be included in the PCR reaction in order to generate an unrelated product that indicates the reaction mixture was set up properly and everything is working correctly *(see* Notes 1–4).

Table 1
The Distribution of the Common β-Thalassemia Mutations[a]

Mutation[b]	Mediterranean			India		Chinese		African American
	Italy	Greece	Turkey	Pakistan	India	China	Thailand	
−88(C → T)	0.4				0.8			21.4
−87(C → G)		1.8	1.2					
−30(T → A)			2.5					
−29(A → G)						1.9		60.3
−28(A → G)						11.6	4.9	
CAP + 1(A → C)					1.7			
CD5(−CT)		1.2	0.8					
CD6(−A)	0.4	2.9	0.6					
CD8(−AA)		0.6	7.4					0.8
CD8/9(+G)				28.9	12.0			
CD15(G → A)				3.5	0.8			
CD16(−C)				1.3	1.7			
CD17(A → T)						10.5	24.7	
CD24(T → A)								7.9
CD39(C → T)	40.1	17.4	3.5	7.9	13.7			
CD41/42(−TCTT)						38.6	46.4	
CD71/72(+A)						12.4	2.3	
IVSI-1(G → A)	4.3	13.6	2.5					
IVSI-1(G → T)				8.2	6.6			
IVSI-5(G → C)				26.4	48.5	2.5	4.9	

IVSI-6(T → C)	16.3	7.4	17.5					
IVSI-110(G → A)	29.8	43.7	41.9					
IVSII-1(G → A)	1.1	2.1	9.7					
IVSII-654(C → T)						15.7	8.9	
IVSII-745(C → G)	3.5	7.1	2.7					
619-bp deletion				23.3	13.3			
Others	4.1	2.2	9.7	0.5	0.9	6.8	7.9	10.6

[a] Expressed as percentage gene frequencies of the total number of thalassemia chromosomes studied.

[b] CD, codon; IVS, intervening sequence; bp, basepairs.

Table 2
Restriction Fragment Sizes (kb) of Various α-Globin Alleles[a]

Allele	α-Gene fragment		ζ-Gene fragment	
	*Bam*HI	*Bgl*II	*Bam*HI	*Bgl*II
αα	14.0	12.6	11.3–10.0[b]	12.6
		7.4	5.9	12.0–10.0[b]
$-\alpha^{3.7}$	<u>10.3</u>	<u>16.0</u>	11.3–10.0[b]	<u>16.0</u>
			5.9	12.0–10.0[b]
$-\alpha^{4.2}$	<u>9.8</u>	7.4	11.3–10.0[b]	12.0–10.0[b]
			5.9	<u>8.7</u>
$-(\alpha)^{20.5}$	<u>4.0</u>	<u>10.5</u>	5.9	<u>10.5</u>
$--^{MED}$	None	None	5.9	<u>13.9</u>
$--^{SEA}$	None	None	<u>20</u>	<u>10.5</u>
			5.9	
$--^{BRIT}$	None	None	5.9	<u>7.8</u>
$--^{SA}$	None	None	5.9	<u>7.0</u>

[a]Characteristic abnormally sized fragments are underscored.
[b]Variable size owing to the ζ hypervariable region.

In most cases the control product is generated from the 3' end of the β-globin gene by primers that span the breakpoints of the 619 bp deletion β-thalassemia mutation. If this deletion gene is present in the target DNA, a 242-bp product instead of the normal 861 bp fragment is generated *(16)*.

2. Materials

1. PCR buffer used in the standard Cetus buffer: 50 m*M* KCl, 10 m*M* Tris-HCl (pH 8.3 at room temperature), 1.5 m*M* MgCl$_2$, 100 µg/mL gelatin. A 10X stock buffer can be prepared by adding together 0.5 mL of 1*M* Tris-HCl, pH 8.3, 1.25 mL 2*M* KCl, 75 µL 1*M* MgCl$_2$, 5 mg of gelatin, and 3.275 mL of distilled water. The stock buffer is heated at 37°C until the gelatin dissolves and then frozen in aliquots.

2. Stock deoxynucleotide mixture 1.25 m*M* each dNTP: Add together 50 µL of a 100-m*M* solution of each dNTP and 3.8 mL of distilled water. The 1.25 m*M* dNTP stock should be stored at –20°C in 0.8-mL aliquots.

   Ready made 100 m*M* dNTP solutions are now easily obtainable commercially (e.g., from Boehringer Mannheim, Mannheim, Germany), although purists may still wish to make up their own stocks from dNTP salts (which are less expensive) as follows: Dissolve to approx 200 m*M*, neutralize carefully with 0.05*M* Tris base to a pH of 7.0 by checking droplets on pH paper, read the optical density of a diluted aliquot at the correct wavelength (259 nm-A, 253 nm-G, 271 nm-C, 260 nm-T), calculate the concentration from the extinction coefficient (for a 1-cm path length: 1.54×10^4-A, 1.37×10^4-G, 9.1×10^3-C, 7.4×10^3-T), and finally adjust to 100 m*M* with distilled water.

Table 3
Oligonucleotide Primers for the Detection of β^S, β^E, β^DPunjab, and β^OArab Mutations as RFLPs

Mutation and affected RE site	Primer sequence, 5'–3'	Annealing temperature, °C	Product size, bp	Absence of site, bp	Presence of site, bp
β^SCD6 (A → T) (Loses *Dde*I site)	ACCTCACCCTGTGGAGCCAC GAGTGGACAGATCCCCAAAGGACTCAAGGA	65 65	443	386 67	201 175 67
β^ECD26 (G → A) (Loses *Mnl*I site)	ACCTCACCCTGTGGAGCCAC GAGTGGACAGATCCCCAAAGGACTCAAGGA	65	443	231 89 56 35 33	171 89 60 35 33
β^D Punjab CD121 (G → C) (Loses *Eco*RI site)	CAATGTATCATGCCTCTTTGCACC GAGTCAAGGCTGAGAGATGCAGGA	65 65	861	861	552 309
β^OArab CD121 (G → A) (Loses *Eco*RI site)	CAATGTATCATGCCTCTTTGCACC GAGTCAAGGCTGAGAGATGCAGGA	65 65	861	861	552 309

175

Table 4
Oligonucleotide Primers Used for Analysis of β-Globin Gene Cluster RFLPs

RFLP	Primer sequence, 5'–3'	Annealing temperature, °C	Product size, bp	Absence of site, bp	Presence of site, bp
ε-HindII	TCTCTGTTGATGACAAATTC	55	760	760	314
	AGTCATTGGTCAAGGCTGACC	55			446
Gγ-XmnI	AACTGTTGCTTTATAGGATTT	55	650	650	450
	AGGAGCTTATTGATAACTCAGAC	55			200
Gγ-HindIII	AGTGCTGCAAAGAAGAAACAACTACC	65	323	323	235
	CTCGCATCATGGGCCAGTGAGCCTC	65			98
Aγ-HindIII	ATGCTGCTAATGCTTCATTAC	55	635	635	327
	TCATTGTGTGATCTCTCTCAGCAG	55			308
5'ψβ-HindII	TCCTATCCATTACTGTTCCTTGAA	55	794	794	687
	ATTGTCTTATTCTAGAGACGATTT	55			107
5'ψβ-AvaII	TCCTATCCATTACTGTTCCTTGAA	55	794	794	442
	ATTGTCTTATTCTAGAGACGATTT	55			352
3'ψβ-HindII	GTACTCATACTTAAGTCCTAACT	55	914	914	480
	TAAGCAAGATTATTTCTGGTCTCT	55			434
β-RsaI	AGACATAATTTATTAGCATGCATG	55	1200	692	692
	CCCCTTCCTATGACATGAACTTAA	55		413	331
				100	100
					82
β-AvaII	GTGGTCTACCCTTGGACCCAGAGG	65	328	328	227
	TTCGTCTGTTCCCATTCTAAACT	65			101
β-HinfI	GGAGGTAAAGTTTTGCTATGCTGTAT	55	475	320	219
	GGGCCTATGATAGGGTAAT	55		155	155
					108

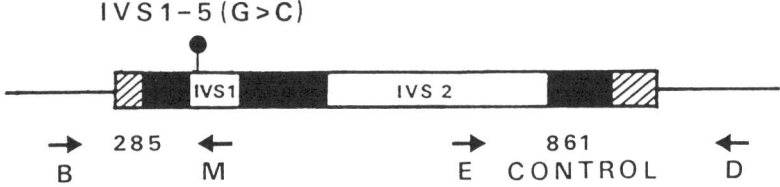

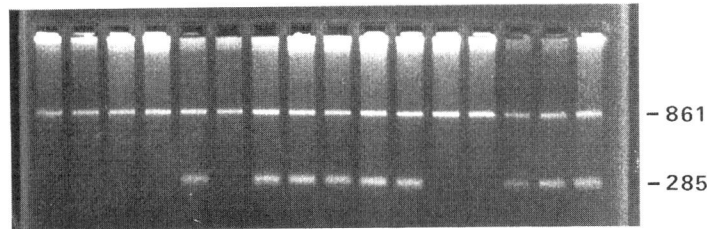

Fig. 1. Diagram showing the β-globin gene and the position of the mutation IVSI-5 (G → C) in the intervening sequence (IVS) 1, together with the positions of the mutant ARMS primer (M) to detect IVSI-5, primer B, and the control pair of primers D and E. The result of screening 16 DNA samples from individuals with β-thalassemia trait with primers A, M, D, and E are shown herein. The 285-bp product seen in nine tracks indicates the presence of IVSI-5 (G → C).

3. PCR reaction mixture stock solution (4 mL) Add together 0.5 mL 10X Cetus buffer, 0.8 mL 1.25 mM dNTP stock solution, and 2.7 mL distilled water.
4. Dilute aliquots of primer stock solutions to make working solutions at a concentration of 1 OD U/mL. The primers are synthesized commercially by OSWEL DNA service (Southampton, UK) and are HPLC purified. Store at –20°C.
5. *Taq* DNA polymerase: AmpliTaq (Applied Biosystems, Warrington, UK) is the gold standard but cheaper thermostable DNA polymerases may be used successfully (e.g., Advanced Biotechnologies, Leatherhead, UK).

3. Methods

3.1. PCR Conditions

For both ARMS-PCR and RFLP-PCR a total reaction volume of 25 μL is used with the following final concentrations: 10 mM Tris-HCl, pH 8.3, 50 mM KCl, 1.5 mM MgCl$_2$, 0.01% gelatin, 0.2 μM each primer, 200 μM each dNTP, 0.1–0.5 μg of genomic DNA, 0.25 U of *Taq* polymerase.

1. Add 20 μL of the PCR reaction mixture into a 0.5-μL Eppendorf tube.
2. Add 1 μL of each required primer (four for ARMS-PCR, two for RFLP-PCR) plus 0.25 U of enzyme per tube. To decrease pipeting errors, the enzyme and

Table 5
Primer Sequences Used for the Detection of the Common β-Thalassemia Mutations by the Allele-Specific Priming Technique[a]

Mutation	Oligonucleotide sequence, 5'–3'	Second primer	Product size, bp	Altered restriction
−88(C → T)	TCACTTAGACCTCACCCTGTGGAGCCTCAT	A	684	+*FokI*
−87(C → G)	CACTTAGACCTCACCCTGTGGAGCCACCCG	A	683	−*Avr*II
−30(T → A)	GCAGGGAGGGCAGGAGCCAGGGCTGGGGAA	A	626	
−29(A → G)	CAGGGAGGGCAGGAGCCAGGGCTGGGTATG	A	625	+*Nla*II
−28(A → G)	AGGGAGGGCAGGAGCCAGGGCTGGGCTTAG	A	624	
CAP+1(A → G)	ATAAGTCAGGGCAGAGCCATCTATTGGTTC	A	597	
CD5(−CT)	TCAAACAGACACCATGGTGCACCTGAGTCG	A	528	−*Dde*I
CD6(−A)	CCCACAGGGCAGTAACGGCAGACTTCTGCC	B	207	−*Dde*I
CD8(−AA)	ACACCATGGTGCACCTGACTCCTGAGCACG	A	520	
CD8/9(+G)	CCTTGCCCCACAGGGCAGTAACGGCACACC	B	225	
CD15(G → A)	TGAGGAGAAGTCTGCCGTTACTGCCCAGTA	A	500	
CD16(−C)	TCACCACCAACTTCATCCACGTTCACGTTC	B	238	
CD17(A → T)	CTCACCACCAACTTCATCCACGTTCAGCTA	B	239	
CD24(T → A)	CTTGATACCAACCTGCCCAGGGCCTCTCCT	B	262	
CD39(C → T)	CAGATCCCAAAGGACTCAAAGAACCTGTA	B	436	+*Mae*I
CD41/42(−TCTT)	GAGTGGACAGATCCCCAAAGGACTCAACCT	B	439	
CD71/72(+A)	CATGGCAAGAAAGTGCTCGGTGCCTTTAAG	C	241	
IVSI-1(G → A)	TTAAACCTGTCTTGTAACCTTGATACCGAT	B	281	−*Bsp*M
IVSI-1(G → T)	TTAAACCTGTCTTGTAACCTTGATACCGAAA	B	281	−*Bsp*M
IVSI-5(G → C)	CTCCTTAAACCTGTCTTGTAACCTTGTTAG	B	285	
IVSI-6(T → C)	TCTCCTTAAACCTGTCTTGTAACCTTCATG	B	286	+*Sfa*N
IVSI-110(G → A)	ACCAGCAGCCTAAGGGTGGGAAAATAGAGT	B	419	

IVSII-1(G → A)	AAGAAAACATCAAGGGTCCCATAGACTGAT	B	634	–HphI
IVSII-654(C → T)	GAATAACAGTGATAATTTCTGGGTTAACGT[b]	D	829	+RsaI
IVSII-745(C → G)	TCATATTGCTAATAGCAGCTACAATCGAGG[b]	D	738	–DdeI
β[s]CD6(A → T)	CCCACAGGGCAGTAACGGCAGACTTCTGCA	B	207	–DdeI
β[C]CD6(G → A)	CCACAGGGCAGTAACGGCAGACTTCTCGTT	B	206	
β[E]CD26(G → A)	TAACCTTGATACCAACCTGCCCAGGGCGTT	B	236	–MnlI

[a]The above primers are coupled as indicated with primer A: CCCCTTCCTATGACATGAACTTAA, B: ACCTCACCCTGTGGAGCCAC, C: TTCGTCTGTTTCCCATTCTAAACT, or D: GAGTCAAGGCTGAGAGATGCAGGA.
[b]The control primers used were primers D plus E: CAATGTATCATGCCTCTTTGCACC (which yield a 861-bp product as shown in Fig. 1) for all the above mutation specific ARMS primers except these two are the [G]γ-HindIII RFLP primers listed in Table 4.

179

Table 6
Primer Sequences Used for the Detection of the Normal DNA Sequence by the Allele-Specific Priming Technique[a]

Mutation	Oligonucleotide sequence, 5'–3'	Second primer	Product size, kb
–87 (C → G)	CACTTAGACCTCACCCTGTGGAGCCACCCC	A	683
CD5 (–CT)	CAAACAGACACCATGGTGCACCTGACTCCT	A	528
CD8 (–AA)	ACACCATGGTGCACCTGACTCCTGAGCAGA	A	520
CD8/9 (+G)	CCTTGCCCCACAGGGCAGTAACGGCACACT	B	225
CD15 (G → A)	TGAGGAGAAGTCTGCCGTTACTGCCCAGTA	A	500
CD39 (C → T)	TTAGGCTGCTGGTGGTCTACCCTTGGTCCC	A	299
CD41/42 (–TCTT)	GAGTGGACAGATCCCCAAAGGACTCAAAGA	B	439
IVSI-1 (G → A)	TTAAACCTGTCTTGTAACCTTGATACCCAC	B	281
IVSI-1 (G → T)	GATGAAGTTGGTGGTGAGGCCCTGGGTAGG	A	455
IVSI-5 (G → C)	CTCCTTAAACCTGTCTTGTAACCTTGTTAC	B	285
IVSI-6 (T → C)	AGTTGGTGGTGAGGCCCTGGGCAGGTTGGT	A	449
IVSI-110 (G → A)	ACCAGCAGCCTAAGGGTGGGAAAATACACC	B	419
IVSII-1 (G → A)	AAGAAAACATCAAGGGTCCCATAGACTGAC	B	634
IVSII-654 (C → T)	GAATAACAGTGATAATTTCTGGGTTAACGC	D	829
IVSII-745 (C → G)	TCATATTGCTAATAGCAGCTACAATCGAGC	D	738
β[S] CD6 (A → T)	AACAGACACCATGGTGCACCTGACTCGTGA	A	527
β[E] CD26 (G → A)	TAACCTTGATACCAACCTGCCCAGGCGTC	B	236

[a]*See* Table 5 legend for details of primers A–D and control primers.

primers in most cases can be mixed together in a separate tube before addition to the reaction mix.

3. Add 1 µL of DNA solution (at 0.1–0.5 mg/mL).
4. Add 30 µL of light paraffin oil and place tubes in a PCR machine.
5. For ARMS-PCR, program for 25 cycles (*see* Note 5) of 94°C for 1 min, 65°C for 1 min, 72°C for 1.5 min, with a final extension period of 3 min at 72°C after the last cycle. For RFLP-PCR, program for 30 cycles of 94°C for 1 min, 55 or 65°C (*see* Table 4) for 1 min, 72°C for 1.5 min, with a final extension period of 3 min at 72°C after the last cycle.

3.2. Analysis of ARMS-PCR Product

1. Remove tubes from the PCR machine and add 5 µL of blue dye (15% ficoll/0.05% bromophenol blue). Mix and spin.
2. Load a 20-µL sample onto a 3% agarose gel and run at 100 V for approx 45 min in Tris-acetate buffer (40 mM Tris-acetate–1 mM EDTA).
3. Stain gel in ethidium bromide solution (0.5 µg/mL) for 15–30 min, visualize bands on a UV light box (312 nm), and photograph with an electronic camera system or a Polaroid camera fitted with an orange filter (e.g., Wratten 22A).

3.3. Analysis of RFLP-PCR Product

1. Remove tubes from PCR machine and add 5–10 U of the appropriate restriction enzyme plus 2 µL of the corresponding 10X buffer.
2. Incubate at 37°C for a minimum of 1 h. Add 5 µL of blue dye, mix, and spin.
3. Load sample onto an agarose gel made of 1.5% agarose and 1.5% NuSieve GTG agarose (FMC) and electrophorese, stain, and photograph as described (*see* Note 6).

4. Notes

1. Both positive and negative controls for each RFLP or mutation being screened always must be amplified and run on the gel alongside the test samples.
2. The relationship of fragment intensities should be constant for all DNA samples of the same genotype. Any deviation to the expected pattern of band intensities should be treated as suspect (e.g., a partial digestion or a false-positive ARMS-PCR result) and the sample retested.
3. As mentioned, sometimes an ARMS primer may produce a positive signal that is less intense relative to the control fragment than expected. If the same faint band is observed in the negative control sample, the result is a false positive. This occurs when either there has been a subtle change of reaction conditions or if the ARMS primer has started to lose its specificity. The latter has occurred occasionally with the stock primer solutions and possibly results from some degradation of the 3' end of the oligonucleotide, in which case the primer has had to be resynthesized.
4. No amplification product may result from the DNA sample being too dilute (reprecipitate in a smaller volume), the DNA being too concentrated (try a 1 in 10 dilution), or the DNA containing impurities. The latter may be overcome by cleaning up the DNA with a repeat phenol extraction, but if the DNA sample is

too small and precious for such treatment, the addition of spermidine to the PCR reaction mixture at a final concentration of 1 mM usually allows amplification to proceed.

5. Always use a limited number of cycles to avoid false-positive results with ARMS primers and also the possibility of amplifying any contaminating maternal DNA in a fetal DNA sample. If, as a last resort, a larger number of cycles is required, amplify diluted DNA controls so that band intensities between samples remain comparable.

6. For the separation of small DNA fragments very similar in size, increase the percentage agarose gel to 4% (3% NuSieve/1% agarose) or even 4.5% (3.5% NuSieve/1% agarose).

7. Finally, before synthesizing a primer, always check the published sequence against the known β-globin DNA sequence for any mistakes or typing errors (authors are the worst proofreaders).

References

1. Baysal, E. (1992) The β and δ thalassemia repository. *Hemoglobin* **16,** 237–258.
2. Flint, J., Harding, R. M., Boyce, A. J., and Clegg, J. B. (1993) The population genetics of the haemoglobinopathies, in *Baillière's Clinical Haematology: Haemoglobinopathies* (Higgs, D. R. and Weatherall, D. J., eds.), Baillière Tindall and W.B. Saunders, London, pp. 215–262.
3. Higgs, D. R. (1993) α-thalassaemia, in *Baillière's Clinical Haematology: The Haemoglobinopathies* (Higgs, D. R. and Weatherall, D. J., eds.), Baillière Tindall and W.B. Saunders, London, pp. 117–150.
4. Higgs, D. R., Pressley, L., Aldridge, B., Clegg, J. B., Weatherall, D. J., Cao, A., et al. (1981) Genetic and molecular diversity in nondeletion HbH disease. *Proc. Natl. Acad. Sci. USA* **78,** 5833–5837.
5. Winichagoon, P., Higgs, D. R., Goodbourn, S. E. Y., Clegg, J. B., Weatherall, D. J., and Wasi, P. (1984) The molecular basis of α-thalassaemia in Thailand. *EMBO J.* **3,** 1813–1818.
6. Vandenplas, S., Higgs, D. R., Nicholls, R. D., Bester, A. J., and Mathew, C. G. P. (1987) Characterization of a new α^0 thalassaemia defect in the South African population. *Br. J. Haematol.* **66,** 539–542.
7. Higgs, D. R., Ayyub, H., Clegg, J. B., Hill, A. V. S., Nicholls, R. D., Teal, H., et al. (1985) α-Thalassaemia in British people. *Br. Med. J.* **290,** 1303–1306.
8. Fischel-Ghodsian, N., Vickers, M. A., Seip, M., Winichagoon, P., and Higgs, D. R. (1988) Characterization of two deletions that remove the entire human ζ-α globin gene complex (--^{THAI} and --^{FIL}). *Br. J. Haematol.* **70,** 233–238.
9. Faa, V., Rosatelli, M. C., Sardu, R., Meloni, A., Toffoli, C., and Cao, A. (1992) A simple electrophoretic procedure for fetal diagnosis of β-thalassaemia due to short deletions. *Prenat. Diag.* **12,** 903–908.
10. Craig, J. E., Barnetson, R. A., Prior, J., Raven, J. L., and Thein, S. L. (1994) Rapid detection of deletions causing δβ thalassemia and hereditary persistence of fetal hemoglobin by enzymatic amplification. *Blood* **83,** 1673–1682.

11. Ristaldi, M. S., Pirastu, M., Rosatelli, C., and Cao, A. (1989) Prenatal diagnosis of β-thalassaemia in Mediterranean populations by dot blot analysis with DNA amplification and allele specific oligonucleotide probes. *Prenat. Diag.* **9,** 629–638.

12. Old, J. M., Varawalla, N. Y., and Weatherall, D. J. (1990) The rapid detection and prenatal diagnosis of β thalassaemia in the Asian Indian and Cypriot populations in the UK. *Lancet* **336,** 834–837.

13. Varawalla, N., Old, J. M., and Fitches, A. C. (1992) Analysis of β-globin gene haplotypes in Asian Indians: Origin and spread of β-thalassaemia on the Indian subcontinent. *Hum. Genet.* **90,** 443–449.

14. Newton, C. R., Graham, A., and Heptinstall, L. E. (1989) Analysis of any point mutation in DNA. The amplification refractory mutation system (ARMS). *Nucl. Acids Res.* **17,** 2503–2516.

15. Kwok, S., Kellogg, D. E., McKinney, N., Spasic, D., Goda, L., Levenson, C., et al. (1990) Effects of primer-template mismatches on the polymerase chain reaction: human immunodeficiency virus type I model studies. *Nucl. Acids Res.* **18,** 999–1005.

16. Varawalla, N. Y., Old, J. M., Sarkar, R., Venkatesan, R., and Weatherall, D. J. (1991) The spectrum of β thalassemia mutations on the Indian subcontinent: the basis for prenatal diagnosis. *Br. J. Haematol.* **78,** 242–247.

10

Automated Genotyping in Diagnosis

Jayne S. Noble, Kim J. Leach, Lucy A. Ellis,
and Graham R. Taylor

1. Introduction

At present automated genotyping in diagnosis involves the detection, digitization, and analysis of labeled DNA using computer software. This chapter describes the use of the Applied Biosystems (Foster City, CA) 373 DNA Sequencer and Genescan 672 software for sizing fluorescently labeled PCR products in a diagnostic molecular genetics laboratory. The Applied Biosystems Genotyper software is not covered since this is not used at present in this laboratory. An outline of the steps involved in automated genotyping, from polymerase chain reaction (PCR) to archiving data, is shown in Fig. 1.

Fluorescently labeled PCR products and size standards are electrophoresed in the same lane through denaturing polyacrylamide gels in the electrophoresis chamber of the 373 DNA Sequencer. An argon ion laser sited a defined distance from the origin of electrophoresis scans the width of the gel. When the fluorescently labeled fragments migrate through the path of the laser, fluorescence is emitted. The fluorescence is refocused onto a photomultiplier tube and the information is digitized and presented for analysis with the 672 software. The emitted fluorescence is detected in 4-wavelength bands for each of two filter sets. Four dyes therefore are detected per lane. One dye is reserved for the size standard, leaving three dyes for the detection and analysis of PCR products. A computer software algorithm creates a calibration curve for the size standard and the PCR products are compared with, and hence sized against, the curve created for each lane.

Two advantages arising from the detection of four dyes per lane are the use of internal lane standards, and the potential for high order multiplexing resulting in high throughput. With the use of internal lane standards, the sample and

From: *Methods in Molecular Medicine: Molecular Diagnosis of Genetic Diseases*
Edited by: R. Elles Humana Press Inc., Totowa, NJ

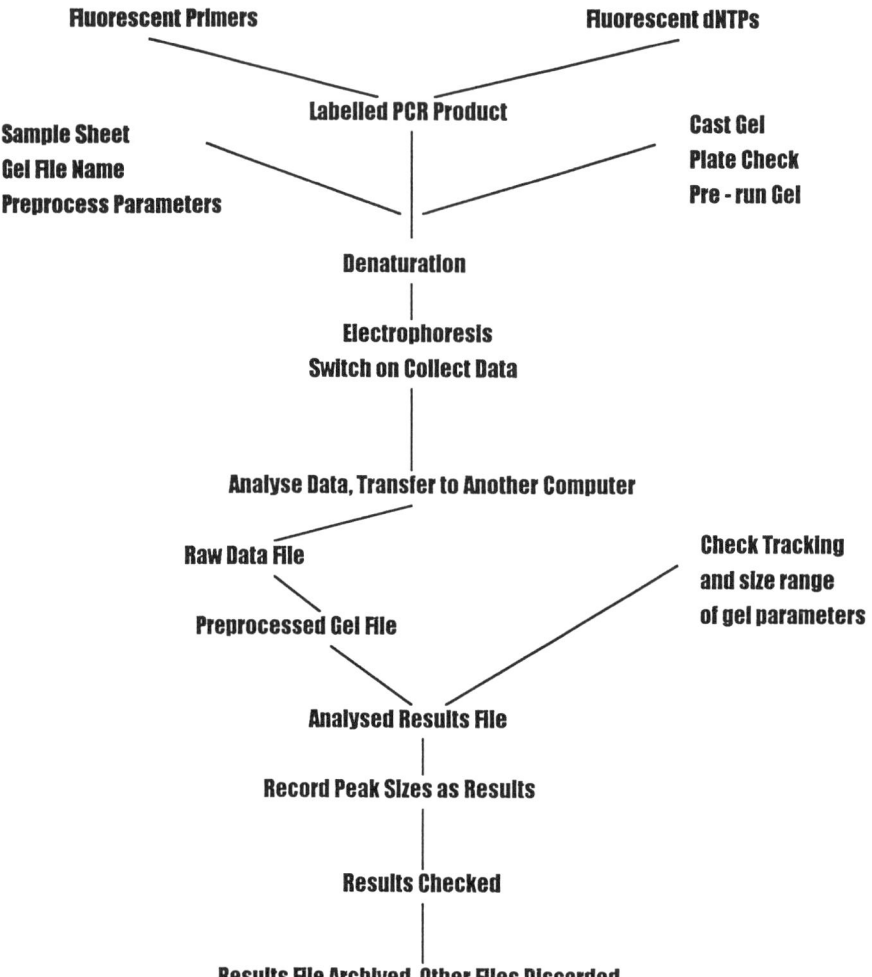

Fig. 1. Overview of the procedure. Labeled PCR products are produced by either incorporation of fluorescent dNTPs or labeled primers. A polyacrylamide gel is cast, scanned, and prerun, and the Genescan collection and analysis files are set up. The PCR products are mixed with a size standard, denatured, and loaded onto the prerun gel. After electrophoresis the collected data is transferred to another Macintosh for analysis. A results file is generated and the PCR products are scored and checked. The results file is then archived.

the standard experience the same electrophoretic environment removing any problems arising from lane to lane and gel to gel variation in mobility. The potential for multiplexing is greater than that for radioactive detection. Different sized products for each dye can be multiplexed and in addition products of similar sizes can also be multiplexed if they are labeled with different dyes. The highest order of multiplexing so far in this laboratory has been of seven microsatellites from within the dystrophin locus.

Further advantages of the system include the elimination of the use of radio-isotopes and the speed at which results can be obtained; less than 4 h compared with at least 16 h for radioactive detection. In addition, since all the products migrate the same distance (i.e., to the laser) before detection, they are all resolved to the same extent so some of the problems associated with reading the larger microsatellites present in a radiolabeled multiplex are reduced.

2. Materials
2.1. PCR

1. *Taq* DNA polymerase (Stratech Scientific, Luton, UK): Store at –20°C.
2. 1X *Taq* DNA polymerase reaction buffer: 10 mM Tris-HCl, pH 9.0, 50 mM KCl, 1.5 mM MgCl$_2$, 0.1% Triton-X 100: A 10X stock is prepared and stored in aliquots at –20°C.
3. dNTP mixture (Pharmacia, Uppsala, Sweden): A 100X stock solution of 20 mM each of dATP, dCTP, dGTP, and dTTP is prepared and stored in aliquots at –20°C.
4. Low G dNTPs (Pharmacia): A 100X stock of solution of 20 mM each of dATP, dCTP, and dTTP and 5 mM dGTP is prepared and stored at –20°C.
5. 7-deaza-2'-dGTP (Pharmacia): Store as supplied, 5 mM (30X stock) at –20°C.
6. Dimethyl sulfoxide (DMSO) (Sigma, St. Louis, MO).
7. Oligonucleotide primers (*see* Section 3.1.1.).
8. Formamide stop solution and gel loader: 0.25 g dextran blue in 250 mL formamide. Deionize and store in aliquots at –20°C.

2.2. Gel Running and Data Analysis

1. Alconex detergent (Aldrich, Milwaukee, WI): Dissolve 5 g in approx 4 L of hot water.
2. 6% Denaturing acrylamide sequencing gel solution (Severn Biotech, Malvern, UK): Store at room temperature in the dark. (Note: Neurotoxin.)
3. TEMED (N,N,N',N'-tetramethylethylenediamine) (BioRad, Hercules, CA): Store at room temperature in the dark.
4. 10% (w/v) Ammonium persulfate (Sigma).
5. 1X TBE buffer: 0.045M Tris-borate, 0.001M EDTA. A 5X stock is prepared and stored at room temperature.
6. Size standards: Genescan-2500 ROX, 2500 TAMRA, 350 ROX, and 350 TAMRA (Applied Biosystems) (*see* Note 1). Store at 4°C.
7. Microcapillary flat tip pipet tips (Sigma).
8. Applied Biosystems 373 DNA Sequencer and Genescan 672 software (Applied Biosystems).
9. Apple Macintosh IIci connected to the 373 DNA Sequencer.
10. Networked Apple Macs for data analysis (*see* Note 2).

2.3. Fluorescent ARMS Assay

Primers: Common primer: 5' GGA CAG AGA CAT ACA TTT CTA TC 3'. Variant primer: 5' FAM-CTT GCT TTC TGA TAT AAT TTG TTT 3'. Wildtype primer: 5' JOE-CTT GCT TTC TGA TAT AAT TTG TTC 3'.

2.4. MutEx Assay

1. Centricon 100 filters (Amicon, Danvers, MA).
2. 1X Exonuclease buffer: 50 mM Tris-HCl, pH 7.6, 7 mM MgCl$_2$, 5 mM DTT. Store at –20°C.
3. MutS protein (United States Biochemicals, Cleveland, OH). Store in aliquots at –80°C. (MutS loses 80% of its activity after two freeze–thaw cycles).
4. T7 DNA polymerase (New England Biolabs, Beverly, MA). Store at –20°C.

2.5. Safety

Consider the following hazards when running gels on the 373 DNA Sequencer.

1. Electrical shock hazard: The 373 DNA Sequencer contains a high voltage power supply. The instrument is designed so that the power supply is disconnected when the door is open. Follow operating procedures as outlined in the user's manual.
2. Laser hazard: The 373 DNA Sequencer contains a laser. Follow operating procedures as outlined in the user's manual to prevent physical harm from radiation exposure.
3. Chemical hazards: Some of the chemicals used with the instrument are hazardous (for example, acrylamide is a neurotoxin). Follow all safety procedures as outlined in the manufacturer's instructions and local rules regarding the use and disposal of such chemicals.

3. Methods

3.1. Labeling Methods

There are several possible ways in which PCR products can be made to fluoresce: using intercalating dyes (ethidium bromide, Yo-Yo, and To-To, Molecular Probes Inc., Eugene, OR), incorporation of fluorescent dNTPs or by the use of labeled primers. Intercalating dyes are not effective in high resolution denaturing conditions and are not discussed further.

3.1.1. Labeled Primers

In spite of their cost disadvantage, fluorescently labeled primers give the best resolution and are easy to use. In addition the option of multiplexing different colors can increase efficiency, offsetting the cost of primer synthesis.

Two sets of primer label are available from Applied Biosystems, using filter set A or B. The original set comprises FAM, JOE, TAMRA, and ROX, seen as blue, green, yellow, and red, respectively, on filter set A. These dyes were coupled to oligonucleotides by an aminolink and required extensive purification, with consequent loss of yield. A second set of labels comprises of 6-FAM, TET, HEX, and TAMRA, which are seen as blue, green, yellow, and red, respectively, on filter set B. 6-FAM, TET, and HEX are each available as amidites and can be attached to the oligonucleotide during synthesis. 6-FAM and FAM can each be detected as blue with filter set A or B, and HEX and JOE have similar fluorescent properties appearing as green on filter set A and yellow on filter set B. The advantages of the amidite dyes is that primers can be used straight off the column following ethanol precipitation, provided high efficiency synthesis was achieved during synthesis. We have successfully carried out multiplex PCR amplifications using ethanol-purified eluate. If necessary further purification can be achieved using an oligonucleotide purification cartridge (Applied Biosystems) or by reverse phase HPLC, but each method loses over 50% of the product.

Fluorescent dyes are unstable in ammonia and should be stored either frozen, as solid, or in 50% glycerol at –20°C. We have maintained stocks of pooled primers (approx 20 pmol/µL of each primer) for multiplex PCR in 50% glycerol for over 12 mo at –20°C. Labeled primers are used in 10-µL reactions at concentrations of between 2.5 and 10 pmol.

3.1.2. Incorporation of Labeled dNTPs

Incorporation of fluorescent dNTPs has the advantage that existing primers can be used. Labeling by incorporation may become the method of choice when very high resolution is not essential. Fluorescein- and rhodamine-labeled dUTP are available from Amersham. Applied Biosystems are developing fluorescently labeled dNTPs for detection of allele expansions by PCR, since the reduced efficiency by which larger alleles are amplified will be compensated by increased levels of incorporation in the expanded alleles.

3.2. PCR

3.2.1. Basic PCR

The essential differences between PCR for fluorescent detection and PCR for radioactive detection are that less primer and fewer cycles are used for fluorescent detection. This has the advantages of faster reaction times and reduced cost.

1. PCR is carried out in a total reaction volume of 10 µL with 2.5–10 pmol of each primer, 1X *Taq* reaction buffer, 200 µM dNTPs, 0.25 U of *Taq* DNA polymerase, and 100 ng of DNA. One of the primers has a fluorescent dye attached to the 5' end (*see* Section 3.1.1.), and the other primer is unlabeled. Hot start PCR *(1)* is always used and between 22 and 25 amplification cycles are carried out.
2. When the reaction is complete an equal volume (10 µL) of formamide-loading buffer is added and the products are either stored at –20°C or used immediately (*see* Note 3).

3.2.2. Multiplex PCR of Microsatellites

For PCR of microsatellites a two-step reaction is used where the annealing and extension steps are carried out at the same temperature *(2)*. To optimize PCR for the multiplex of microsatellites:

1. Various annealing/extension temperatures are tried and the temperature at which all the microsatellites amplify sufficiently is chosen.
2. Initially the same concentration of each primer is used. The concentration of the primers then is adjusted so that the peak heights of the PCR products for each primer pair are of similar intensities (*see* Note 4).

3.2.3 PCR of Trinucleotide Repeats

For the amplification of the trinucleotide repeats associated with fragile X syndrome, myotonic dystrophy, and Huntington's disease (HD), the following modifications to the PCR conditions are made (*see* Note 5).

1. DMSO is added to the reaction buffer to a final concentration of 10% (v/v).
2. Low G dNTPs and 7-deaza-2'-dGTP are added to the reaction mixture instead of the standard dNTP mix for amplification of the trinucleotide repeats associated with fragile X syndrome and HD.
3. A 10-min denaturation step before the start of the cycles is used for amplification of the trinucleotide repeats associated with fragile X syndrome and HD.

3.3. Plate Cleaning and Gel Casting

Plate cleaning and gel casting is carried out as described in the user's manual. It is essential that the plates are as clean as possible; any particles (dust, acrylamide, grease) that may fluoresce must be removed (*see* Note 6). Three different sizes of glass plates, 6-, 12-, and 24-cm well-to-read lengths and two sizes of comb, 24 or 36 wells, are available for use (*see* Note 7). Approximately 35 mL of 6% acrylamide gel solution with 250 μL of 10% APS and 25 μL of TEMED are used for a 12-cm well-to-read gel (*see* Note 8). The gel can be used 1 h after casting.

3.4. Gel Running

3.4.1. Setting Up the Genescan Collection and Analysis Software

The Genescan 672 software is divided into two programs, Genescan (GS) Collection and Genescan (GS) Analysis. The two programs are linked by the name of the run. The former is responsible for collecting data generated during a run, this information is stored in a raw gel file. For each run, GS Analysis is set up to process the data from that particular gel, which is then transferred into a gel file and, on further analysis a results file is created.

The computer linked to the 373 DNA Sequencer can be programed to automatically open the GS Collection and Analysis files on startup (*see* Note 9).

Once these files are open the essential steps for collection are:

1. Name the collection file.
2. Set the run time.

The GS Analysis program initially preprocesses the raw gel data to produce a gel file that subsequently can be analyzed. The program launches automatically at the end of the run, therefore, the preprocess parameters have to be set up before the start of the run.

The essential steps are:

1. Set up and fill in the sample sheet.
2. Define the preprocessing parameters, including the matrix standards (*see* Section 3.4.2.).

All the above steps are carried out as described in the user's manual (*see* Note 10).

3.4.2. Matrix Standards

On preprocessing, 672 GS software converts fluorescent signals to different colored peak intensities by comparing the signals detected with Matrix standards (Applied Biosystems). Matrix standards are obtained by loading the 373 with standard reagents labeled with each of the different fluorochromes. The original dye-primer sequencing set of FAM, JOE, TAMRA, and ROX were the first dyes available and are used on early GS applications. They can be preprocessed using the instrument matrix standard (which was actually designed for sequencing) but ideally a matrix file should be set up for the GS rather than sequencing application. Newer primers usually will be made by the use of fluorescent amidites. These are currently available as 6-FAM, HEX, and TET.

3.4.2.1. DYE PRIMER MATRIX STANDARDS

These are FAM, JOE, TAMRA, and ROX and use filter wheel A. ROX usually is reserved for size standards.

1. Before use, heat the samples to 50°C for 10 min, mix well, and centrifuge briefly.
2. Mix 2.5 µL of matrix standard with 2.5 µL of formamide, denature at 90°C for 2 min, chill on ice, and load.
3. The matrix calculation is performed as an option on the 672 analysis program.

3.4.2.2. FLUORESCENT AMIDITE MATRIX STANDARDS

These are 6-FAM, TET, HEX, and TAMRA and use filter wheel B. TAMRA usually is reserved for size standards. Load and calculate as described (*see* Note 11).

3.4.3. Setting Up the 373

The electrophoresis parameters, including run time and the filter set corresponding to the dyes being used, must be selected prior to electrophoresis. These are selected as described in the user's manual.

3.4.4. Preparing the Gel for Loading

Once the gel has set, it can be placed in the 373 electrophoresis chamber and prepared for loading. This is carried out as described in the user's manual. The plates are scanned by the laser prior to loading to check that there are no signals produced by particles fluorescing on the plates or in the gel.

The steps are as follows:

1. Scan the plates.
2. Clean if required (*see* Note 12).
3. Assemble the buffer chambers, remove the comb, and add 1X TBE running buffer.
4. Prerun the gel for at least 10 min prior to loading (*see* Note 13).

3.4.5. Sample Preparation and Gel Loading

The samples are mixed with an internal lane standard prior to loading (*see* Note 1).

1. Mix 4 µL of PCR product containing loading buffer with 1 µL of standard.
2. Heat to 95°C for 2 min to denature.
3. Cool on ice.
4. Stop the prerun on the 373.
5. Flush the wells with running buffer.
6. Load 1.5 µL of denatured sample per well using a microcapillary flat tip pipet tip.
7. Start the run on the 373.
8. Start data collection on the Apple Macintosh.

3.5. Data Analysis

3.5.1. Creating the Results File

3.5.1.1. GEL ANALYSIS

The preprocessing that occurs immediately after a run automatically creates a gel file that, on subsequent analysis, allows the results file to be examined. Both these files are placed in a folder that is identified by the run name and date.

All the unprocessed information, received direct from the 373, is stored in a raw gel file. If necessary, this can be repreprocessed with newly defined preprocess parameters by double clicking the raw gel file. The gel file is then placed in a new folder of the same title appended with .1, .2, and so on for each new folder. This function allows alteration of the gel file, for example, to allow previously cut off size standards to be included in the analysis.

After preprocessing, an analysis control panel is displayed. Before analyzing the lanes on the gel check that:

1. The lanes are tracked correctly.
2. The size standards have been assigned correctly (if automatically defined).

Both these functions are made easier by adjusting the gel contrast (gel menu), which makes the red dye of the standards and the dyes of the PCR products easier to visualize. These are carried out as described in the user's manual.

We use the third-order least squares method to size PCR products, as previously described. This sizing method gives accurate and reproducible results; we have found that sizes are generally within 1 base for duplicates both within and between gels *(3)*. It is important to make sure that at least one standard band passes the laser after the largest PCR product to enable accurate size calculation.

3.5.1.2. Electrophoretogram Results

Once the lanes have been analyzed the electrophoretogram results can be examined and used to score peak sizes. Failure to size peaks is usually due to an anomaly in the size standards of that particular lane. This can be confirmed by selecting "define new" on the analysis panel and naming the lane in question. The values can be altered if necessary, for example:

1. If a split peak has occurred: The minor peak generated can be assigned as zero and this lane is then reanalyzed alone.
2. If a lane has a high background level for the red dye, creating false peaks in the size standards: The threshold level for recognition of this color can be increased in the "maximum peak heights per dye" section of the analysis parameters. Simply increase the value for red to above the default value of 50 (i.e., to 150–200) and reanalyze this lane alone.

3.5.1.3. Helpful Features

1. Electrophoretograms are automatically scaled to the size of the largest peak. The Data Scaling application in the "view" menu allows smaller peaks to be examined.
2. Peaks that are close together can be resolved using the Zoom application also in the "view" menu.
3. In order to compare lanes (e.g., to look for sample carryover) they can be superimposed. Altering the color of one of the lanes then allows easy visualization.

All of the preceding features are described in the user's manual.

3.5.1.4. Problems Encountered

1. Overloading or overamplification of samples: This may produce broad peaks that cannot be sized, because the program splits the broad peak into several peaks with different sizes. This problem can be overcome by diluting the sample (e.g., 1 in 5) in loading buffer. Overamplification also generates extra peaks in addition to the main product.

2. With the new dyes (6-FAM, TET, HEX, and TAMRA) TAMRA is reserved for size standards in most cases. When used as a primer label (coupled via an aminolink) we have found that it can be unstable and cause artifactual peaks. The effect can be reduced by ethanol precipitation of the primers leaving free TAMRA in solution. For this reason we prefer not to use TAMRA-labeled primers.

3. Some microsatellites (D15S113 [*see* Section 3.7.7.] and F8C IVS13 [*see* Section 3.7.6.]) have been found to be prone to a sizing artifact whereby PCR products differ by 1 base (Fig. 2). It is possible that this artifact is caused by the terminal transferase-like activity of *Taq* polymerase. This artifact makes allele assignment within families difficult and there is a danger that results could be misinterpreted because of it. If this occurs information is not used from the markers.

3.5.2. Scoring Results, Checking Procedures, and Quality Control

The operator who has set up the run reads the result initially (*see* Note 14). The scoring of the alleles is then checked independently. The following factors are taken into account for both scoring and checking.

1. Peak height: A minimum peak height of 50 is used. If the peak height is low (50–150) the electrophoretograms from the two neighboring lanes are taken into consideration to exclude the possibility of lane-to-lane contamination. If the peak height of the majority of the samples on the gel is high (3000–4000) the samples with low peak heights (50–150) are repeated.

2. Negative control: If there is slight contamination of the negative control the peak height of the preceding lane is taken into consideration (*see* Note 15).

3. Other controls: For example, a delta F508 heterozygote control is included for each delta F508 PCR.

4. Sample information: The names on the lane and on the PCR worksheet are cross-checked to ensure the correct result is recorded on the PCR worksheet.

3.5.3. Archiving Data

Once all the analysis is complete (including the checking of results) a file is prepared for storage on an optical disc. The raw gel file, sample sheet, and processed gel file are deleted and the results file is archived so that a record of the results is always available from any run.

3.6. Detection of Mutations

Detection of mutations is becoming an essential part of the core work of Clinical Molecular Genetics. Many of the popular methods (SSCP, DGGE, chemical cleavage of mismatches) have been adapted for fluorescent analysis. Of these, probably chemical cleavage has produced the most impressive results so far, since both strands can be labeled and essentially all mutations should be revealed *(4)*. Nevertheless, the method is labor intensive and uses toxic chemicals. We have developed a technique that should give analogous results, using enzymatic procedures (*see* Section 3.6.2.) *(5)*. For easy detection of known mutations, we have used competitive priming using differentially labeled primers.

3.6.1. Fluorescent Detection of Known Mutations
Using Competitive Hybridization and Priming (Fluorescent ARMS)

The ARMS technique *(6)* in its usual format requires two sets of tubes to monitor amplification using primers designed to detect wild-type and mutant sequences (*see* Chapter 5).

Designing reliable primers and optimizing conditions can be difficult for conventional ARMS tests. By including both wild-type and mutant primers labeled with different fluorochromes in the same reaction, the test becomes much more robust. This is presumably because the primers compete with each other not only at the primer extension step, but also at the hybridization step. The increase in specificity is so marked that the usual strategy of deliberately mismatching the 3' position is not essential. The method described here was adapted to detect a sequence polymorphism in human hMSH2 *(7)*.

1. Carry out PCR in a total reaction volume of 20 μL with 10 pmol of all three primers, 1X *Taq* reaction buffer, 200 μM dNTPs, 1.25 U *Taq* DNA polymerase (essential to have no 3'–5' proofreading activity), and 50 ng of DNA.
2. Use hot start PCR and set the annealing and extension steps to the same temperature.

A single peak is seen at 285 bases (Fig. 3); either green for wild-type or blue and green for variant/wild-type heterozygotes. Variant homozygotes (so far not seen) would appear as blue peaks only.

3.6.2. Detection of Unknown Mutations Using the MutEx Assay

The MutS-Exonuclease (MutEx) assay depends on the ability of the mismatch binding protein that attaches to heteroduplex molecules at the site of mismatches (point mutation or 1–4 base insertion/deletions) and protects the molecule from processive exonuclease attack *(5)*.

1. Conduct PCR as normal and check for the presence of a product using agarose gel electrophoresis.
2. Exchange the PCR buffer including dNTPs for exonuclease buffer by centrifugal dialysis (Centricon 100).
3. Form heteroduplexes by heating to 95°C then cooling to 65°C at 1°C every 40 s.
4. Add 4 pmol (5 μL) MutS to 2 pmol of heteroduplex DNA on ice in a final volume of 12 μL. The magnesium concentration is adjusted to 8 m*M*.
5. After 15–60 min on ice add 10–15 U of T7 DNA polymerase and leave the tubes on ice for a further 1 min.
6. Transfer the tubes to a 37°C water bath for 3 min.
7. Add an equal volume of formamide loading buffer and store the samples either at –20°C or denature and load immediately onto a gel as described previously.

The results show clear peaks corresponding to within 20 bases of the mutation with low background.

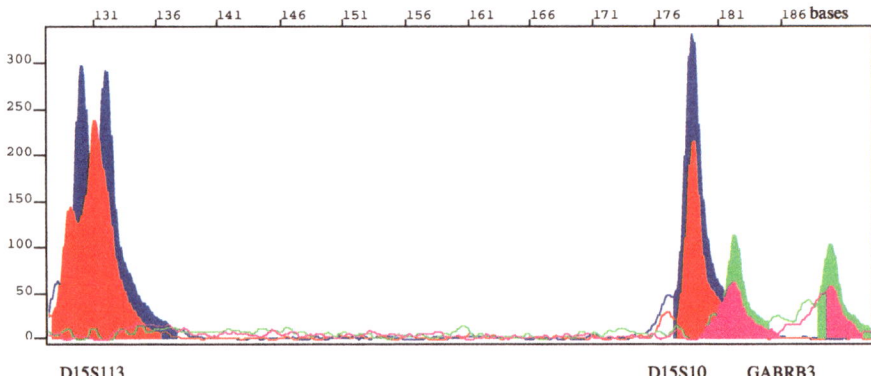

Fig. 2. Electrophoretogram of the sizing artifact observed with D15S113. The PCR products from separate amplifications of one individual have been superimposed. The red and pink peaks are from one amplification and the blue and green peaks are from the other. The PCR products from D15S10 and GABRB3 are identical in size and superimpose exactly. The PCR products from D15S113 are not identical in size and do not superimpose exactly; the alleles vary in size by 1 base.

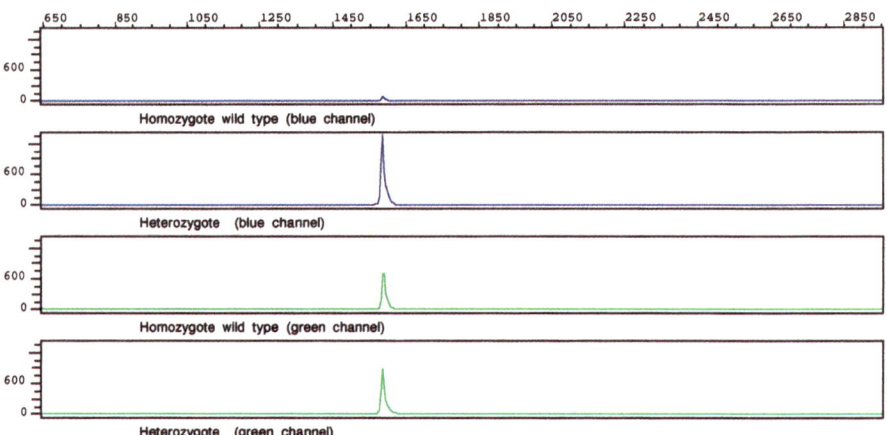

Fig. 3. Electrophoretograms of PCR products obtained with Fluorescent ARMS. A single peak (285 bases) is seen in the green channel only for homozygote wild-type and a single peak (285 bases) is seen in both the blue and the green channels for variant/wild-type heterozygote.

3.7. Applications: The Use of the 373 DNA Sequencer and Genescan 672 Software in the Diagnostic Molecular Genetics Laboratory

The use of the 373 DNA Sequencer and GS 672 software in the diagnostic molecular genetics laboratory allows for rapid automated genotyping. Two approaches are used routinely:

1. The detection of known mutations (deletions, trinucleotide repeat expansions).
2. Linkage analysis using highly polymorphic microsatellites markers *(8)*.

Protocols for the diagnosis of cystic fibrosis, Duchenne muscular dystrophy, myotonic dystrophy, fragile X syndrome, HD, Hemophilia A, Prader-Willi syndrome, Angelman syndrome, familial adenomatous polyposis, and familial breast/ovarian cancer have been developed. A protocol has also been established for identity testing.

3.7.1. Cystic Fibrosis

A multiplex reaction is used which contains primers for the region spanning the delta F508 deletion in exon 10 of the cystic fibrosis transmembrane regulator (CFTR) gene *(9)* and the intron 8 *(10)* and intron 17 b microsatellites *(11)* (Fig. 4). The microsatellites are useful for linkage analysis if delta F508 is not the mutation present in the family.

3.7.2. Duchenne Muscular Dystrophy

A multiplex reaction is used that contains primers for microsatellites within and flanking the dystrophin gene. The microsatellites flanking the dystrophin gene are 3'CA, 5'DYS I, and 5'DYS II and the intragenic microsatellites are STR44, STR45, STR49, and STR50 (in introns 44, 45, 49, and 50, respectively) *(12–14)*. Microsatellites with PCR products of similar sizes are labeled with different dyes allowing unambiguous detection (Fig. 5). The microsatellites are used for prenatal diagnosis where no deletion is present in the family and for carrier detection by linkage analysis. The intragenic microsatellites have proved to be useful for determining carrier status in at-risk females from either apparent noninheritance of alleles or heterozygosity at a deleted site previously characterized in the proband.

3.7.3. Myotonic Dystrophy

Primers to amplify the CTG triplet repeat present in the Myotonin gene are used *(15)*. Alleles within the unexpanded range and minimally expanded alleles are detected. Minimal expansions are less intense than unexpanded alleles and show stuttering (peaks 3 bases apart) of the repeated unit (Fig. 6). (Larger expansions are detected by Southern blotting.) PCR is used as a screen to identify most unaffected individuals (two unexpanded alleles) and only individuals with one unexpanded allele are analyzed with Southern blotting.

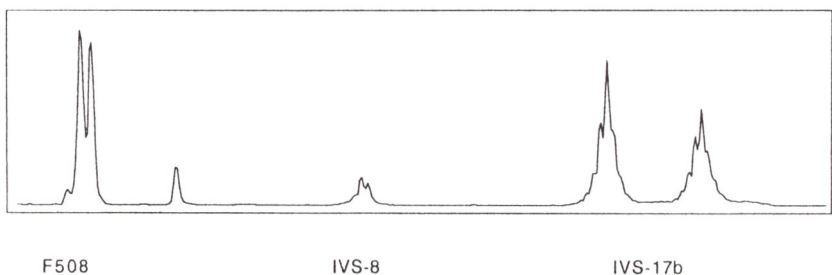

F508   IVS-8   IVS-17b

Fig. 4. Electrophoretogram of PCR products from the CFTR multiplex. The individual is heterozygous for the delta F508 deletion (96 and 99 bases) and heterozygous for alleles of the IVS-8 and IVS-17b microsatellites.

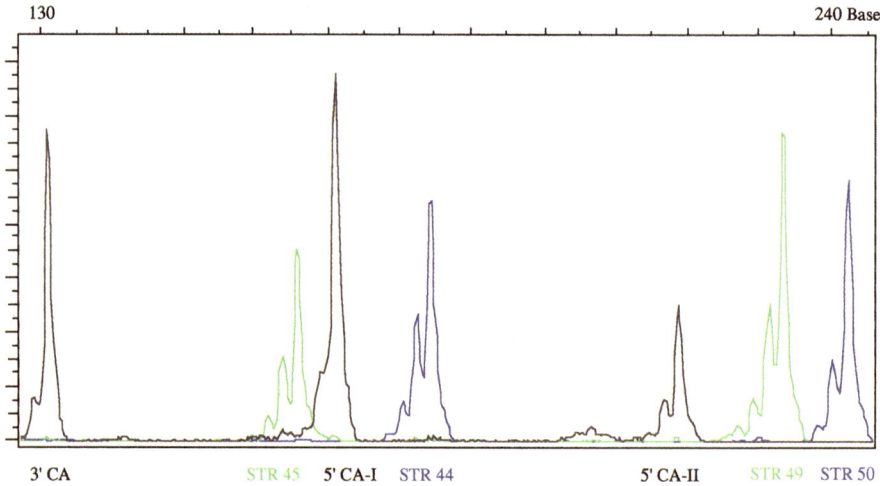

Fig. 5. Electrophoretograms of PCR products from the DMD microsatellite multiplex. The electrophoretograms obtained from each channel have been superimposed. The blue channel shows the alleles from STR44 and STR50, the green channel alleles from STR45 and STR49 and the yellow channel alleles from the flanking markers 3'CA, 5'DYSI, and 5'DYSII.

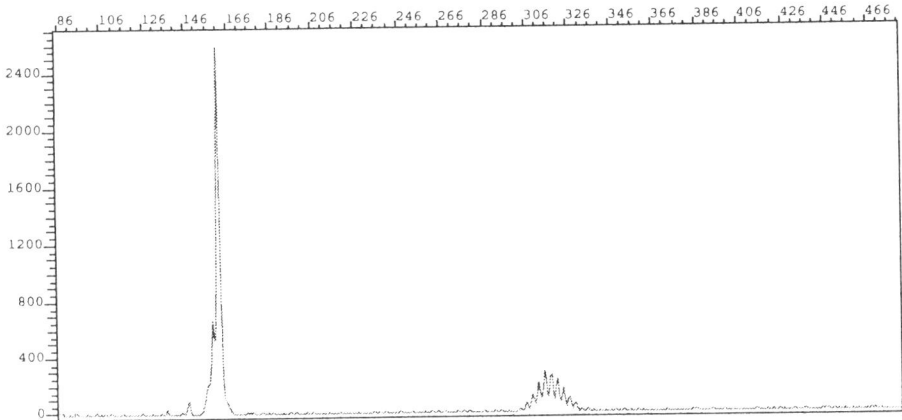

Fig. 6. Electrophoretogram of PCR products from the CTG repeat present in the Myotonin gene. The first peak is from an unexpanded allele (about 17 repeats) and the second peak is from an expanded allele (about 68 repeats). The expanded allele is less intense than the unexpanded allele and shows stuttering, with peaks 3 bases apart, of the repeated unit.

3.7.4. Fragile X Syndrome

Primers to amplify the CGG triplet repeat associated with the fragile X syndrome are used *(16)*. Alleles within the normal range, 6–56 repeats, are detected. Expanded alleles above approx 70 repeats will not be detected and Southern analysis is used to detect these. As with myotonic dystrophy, PCR is used to screen out most unaffected individuals (one unexpanded allele in males and two in females) prior to Southern analysis.

3.7.5. Huntington Disease

Primers to amplify the CAG triplet repeat present in the HD gene are used *(17)*. Both unexpanded and expanded alleles are detected (the expansions are smaller than those associated with myotonic dystrophy and fragile X syndrome) and PCR is used for confirmation of diagnosis and predictive testing.

3.7.6. Hemophilia A

Primers to amplify the microsatellite present in intron 13 of the factor VIII gene are used for carrier detection by linkage analysis *(18)*.

3.7.7. Prader-Willi and Angelman Syndrome

A multiplex reaction is used to amplify five microsatellites that span the region of chromosome 15, 15ql 1-13, where the loci for these two disorders lie. The markers are D15S113, D15S10, D15S11, GABRB3, and GABRA5 *(19–23)*. Haplotype construction in the affected individual and their parents can allow the detection of deletions and uniparental disomy.

3.7.8. Familial Adenomatous Polyposis

A multiplex reaction is used to amplify four microsatellites CB83, CB26, DP1, and MCC *(24–27)*. High-risk haplotypes can be established within families allowing predictive tests for at-risk family members.

3.7.9. Familial Breast/Ovarian Cancer

Primers for three microsatellites THRA1, D17S857, and D17S579 that are in the region of chromosome 17q where the BRCA1 gene is located are used *(28–30)*. These primers are not multiplexed as they amplify under different conditions. High-risk haplotypes can be established within families allowing predictive tests for at-risk family members.

3.7.10. Identity Testing

A multiplex reaction has been designed for use in cases when inheritance or sample mix-up is being queried. The multiplex consists of five primer pairs that amplify D21S11, D13S308, AMGL, and MBP on chromosome 18 *(31–34)*. The AMGL marker is used to confirm the sex of the sample. The other highly polymorphic markers are used to clarify the identity of the sample. These markers are trinucleotide and tetranucleotide repeats (*see* Note 16).

4. Notes

1. The Genescan-2500 ROX and Genescan-2500 TAMRA standards are used routinely. These have been developed for use with 6% denaturing polyacrylamide gels and detect products in the range 50–500 bases. Further standards are also available; the Genescan-350 ROX and 350 TAMRA standards have been used recently. These standards contain fragments ranging in size from 50–350 bases and are useful for detecting shorter PCR products, for example, the delta F508 deletion. In addition, the use of a standard with the largest fragment of 350 bases allows the option of reusing the polyacrylamide gel once the largest fragment has migrated past the laser. The choice of standard depends on the fluorescent dyes used in the PCR and the size of the PCR products. In addition sufficient points are needed on the calibration curve for accurate sizing; at least one point above the size of the largest product to be detected is necessary. We have found that third order least squares approximation for calculating the standard curve works adequately. Mix the standards thoroughly before use.

2. In order to fully support the Genescan software and analyze all the data generated, we found that an additional Macintosh Quadra computer was necessary, along with a color printer and read/write optical disk drive for archiving data. More recently, a third Quadra has been added to the network, with all the computers linked up by ethernet for rapid transfer. Potential users are advised to discuss computer options with Applied Biosystems, since the product range of both Applied Biosystems and Apple Computers are subject to frequent changes.

3. We have stored PCR products in loading buffer at –20°C for up to 2 wk with no effect on stability. However, PCR products mixed with size standards are not stored at –20°C.

4. In a multiplex reaction some PCRs are intrinsically less efficient than others in reaction conditions that are suboptimal for some primer pairs.

5. The trinucleotide repeats associated with these conditions are G-C rich. This affects the efficiency of the PCR owing to secondary structure of the DNA fragments. Reagents which reduce the effect of the secondary structure such as DMSO and 7-deaza dGTP are therefore added to the reaction mixture. We have found that the DNA must be in solution and samples are occasionally heated to 55°C prior to amplification if a result is urgently needed.

6. When the plates are submerged in the Alconex solution, gently rubbing the surface of the plates with the fingertips is enough to dislodge any grease. To speed up plate drying, a hairdryer can be used. Tape the plates together so that the same sides of the plates are always on the inside.

7. The well-to-read length (the distance the fragment migrates before being detected by the laser) can be varied to suit the resolution desired. A 6-cm well-to-read length will give 2 base resolution in 1.5 h and a 24-cm well-to-read length will give 1 base resolution in 5 h. A well-to-read length of 12 cm was found to be adequate for most applications, including microsatellites and trinucleotide repeats. The optimal run time should also be taken into consideration. The use of the 12-cm well-to-read plates allows up to three runs per day. We have found that by using a 36-well comb several PCR reactions can be run on the same gel; that is, diseases can be batched together.

8. Any air bubbles in the gel can be allowed to rise to the surface of the gel by holding the gel in a vertical position. They can also easily be removed using a "bubble-getter" (Promega, Madison, WI) or by gently tapping the gel plates. Drawing the gel solution into a 30-mL syringe and injecting it between the plates allows more even casting and prevents overflow.

9. The GS Collection and Analysis files both have alias files. By dragging these files into the start-up alias icon they are both automatically opened when the computer is switched on and the GS Collection tiles for map, scan, and gel are displayed.

10. The GS quick reference card is very useful when setting up the Collection and Analysis programs

11. JOE and HEX have similar fluorescent characteristics, and can be interchanged provided that very accurate quantitation is not essential. They appear as green on filter set A and yellow on filter set B. FAM and 6-FAM are also similar, both appear as blue on filter A or B.

12. Scan the plates prior to adding the running buffer to the buffer chambers so they can be easily removed if necessary. If the plates are dirty the easiest way to clean them is to wipe across the region that is scanned by the laser with laboratory tissue moistened with distilled water. Start in the middle of the plate and wipe toward the edges. If this does not remove the dirt take the plates out of the 373 and wash the outer surface with running tap water, rinse with distilled water, and dry. Repeat the plate check.

13. With practice, loading the gel is relatively easy, however, it can be difficult to see the wells. Loading buffer can be run into the gel wells prior to prerunning the gel. This makes the wells much easier to see for sample loading.

14. We have found that this is best done by showing the desired electrophoretogram and selecting with the mouse the peak being scored. The size of the peak is highlighted in the table and this data can then be recorded on the worksheet. The average of the duplicates is taken and recorded. (The size is given in bases but we actually record the result as basepairs.) Printing the data for each electrophoretogram proved uneconomical with respect to the amount of paper used and also, "eyeballing" the size of the peak, among all of the data in the table, was not always easy.

15. Contamination is generally carry over from loading of the previous lane. The negative control is accepted if the PCR products are identical to those in the preceding lane and if the peak height is <10% of that of the preceding lane.

16. Slippage synthesis of simple sequence DNA is a well-known phenomenon *(35)* and probably explains why microsatellites are polymorphic. PCR products are also subject to slippage synthesis during amplification which produces artifact (shadow) bands. For dinucleotide repeats these shadow bands produce a two-base ladder and with trinucleotide repeats a three-base ladder is seen. However, tetranucleotide repeats are far less prone to this artifact and almost no laddering is seen. Tetranucleotide STRs therefore are much more robust since not only is less laddering seen, but the alleles are separated by four bases instead of two and therefore are easier to resolve.

Acknowledgements

We thank Nigel Hall, Mark Robinson, Janet Hughes, and Virpi Laitinen for their valuable contributions to the work described here. We also thank Bob Mueller for his encouragement with this work.

The 373 DNA Sequencer was purchased through the kind generosity of the George John Livanos Charitable Trust.

References

1. Horton, R. M., Hoppe, B. L., and Conti-Tronconi, B. M. (1994) Ampligrease: hot start PCR using petroleum jelly. *BioTechniques* **16,** 42,43.
2. Noble, J. S., Taylor, G. R., Stewart, A. D., Mueller, R. F., and Murday, V. A. (1991) A rapid PCR-based method to distinguish between fetal and maternal cells in chorionic biopsies using microsatellite polymorphisms. *Dis. Markers* **9,** 301–306.
3. Taylor, G. R., Noble, J. S., and Mueller, R.. F. (1994) Automated analysis of multiplex microsatellites. *J. Med. Genet.,* **31,** 937–943.
4. Harris, I. I., Green, P. M., Bentley, D. R., and Giannelli, F. (1994) Mutation detection by fluorescent chemical cleavage: application to haemophilia B. *PCR Methods Applic.* **3,** 268–271.
5. Ellis, L. A., Taylor, G. R., Banks, R., and Baumberg, S. (1994) MutS binding protects heteroduplex DNA from exonuclease digestion *in vitro*: a simple method for detecting mutations. *Nucleic Acids Res.* **22,** 2710,2711.

6. Newton, C. R., Graham, A., Heptinstall, L. E., Powell, S. J., Summers, C., Kalsheker, N., Smith, J. C., and Markham, A. F. (1989) Analysis of any point mutation in DNA. The amplification refractory mutation system (ARMS). *Nucleic Acids Res.* **17,** 2503–2516.
7. Hall, N. R., Taylor, G. R., Finan, P. J., Kolodner, R. D., Bodmer, W. F., Cottrell, S. E., et al. (1994) Intron splice acceptor site sequence variation in the HNPCC gene hMSH2. *Eur. J. Cancer* **30A,** 1550–1552.
8. Weber, J. L. and May, P. E. (1989) Abundant class of DNA polymorphisms which can be typed using the polymerase chain reaction. *Am. J. Hum. Genet.* **44,** 388–396.
9. Taylor, G. R., Noble, J. S., Hall, J. L., Quirk, P., Stewart, A. D., and Mueller, R. F. (1989) Rapid screening for delta F508 in cystic fibrosis. *Lancet* **II,** 1345.
10. Estivill, X., Morral, N., Casala, T., and Nunes, V. (1991) Prenatal diagnosis of cystic fibrosis by multiplex PCR of mutation and microsatellites. *Lancet* **338,** 458.
11. Zielenski, J., Markiewicz, D., Rinisland, R., Rommens, J. M., and Tsui, L.-C. (1991) A cluster of highly polymorphic dinucleotide repeats in intron 17b of the CFTR gene. *Am. J. Hum. Genet.* **49,** 1256–1261.
12. Beggs, A. H. and Kunkel, L. M. (1990) A polymorphic CACA repeat in the 3' untranslated region of dystrophin. *Nucleic Acids Res.* **18,** 1931.
13. Feener, C. A., Boyce, F. M., and Kunkel, L. M. (1991) Rapid detection of CA polymorphisms in cloned DNA: application to the 5' region of the dystrophin gene. *Am. J. Hum. Genet.* **48,** 621–627.
14. Clemens, P. R., Fenwick, R. G., Chamberlain, J. S., Gibbs, R. A., deAndrade, M., Chakraborty, R., and Caskey, C. T. (1991) Carrier detection and prenatal diagnosis in Duchenne and Becker muscular dystrophy families, using dinucleotide repeat polymorphisms. *Am. J. Hum. Genet.* **49,** 951–961.
15. Brook, J. D., McCurrah, M. E., Harley, H. G., Buckler, A. J., Church, D., Aburatani, H., et al. (1992) Molecular basis of myotonic dystrophy: expansion of a trinucleotide (CTG) repeat at the 3' end of a transcript encoding a protein kinase family member. *Cell* **68,** 799–808.
16. Fu, Y-H., Kuhl, D. P. A., Pizzuti, A., Pieretti, M., Sutcliffe, J. S., Richards, S., et al. (1991) Variation of the CGG repeat at the Fragile X site results in genetic instability: resolution of the Sherman paradox. *Cell* **67,** 1047–1058.
17. The Huntington's Disease Collaborative Research Group (1993) A novel gene containing a trinucleotide repeat that is expanded and unstable on Huntington's disease chromosomes. *Cell* **72,** 971–983.
18. Lalloz, M. R. A., McVey, J. H., Pattinson, J. K., and Tuddenham, E. G. (1991) Haemophilia A diagnosis by analysis of a hypervariable dinucleotide repeat within the factor VIII gene. *Lancet* **338,** 207–211.
19. Mutirangura, A., Greenberg, F., Butler, M. G., Malcolm, S., Nicholls, R. D., Chakravarti, A., and Ledbetter, D. H. (1993) Molecular dissection of the Prader-Willi/Angelman syndrome region (15q11-13) by YAC cloning and FISH analysis. *Hum. Mol. Genet.* **1,** 417–425.
20. Lindeman, R., Kouts, S., Woodage, T., Smith, A., and Trent, R. J. (1991) Dinucleotide repeat polymorphism at D15S10 in the Prader-Willi chromosome region (PWCR). *Nucleic Acids Res.* **19,** 5449.

21. Mutirangura, A., Kuwano, A., Ledbetter, S. A., Chinault, A. C., and Ledbetter, D. H. (1992) Dinucleotide repeat polymorphism at the D15S11 locus in the Angelman/Prader-Willi region (AS/PWS) of chromosome 15. *Hum. Mol. Genet.* **1,** 139.

22. Mutirangura, A., Ledbetter, S., Kuwano, A., Chinault, A. C., and Ledbetter, D. H. (1992) Dinucleotide repeat polymorphism at the $GABA_A$ receptor β3 (GABRB3) locus in the Angelman/Prader-Willi region (AS/PWS) of chromosome 15. *Hum. Mol. Genet.* **1,** 67.

23. Glatt, K. A., Sinnett, D., and Lalande, M. (1992) Dinucleotide repeat polymorphism at the $GABA_A$ receptor α5 (GABRA5) locus at chromosome 15q11-q13. *Hum. Mol. Genet.* **1,** 348.

24. Breukel, C., Tops, C., van Leeuwen, C., van der Klift, H., Fodde, R., and Khan, M. P. (1991) AT repeat polymorphism at the D15S122 locus tightly linked to adenomatous polyposis coli (APC). *Nucleic Acids Res.* **19,** 6665.

25. van Leeuwen, C., Tops, C., Breukel, C., van der Klift, H., Fodde, R., and Khan, P. M. (1991) CA repeat polymorphism at the D15S299 locus linked to adenomatous polyposis coli (APC). *Nucleic Acids Res.* **19,** 5805.

26. Spirio, L., Joslyn, G., Nelson, L., Leppert, M., and White, R. (1991) A CA repeat 30–70 kb downstream from the adenomatous polyposis coli (APC) gene. *Nucleic Acids Res.* **19,** 6349.

27. van Leeuwen, C., Tops, C., Breukel, C., van der Klift, H., Deaven, L., Fodde, R., and Khan, P. M. (1991) CA repeat polymorphism within the MCC (mutated in colorectal cancer) gene. *Nucleic Acids Res.* **19,** 5805.

28. Bowcock, A. M., Anderson, L. A., Friedman, L. S., Black, D. M., Osbourne-Lawrence, S., Rowell, S. E., Hall, J. M., et al. (1993) THRA1 and D17S183 flank an interval of <4cM for the breast-ovarian cancer gene (BRCA1) on chromosome 17q21. *Am. J. Hum. Genet.* **52,** 718–722.

29. Anderson, L. A., Friedman, L., Osbourne-Lawrence, S., Lynch, E., Weissenbach, J., Bowcock, A., and King, M.-C. (1993) High-density genetic map of the BRCA1 region of chromosome 17q12-q21 *Genomics* **17,** 618–623.

30. Hall, J. M., Friedman, L., Guenther, C., Lee, M. K., Weber, J. L., Black, D. M., and King, M.-C. (1992) Closing in on a breast cancer gene on chromosome 17q. *Am. J. Hum. Genet.* **50,** 1235–1242.

31. Sharma, V. and Litt, M. (1992) Tetranucleotide repeat polymorphism at the D21S11 locus. *Hum. Mol. Genet.* **1,** 67.

32. Haddad, L. A. and Pena, S. D. J. (1993) CAT repeat polymorphism in a human expressed sequence tag (EST0044) (D13S308). *Hum. Mol. Genet.* **2,** 1748.

33. Sullivan, K. M., Mannucci, A., Kimpton, C. P., and Gill, P. (1993) A rapid and quantitative DNA sex test: fluorescence-based PCR analysis of X-Y homologous gene amelogenin. *BioTechniques* **15,** 636.

34. Polymeropoulos, M. H., Xiao, H., and Merril, C. R. (1992) Tetranucleotide repeat polymorphism at the human myelin basic protein gene (MBP). *Hum. Mol. Genet.* **1,** 658.

35. Schlotterer, C. and Tautz, D. (1992) Slippage synthesis of simple sequence DNA. *Nucleic Acids Res.* **20,** 211–215.

11

Genetic Counseling and Molecular Testing

Lauren Kerzin-Storrar

1. Introduction

The provision of genetic counseling should be an integral component to molecular diagnostic testing for two important reasons: The potential impact (medical and psychosocial) for the individual being tested and for their family is great *(1)* and ensuring informed choice is crucial as uptake of genetic testing varies between conditions and may be <10% *(2–4)*. Many people, once counseled, choose not to be tested, and this choice might be lost if counseling is not provided. Genetic counseling is comprehensive and includes:

1. Diagnosis and discussion of prognosis;
2. Explanation of the mode of inheritance and recurrence risks;
3. Discussion of options, including reproductive and testing;
4. Facilitating decision making; and
5. Support toward adjusting to the genetic implications.

Genetic counseling is usually provided by medically trained clinical geneticists together with nonmedical genetic counselors. In North America, most nonmedical genetic counselors have a masters degree in genetic counseling or nursing; in the United Kingdom most are specialist nurses without formal training, although there is now an MSc course in genetic counseling at the University of Manchester open to nursing and science graduates *(5,6)*. Genetic counseling services are organized on a regional basis in the United Kingdom where each Regional Genetic Service runs pediatric, adult, and reproductive clinics primarily for families at increased risk. However, screening at the population level now means that elements of genetic counseling are being provided in other specialty clinics, as well as in general practice and community-based centers *(7,8)*. In North America, regional services based in teaching hospitals

From: *Methods in Molecular Medicine: Molecular Diagnosis of Genetic Diseases*
Edited by: R. Elles Humana Press Inc., Totowa, NJ

are also common, although smaller hospitals and clinics may also provide a genetic counseling service, along with disease-specific clinics.

Advances in molecular technology, and the potential for diagnostic, predictive, carrier, and prenatal testing, has brought with it a large increase in workload for those providing genetic counseling, but has also reinforced the need for such counseling to be associated with the laboratory provision of a genetic test. It was probably fortunate that the first uses of molecular testing depended on linkage, as this necessitated close collaboration between those working in the laboratory and those in contact with the families, not only to clarify pedigrees and obtain appropriate blood samples, but also so that genetic counselors could develop techniques for explaining complex tests to families in a clear and effective way. Although mutation testing may be more straightforward in concept, there are still many advantages to retaining the model of Regional Genetic Services, which provide genetic counseling and laboratory services "under one roof." This is not always possible, for example, where a laboratory offers a supraregional service, or a single disease service where samples come from clinicians in many centers, however, at the very least, clinicians, genetic counselors, and clinical molecular geneticists need to talk to one another!

The implications and protocols for DNA-based testing differ according to the type of test, and this chapter, therefore, considers diagnostic, presymptomatic, carrier, and prenatal testing separately before addressing more general issues pertaining to genetic registers, ethical considerations, and the emotional impact for laboratory staff.

2. Diagnostic Testing

A diagnostic test is one which confirms that an affected individual is suffering from a named condition. This implies that the patient is showing symptoms, and the diagnostic test is often used to confirm a clinical diagnosis. In a clinical DNA laboratory, samples may be received on boys or men with muscular dystrophy, infants with cystic fibrosis, adults with Huntington's disease, and so on. In some instances the diagnosis may be firm before DNA testing, whereas in other instances the DNA test is being used to exclude one of several possible diagnoses.

Diagnostic samples will often be received from clinicians outside genetics, and indeed genetic counseling would not be appropriate if a genetic condition has not yet been confirmed. However, where a molecular diagnosis is then made, the laboratory report might include a statement indicating the genetic implications of the diagnosis with the suggestion of referral of family members for genetic counseling.

Although diagnostic samples are largely not problematic from the point of view of pre-test counseling, it is important that laboratory staff are happy that referring clinicians do clearly indicate that this is a genuine diagnostic request for an individual already showing symptoms to avoid mistakenly performing a presymptomatic test. Because of the serious implications of presymptomatic tests for Huntington's disease and other late onset neurological disorders (*see* Section 3.), some laboratories now require an accompanying consent form for Huntington's diagnostic tests, based on the form originally devised by the late Professor Harding at the Institute of Neurology, London (*see* Fig. 1).

3. Presymptomatic Testing

Molecular testing is a powerful tool for predicting the future health of an individual, a whole family, or potentially whole populations. Predicting illness in advance of symptoms is relatively new to medicine and little was known about the impact of this use of DNA technology. Concerns were therefore high, and most predictive test programs began as research projects where both pre-test counseling and assessment of long term sequelae has been incorporated into study design.

Uptake of presymptomatic testing is very low among those at risk of Huntington's disease *(2)*, but much higher for conditions such as adult polycystic kidney disease *(3,4)*, and familial adenomatous polyposis coli *(4)*. The important message is that many at-risk individuals prefer to remain at risk, and it is therefore imperative that a presymptomatic test is only performed after informed consent is obtained. Laboratories may assume that this has been dealt with by the referring clinician, but guidelines are often helpful.

Because of the concerns related to Huntington's disease (given its particular combination of distressing features and lack of effective treatment), national and international protocols *(9)* have been drawn up for predictive testing. These include the extent of pre- and post-test counseling, and a number of procedural assurances including completion of a consent form (Fig. 2). A particular point of relevance for laboratory staff is the arrangement for communicating results. An appointment for the results session is made when the blood sample is obtained. Because of the unacceptable distress caused in these highly emotive situations if results are not available for the designated appointment, both the laboratory staff and the genetic counselors should agree on a suitable time period. Laboratory staff should be informed of the result appointment date so that any problems encountered in obtaining a result can be communicated to clinical staff in advance of the appointment. The at-risk individual requesting the test is informed that they may change their mind right up until they arrive for their result, and it is therefore preferable that clinical staff in direct communication with the patient are not made aware of the result until just before they see the patient. This can be achieved by the report being issued in a sealed envelope, and laboratory staff respecting the need for discretion if a result is obtained well in advance of the result session.

CONSENT FORM

DIAGNOSTIC TESTING FOR THE HUNTINGTON'S DISEASE MUTATION

I understand that it is possible to have a test to see whether or not I/my relative have/has Huntington's disease, and I wish to proceed with this test.

I understand that the test will show one of the following:

1) That I/he/she do/does have this condition, and that my children may be at risk of carrying the abnormal gene

2) That I/he/she do/does not have/has HD

3) That the result is difficult to interpret

NAME (block capitals)..

ADDRESS ....

....

....

DATE ....   HOSPITAL NO ....

Signature of patient ....

Signature of spouse/partner ....(not essential but preferred if applicable)

OR Signature of next of kin ....
(if patient is unable to give informed consent)

For medical staff:

I have explained the principles and implications of HD testing to the above, as detailed in the supplied information sheet, and have sent a copy of this form to the DNA laboratory. I have reason to believe that he/she has HD, as opposed to being at risk with (or without) unrelated symptoms.

Signature ....

Name in capitals......................................

Fig. 1. Example of a consent form for use with diagnostic test requests.

PREDICTIVE TEST CONSENT FORM

I ....,

OF...

....

....

hereby consent to undergo presymptomatic testing for Huntington's disease. I wish
to be informed of the result of the test. I confirm that I discussed the implications of this
with .... and that the potential disadvantages of the test
have been explained to me.

I agree/do not agree for my family doctor (Dr ....) to be informed of
the result. I understand that the result of the test will not be conveyed to any other
person without my explicit permission.

Signed ....   Date ....

Fig. 2. Example of a consent form for predictive testing.

Whether the particular case of Huntington's disease can be extended to
presymptomatic testing for other conditions is currently being investigated in
studies looking at testing for familial adenomatous polyposis coli, dominant
breast and ovarian cancer, and other conditions. Although the potential for prevention and treatment of symptoms will influence recommendations made for
the appropriate use of presymptomatic tests, it is unlikely that any presymptomatic testing should be performed without some pre-test counseling, formal
consent, and arrangements for follow-up.

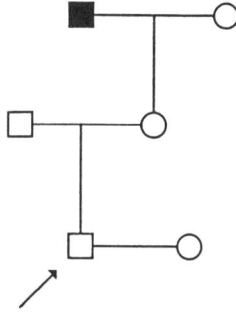

Fig. 3. Predictive test request for a dominant condition from an individual at <50% risk.

The particular problems that arise when presymptomatic testing is requested for individuals at <50% risk where there are living intervening relatives (*see* Fig. 3), or for children in late onset disorders, is discussed in the next section.

4. Carrier Testing

Testing for heterozygote carrier status for autosomal and X-linked recessive conditions is probably the most common type of request for molecular testing. Heterozygote carrier testing may be performed on:

1. Presumed obligate carriers (parents of a known affected child, usually with a view to prenatal diagnosis in future pregnancies);
2. Those at increased risk because of a family history (cascade screening);
3. Those at increased risk because of their ethnic background (targeted population screening); and
4. Those at no special risk (population screening).

Genetic counseling surrounding carrier tests will obviously vary according to which of these situations apply. Although identification of heterozygote carrier status does not usually have serious health implications, psychological sequelae to discovering that one carries an "abnormal" gene has been documented. Studies of carriers identified on population screening for the hemoglobinopathies *(8)*, Tay Sachs disease *(10,11)*, and cystic fibrosis *(7,12)* suggest that carrier status can affect psychological well-being; decisions regarding marriage and choice of partner; and stigmatization from noncarriers, insurance companies, and employers. Many of these adverse effects may be the result of poor understanding (both in carriers and in society) about the carrier state, and underline the importance of both pre- and post-test counseling.

Uptake of carrier testing for females in families with X-linked conditions is usually high, perhaps because of the significant implications for reproduction as well as the severity of many X-linked conditions (e.g., Duchenne muscular dystrophy, fragile-X, Menkes' disease, X-linked hydrocephalus), but is also high for less severe conditions where subsequent uptake of prenatal diagnosis is lower (e.g., Becker muscular dystrophy, hemophilia). Historically, molecular testing for many X-linked conditions has involved ongoing studies using new techniques as they develop particularly because of the complexities of identifying a heterozygote gene carrier. Continued testing after initial test results has important counseling implications. Does the woman know that further tests will be performed and that these may clarify the initial results, but may also change her situation significantly? The clinical laboratory should have an explicit understanding with clinical staff about whether ongoing tests should be automatically performed, or whether the patient should be contacted first. An ideal approach to this is the development of a Regional Genetic Register service where families are regularly reviewed by clinical and laboratory staff, and families expect regular updates on their situation *(13)* (*see* Section 7.).

5. Prenatal Testing

One of the aims of carrier, and to a lesser extent presymptomatic/diagnostic testing, is to be in a position to offer prenatal testing to those individuals at significant risk. Indeed the possibility of an accurate molecular prenatal test has had a dramatic impact on many families' reproductive plans. Before accurate prenatal molecular tests were possible, many parents of children with spinal muscular atrophy and cystic fibrosis chose not to have any further pregnancies, and many sisters/mothers/aunts/cousins of boys with Duchenne muscular dystrophy experienced the trauma of a midtrimester termination of a male fetus. For these families, the option of prenatal diagnosis has been a prerequisite for embarking on a pregnancy. Indeed many healthy children have been born who would otherwise have been terminated in utero, or never been conceived, if prenatal testing had not been possible. Nevertheless, prenatal diagnosis and the associated option of termination of pregnancy can have considerable psychological sequelae for pregnant women and their partners *(14)*.

Although prenatal diagnosis is now possible for an ever-increasing range of Mendelian conditions, uptake varies considerably between conditions. In general, requests for prenatal diagnosis are most common for disorders with onset in infancy/childhood, with more severe prognosis and little prospect for treatment; whereas prenatal diagnosis is less likely to be requested for conditions with late onset, less severe symptoms, and some prospect of treatment. Very few women at high risk of having a son with Duchenne muscular dystrophy will take the risk, whereas most people at risk of transmitting adult polycystic kidney disease accept the risk to their children without availing themselves of prenatal diagnosis *(3,4)*. However, for each disorder, individual couples will make different decisions. Of two pregnant couples with the same family history and same risk of recurrence, one may choose prenatal diagnosis and termination of an affected fetus whereas the other may carry on with the pregnancy without testing.

Decision making can be particularly difficult where the severity of the condition is variable, such as in neurofibromatasis and myotonic dystrophy. Requests for prenatal diagnosis for these conditions are infrequent, but surveys of these patients suggest that uptake would be higher if molecular diagnosis were a better indicator of phenotype *(15,16)*. Decision making also may be complicated when molecular diagnosis is by linkage, leaving a residual risk. Residual risks of <5% are often, but not always, acceptable to patients, and the use of flanking markers to reduce the residual risk may be requested. It is also important to point out here that making the decision to have prenatal diagnosis does not imply a decision to terminate a high-risk fetus; some couples choose prenatal diagnosis in order to prepare themselves for an affected child.

These issues make clear the necessity for pre- and post-test counseling. The majority of molecular prenatal diagnoses will be to couples with a family history, although some tests for the hemaglobinopathies, Tay Sachs disease, and cystic fibrosis will be the result of population-based carrier screening. Couples at known high risk should have access to genetic counseling via the relevant genetic service.

Communication between clinical staff and the laboratory carrying out the prenatal testing is important in two regards. First, laboratory staff need to be clear precisely what tests are being requested: for example, should flanking markers be used and if so, has the patient been made aware of the possibility of an ambiguous result owing to recombination between the markers; and is the sample for a Huntington's disease prenatal test for mutation testing, or exclusion testing only using linkage? Second, it is crucial that laboratory and clinical staff are clear about the timing of results of tests. The majority of molecular prenatal testing will be on chorionic villus samples (CVS), and the laboratory would expect to have some advance notice of the samples' arrival. Because of the controversy over CVS being possibly associated with a small increased risk of limb abnormalities when carried out before 10 wk of pregnancy *(17)*, many centers now opt for CVS at 10–11 wk. One of the important advantages of CVS to couples at high genetic risk has been its availability in the first trimester to enable, where necessary, a transcervical termination of pregnancy under general anesthetic. However, as this method of termination can usually only be performed safely until 14 wk gestation there will be limited time available following CVS to complete molecular tests. Diagnosis later than this may lead to termination by induction of labor.

6. Ethical Considerations

Ethical issues surrounding genetic testing have been the source of considerable debate and the subject of many reports over recent years *(18–20)*, and would not appropriately be considered in detail here. There are however, three issues of relevance to clinical molecular genetic laboratories worth highlighting: consent, testing children, and inadvertent discovery of genetic information.

As mentioned in Section 3. on predictive testing, international guidelines *(9)* have ensured that a written consent form is completed by the patient and his or her doctor before a Huntington's disease predictive test is carried out. Currently in the United Kingdom consent forms are not routinely required for all genetic tests, although some centers have begun to introduce these. Laboratories may choose to assume, on receiving a sample from a clinician, that consent has been obtained from the patient verbally or in a written form filed in the patient's clinical notes. Alternatively, laboratories may decide to require that a consent form be included as part of the request card accompanying the sample. Consent forms for genetic testing would normally include a clear statement of the purpose for which the sample has been taken, and the signatures of the patient and the health professional who has discussed the possible implications of the test with them (including implications for other family members). It is particularly important that laboratory staff are made aware of whether consent has been given for clinical testing, research purposes, or for storage only.

The pros and cons of genetic testing in children is under debate. A working party of the UK Clinical Genetics Society *(20)* published preliminary recommendations in 1994 which were only partly endorsed by the UK Genetic Interest Group, an umbrella organization speaking for families affected by genetic disease *(21)*. There is general consensus that diagnostic testing for a child showing symptoms of a genetic condition, or predictive testing where this would lead to early treatment, is not problematic, and that predictive testing for late onset disorders without early treatment options (e.g., Huntington's disease) is not usually appropriate. There is considerably less agreement on whether heterozygote carrier testing should be done in children. A survey of clinical molecular genetic laboratories in the United Kingdom by the Clinical Genetics Society working party showed that laboratories do regularly receive samples from children for carrier testing for cystic fibrosis and other recessive disorders, commonly from pediatricians, and that most laboratories do not have guidelines for these requests. The clinical and laboratory geneticists in our department in Manchester have jointly decided that, locally, carrier testing in children should be discouraged.

It is in the nature of molecular genetic testing that unsolicited information about family members may be discovered inadvertently. Nonpaternity can be identified through family testing and may exclude an individual from being at genetic risk. Diagnosis can be revealed by implication from testing individuals in a family linked through a relative who has not requested testing (such as in the example shown in Fig. 3). Heterozygote carrier status on an unborn baby will be revealed when testing a prenatal sample for the primary purpose of diagnosing a (homozygous) affected pregnancy. Laboratory guidelines for generating and reporting this information should be considered carefully and after discussion with clinical colleagues.

7. Genetic Registers

Regionally organized genetic family registers provide a mechanism for extending access to genetic counseling to all individuals at significant risk of chosen disorders, as well as a system for maintaining long-term contact with these families. Relatives of probands referred to the genetic service are proactively offered genetic counseling and continuing follow-up *(4)*. Relatives are only contacted after careful discussion with the proband, and where appropriate, the general practitioner. Individuals are only included on the register with their explicit permission after genetic counseling. It is essential to preserve confidentiality and privacy for family members, and information included on the register must not be divulged to third parties without the explicit agreement of the individual concerned. Because of the sensitive nature of the information held on extended families, it has been recommended that genetic registers should normally be organized regionally rather than nationally or internationally. Disorders chosen for the register approach are usually ones where the implications extend through the generations; autosomal dominant conditions such as Huntington's disease, neurofibromatosis, adult polycystic kidney disease, familial adenomatous polyposis coli, and other dominant cancers; X-linked disorders such as Duchenne and Becker muscular dystrophies and fragile X; and the balanced chromosome translocations. Genetic counseling and annual contact is provided by the clinical genetic team. This family-centered approach is ideal for molecular testing because it facilitates collection and storage of samples from appropriate relatives in extended kindreds *(13)*. Because families agree to long-term follow-up, they are prepared to receive updated laboratory results and to provide additional samples if needed. A further advantage of this approach is that proactive counseling and testing usually from the teens onward decreases requests for family testing urgently in pregnancy. When the molecular laboratory and the genetic register service are based in the same place, close collaboration can focus resources on prioritizing molecular testing for those individuals for whom it is most relevant. At a practical level, integrating laboratory and clinical register databases may be helpful, as well as regular working meetings between laboratory and clinical register staff.

8. Personal Issues for Laboratory Staff

Clinical scientists are commonly asked to provide blood samples for use as controls or in developing new techniques in the laboratory. Similarly, students and junior staff are often set to do their own karyotype and cystic fibrosis gene screen. This should be approached with caution where information of potentially clinical significance could be generated. The basic premise that genetic testing should not be done without some element of pre-test counseling, is just as applicable to laboratory scientists who are, after all, human first and scientists second!

Although the need for providing emotional support to staff working in the health services is being increasingly acknowledged *(22)*, this has been focused primarily on staff involved directly in patient care. Little attention is paid to the feelings of laboratory staff who may be under continual pressure to generate urgent test results which have serious clinical significance. This is of particular relevance in clinical molecular genetic laboratories where test results may lead to terminations of pregnancy or presymptomatic diagnosis of serious genetic diseases. Clinical staff are trained in "breaking bad news" to patients, but laboratory scientists may also experience an element of the stresses of giving bad news when in the position of communicating results verbally to clinical staff closely involved with the patient. Laboratory staff should be encouraged to discuss the emotional demands of their work, and this could be incorporated into laboratory meetings, as well as through informal contact with clinical colleagues.

9. Summary

Molecular genetic testing can provide powerful information about disease and risk of disease, both pre- and postnatally, for individuals and their nuclear and extended families. Because of the potential psychological as well as medical implications of genetic testing, counseling before and after testing must be available as an integral component of the testing service, and the right to make a choice not to have a genetic test must be an option. Communication between the clinical molecular genetic laboratory and clinical colleagues providing genetic counselling is essential to ensure that molecular genetic advances bring the best possible benefits with the least possible harm. Clinical molecular geneticists should contribute to discussion and debate about the human implications of their work.

References

1. Andrews, L. B., Fullarton, J. E., Holtzman, N. A., and Motulsky, A. G. (eds.) (1994) *Assessing Genetic Risks: Implications for Health and Social Policy,* National Academy Press, Washington, DC.
2. Craufurd, D., Kerzin-Storrar, L., Dodge, A., and Harris, R. (1989) Uptake of presymptomatic predictive testing for Huntington's disease. *Lancet* **2,** 603–605.
3. Hodgkinson, K. A., Kerzin-Storrar, L., Watters, E. A., and Harris, R. (1990) Adult polycystic kidney disease: knowledge, experience and attitudes to prenatal diagnosis. *J. Med. Genet.* **27,** 552–558.
4. Kerzin-Storrar, L., Khan, A. A., Watters, E. A., Craufurd, D., et al. (1991) A regional genetic family register. *Am. J. Hum. Genet.* **49,** 42.
5. Walker, A. P., Scott, J. A., Biesecker, B. B., Conover, B., Blake, W., and Djurdjinovic, L. (1990) Report of the 1989 Asilomar meeting on education in genetic counselling. *Am. J. Hum. Genet.* **46,** 1223–1230.
6. Kerzin-Storrar, L. (1993) A new MSc course in genetic counselling for non-medical co-workers in clinical genetics. *J. Genet. Counselling* **2,** 44.
7. Harris, H., Scotcher, D., Hartley, N., Wallace, A., Craufurd, D., and Harris, R. (1993) Cystic fibrosis carrier testing in early pregnancy by general practitioners. *Br. Med. J.* **306,** 1580–1583.
8. Wooldridge, E. Q. and Murray, R. F. (1989) The health orientation scale: a measure of feeling about sickle cell trait. *Soc. Biol.* **35,** 123–136.
9. Tyler, A., Walker, R., Went, L., and Wexler, N. (1994) Guidelines for the molecular genetics predictive test in Huntington's disease. Clinical practice in medical genetics. *J. Med. Genet.* **31,** 555–559.
10. Zeesman, S., Clow, C. L., Cartier, L., and Scriver, C. R. (1984) A private view of heterozygosity: eight-year follow-up on carriers of Tay-Sachs gene detected by high school screening. *Am. J. Med. Genet.* **18,** 769–778.
11. Marteau, T. M., van Duijn, M., and Ellis, I. (1992) Effects of genetic screening on perceptions of health: a pilot study. *J. Med. Genet.* **29,** 24–26.
12. Mitchell, J., Scriver, C. R., Clow, C. L., and Kaplan, F. (1993) What young people think and do when the option for cystic fibrosis carrier testing is available. *J. Med. Genet.* **30,** 538–542.
13. Read, A. P., Kerzin-Storrar, L., Mountford, R. C., Elles, R. G., and Harris, R. (1986) A register based system for gene tracking in Duchenne muscular dystrophy. *J. Med. Genet.* **23,** 581–586.
14. Abramsky, L. and Chapple, J. (eds.) (1994) *Prenatal Diagnosis: The Human Side,* Chapman and Hall, London.
15. Benjamin, C. M., Colley, A., Donnai, D., Kingston, H., Harris, R., and Kerzin-Storrar, L. (1993) Neurofibromatosis type 1: knowledge, experience, and reproductive decisions of affected patients and families. *J. Med. Genet.* **30,** 567–574.
16. Faulkner, C., Clancy, T., and Kingston, H. (1995) A study investigating the knowledge, views and experience of myotonic dystrophy (MD) among a group of affected women (poster, autumn 1995), Clinical Genetics Society, London.

17. Firth, H. V., Boyd, P. A., Chamberlain, P. F., MacKenzie, I. Z., Morriss-Kay, G. M., and Huson, S. M. (1994) Analysis of limb reduction defects in babies exposed to chorionic villus sampling. *Lancet* **343,** 1069–1071.

18. Nuffield Council on Bioethics (1993) *Genetic Screening: Ethical Issues,* Author, London.

19. Clarke, A., Fielding, D., Kerzin-Storrar, L., Middleton-Price, H., Montgomery, J., Payne, H., Simonoff, E., and Tyler, A. (1994) The genetic testing of children: report of a working party of the Clinical Genetics Society (U.K.). *J. Med. Genet.* **31,** 785–797.

20. Dalby, S. (1995) GIG response to the UK Clinical Genetics Society report "The genetic testing of children." *J. Med. Genet.* **32,** 490–494.

21. British Medical Association (1995) *The BMA's Views on Genetic Testing,* Author, London.

22. Friedrich, E. (1994) Caring for the carers, in *Prenatal Diagnosis: The Human Side* (Abramsky, L. and Chapple, J., eds.), Chapman and Hall, London, pp. 202–212.

12

Molecular Approaches to the Detection of Deletions and Uniparental Disomy in Prader-Willi and Angelman Syndromes

John F. Harvey and John A. Crolla

1. Introduction

The chromosomal region 15q11→q13 exhibits one of the best characterized examples of genomic imprinting in humans in that biparental inheritance of this region is essential for normal development. Prader-Willi syndrome (PWS) and Angelman syndrome (AS) are clinically distinct neurogenetic disorders caused by the loss of function of the paternal (PWS) or maternal (AS) contribution of closely apposed genes within 15q11→q13.

In approx 75%, of PWS patients, the loss of the paternal allele(s) is caused by deletion, or very rarely, by translocations involving breakpoints in 15q11→q13, whereas the remaining 25% present with maternal uniparental disomy (UPD). By contrast, whereas ~60% of AS patients have maternal deletions, only 4% have paternal UPD and the remainder have no detectable abnormalities *(1)*.

Historically, the diagnosis of PWS and AS depended on the use of conventional cytogenetic methods for the detection of interstitial deletions or other structural anomalies involving bands 15q11→q13. However, conventional microscopic diagnosis of interstitial deletions particularly in this region is notoriously difficult, and both false-positive and negative results have been demonstrated. Furthermore, cytogenetic analysis *per se* cannot identify cases of UPD. The identification and cloning of 15q11→q13 specific probes for use in polymerase chain reaction (PCR)-based microsatellite CA repeat analysis [(CA)n], Southern blotting, and fluorescence *in situ* hybridization (FISH) studies now make possible the implementation of combined conventional cytogenetic, molecular cytogenetic, and DNA approaches to the diagnosis of the majority of PWS and AS patients caused by deletion or UPD.

From: *Methods in Molecular Medicine: Molecular Diagnosis of Genetic Diseases*
Edited by: R. Elles Humana Press Inc., Totowa, NJ

In order to harness this battery of techniques to their best advantage, we have developed a sequential strategy for deletion and UPD detection. Initially all PWS/AS referrals are examined with conventional cytogenetic analysis to exclude a structural abnormality of any chromosome. Screening for deletions in proximal 15q is carried out using FISH with cosmid probes cloned from the PWS/AS critical regions *(2)*, a strategy that will successfully diagnose the majority (but not all) PWS and AS patients with deletions. If a deletion is detected, no further action is required and a report can be issued. If no deletion is seen, however, further samples from the proband and both parents are required so that DNA analysis can be employed to diagnose/exclude UPD.

Two main molecular approaches are used. The first is PCR-based (CA)n repeat analysis *(3)*, which is both rapid (2 d) and highly informative, but requires parental DNA for the correct interpretation of the results. The second is the slower (1–2 wk) Southern blotting approach using the probe PW71b(D15S63), which exploits the differential methylation patterns within this imprinted region *(4,5)*.

The vast majority of classical PWS and ~65% of AS patients will be confirmed using these combined molecular approaches. However, it should be noted that a number of rare methylation mutations and locus-specific microdeletions patients have been reported in the literature *(6,7)*, and particularly in cases with clearly defined PWS/AS phenotypes where UPD and deletions have been excluded, more specialist investigations may be required to make a definitive diagnosis.

2. Materials

Many of the reagents, including the probes for FISH studies, are available commercially. Any reagents prepared in the laboratory should be made up with analytical-grade reagents, and ultrapure (or similar grade) water. The FISH protocol given below assumes the use of commercially available digoxigenin-labeled probes for the PWS/AS region and their detection using fluorescein isothiocyanate (FITC) conjugated reagents. Please note that although the detection method described here differs slightly from that recommended by the probe manufacturer, it nevertheless gives reliable and reproducible results in this laboratory.

2.1. FISH Analysis

2.1.1. Slide Preparation and Denaturation

1. Methanol.
2. Glacial acetic acid.
3. 70% Industrial methylated spirits (IMS).

4. 2X SSC: Prepare from 20X SSC stock: $3M$ NaCl and $0.3M$ trisodium citrate (*see* Note 1).
5. RNase A: 10 mg/mL RNase in RNase buffer: 10 mM Tris and 15 mM NaCl at pH 7.5 (*see* Note 2).
6. Formamide: **caution** (*see* Note 3).
7. Water bath at 72°C.
8. Glass microscope slides.
9. Microfuge.

2.1.2. Hybridization

1. Commercial probe mixtures of D15S11, GABRB3, and/or SNRPN (ONCOR probes supplied by Alpha Laboratories, Eastleigh, UK) (*see* Notes 5 and 6).
2. 2X SSC.
3. 70, 90, and 100% IMS solutions at room temperature.
4. 70% IMS at –20°C.
5. Water bath at 37°C.
6. Humidified incubation chamber for slides, e.g., a plastic lunch box with a sealable lid, containing 5 mL of 2X SSC in the base for humidification (*see* Note 7).
7. Suitable slide rack for holding slides in transverse position during hybridization.
8. Rubber solution (Dunlop, UK).
9. 22 × 22-mm Glass coverslips.
10. 20-, 100-, and 1000-µL micropipets (Gilson, Anachem, Bedfordshire, UK).

2.1.3. Posthybridization Stringent Washing and Detection

1. 20X SSC.
2. 2X SSC.
3. 4X SSC/Tween-20 wash solution: 4X SSC and 0.05% Tween-20 (*see* Note 8).
4. 1% Boehringer block solution (Boehringer Mannheim, Lewes, UK) (*see* Note 9).
5. Antidigoxigenin (mouse monoclonal) diluted 1:500 in 1% Boehringer block solution (*see* Note 10).
6. Antimouse-FITC (made in rabbit) (Sigma, Poole, UK) diluted 1:500 in 1% Boehringer block solution (*see* Note 10).
7. Antirabbit-FITC (made in goat) (Sigma) diluted 1:500 in 1% Boehringer block solution (*see* Note 10).
8. Antifade solution (Vector, UK) (see Note 11).
9. Propidium iodide (PI): 0.05 mg/mL (Sigma).
10. Epifluorescent UV microscope (e.g., Carl Zeiss, Axiostop, Germany) fitted with suitable barrier and excited filters (Carl Zeiss filter combination 15 or Pinkel 83 series filter set. Chroma Technology Corps., Brattleboro, VT) for the visualization of the probe (green-FITC) and red chromosomal (PI) signals.
11. Water bath at 42°C.
12. *Either* 24 × 50-mm glass coverslips (*see* Note 12) *or* Shandon plastic coverplates (Shandon Life Sciences, Basingstoke, UK) (*see* Note 12).

2.2. DNA Extraction

1. 50-, 15-, and 1.5-mL (Eppendorf) disposable centrifuge tubes (Sarstedt, Leicester, UK).
2. Refrigerated microfuge and bench-top centrifuges (Sorvall refrigerated microfuge RMC 14 and a refrigerated bench-top centrifuge RT6000B with an H-1000B swinging bucket rotor).
3. Crushed ice and double-distilled water supplies.
4. Sucrose lysis buffer: $0.32M$ sucrose, 10 mM Tris-HCl, 5 mM MgCl$_2$, 1% Triton X-100, pH 7.5. Make to 1 L.
5. Resuspension buffer: $0.075M$ NaCl, $0.024M$ EDTA, pH 8.0. Make to 1 L.
6. Proteinase K at 50 mg/mL.
7. Sodium dodecyl sulfate (SDS) (as a 20% [w/v] ready-made stock by Amresco from CamLab, Cambridge UK).
8. TE: 10 mM Tris-HCl, 1 mM EDTA, pH 8.0.
9. Ethanol 99.7–100% (v/v).

2.3. CA Repeat Analysis

1. Vertical "sequencing gel" electrophoresis apparatus with 3000-V power supply (Bio-Rad Labs, Ltd., Hamel Hampstead, UK, Sequi-Gen Sequencing Cell and Power-Pac 3000).
2. Thermal cycler and thin-walled reaction tubes (0.5 mL) (Perkin Elmer, Applied Biosystems Ltd., Warrington, UK).
3. Stock 5X Tris/borate/EDTA (5X TBE): $0.445M$ Tris borate and $0.01M$ EDTA, pH 8.3, commercially available (Sigma).
4. Stock acrylamide/bis-solution: 40% (w/v) acrylamide-2.1% (w/v) bis:acrylamide— ratio 19:1, commercially available (Severn Biotech Ltd., Kidderminster, UK). Store at 4°C.
5. N,N,N',N',-tetramethyleneethylenediamine (TEMED): Store at 4°C.
6. Ammonium persulfate (APS): Dissolve 1 g in 10 mL distilled water. Freeze as 800-μL aliquots at −20°C
7. Urea (Sigma).
8. Stop buffer: A 10-mL solution of 45% formamide, 20 mM EDTA, 0.05% bromophenol blue, 0.05% xylene cyanole.
9. Siliconizing solution (Acrylease by Stratagene, Cambridge, UK).
10. Redivue [γ^{32}P]ATP at 3000 Ci/mmol Amersham International (Amersham, Slough, UK). Store at 4°C. **Caution** (*see* Note 22).
11. T4 Polynucleotide kinase and 10X enzyme buffer as provided by enzyme manufacturers (CamBio, Cambridge, UK). Store at −20°C.
12. *Taq* DNA-polymerase and Mg-free 10X enzyme buffer as provided by enzyme manufacturers (Promega, Southampton, UK). Store at −20°C.
13. Stock 25-mM MgCl$_2$ solutions (Promega). Store at −20°C.
14. Stock of four, 100 mM dNTPs (Promega). Store at −20°C.
15. Mineral oil, light white oil (if required) (Sigma).

Table 1
Oligonucleotide Primers Used in the Multiplex PCR Reaction

Probe	Locus	Primer sequence	Size, bp
4-3 RCA	D15S11	F 5'-GACATGAACAGAGGTAAATTGGTGG-3'	243–263
		R 5'-GCTCTCTAAGATCACTGGATAGG-3'	
GABRB3CA	GABRB3	F 5'-CTCTTGTTCCTGTTGCTTTCAATACAC-3'	181–201
		R 5'-CACTGTGCTAGTAGATTCAGCTC-3'	
AFM200wb4	D15S122	F 5'-GATAATCATGCCCCCCA-3'	143–159
		R 5'-CCCAGTATCTGGCACGTAG-3'	
LS6-1CA	D15S113	F 5'-CATGTACTGTTTTATCCCTGTGTGGC-3'	130–140
		R 5'-CTGCTGCTTATACTCTTTCTCTATTC-3'	

16. Oligonucleotide dinucleotide repeat primers, 4-3RCA(D15S 11) *(8)*, AFM200wb4 (D15S122) *(9)*, LS6-1CA(D15S113) *(3)*, and GABRB3CA *(10)* for multiplex PCR (Oswel DNA Service, Southampton, UK) (*see* Table 1).
17. Autoradiography cassettes: with intensifying screens.
18. X-ray film: for example, Kodak X-Omat AR5 (Kodak, Cambridge, UK).

2.4. Methylation Analysis

1. Horizontal gel electrophoresis apparatus with $20 \times 20/24$ cm gel formers and combs (Bethesda Research Labs, Cambridge, UK) and 300-V power supply (Northumbria Biologicals Ltd., Cramlington, UK).
2. Agarose (Appligene, Durham, UK).
3. 5 mg /mL Ethidium bromide. **Caution** (*see* Note 20).
4. UV transilluminator. UV protective visor and goggles. **Caution** (UV Products Inc., San Gabriel, CA).
5. CU-5 Polaroid camera and hood with Kodak Wratten 22A or 23A red filter (Kodak) and B and W 667 Polaroid film (Polaroid, St. Albans, UK).
6. Restriction enzymes *Hpa*II and *Hin*dIII and appropriate buffer as recommended by the manufacturer (Boehringer Mannheim).
7. Spermidine/MgCl$_2$: mix of equal volumes of 120 m*M* spermidine and 100 m*M* MgCl$_2$ (Sigma).
8. Denaturation solution (DN): 0.5*M* NaOH, 1*M* NaCl.
9. Neutralization solution (N): 1*M* Tris-HCl, 1.5*M* NaCl, pH 8.0. Ready-made powdered blend (Sigma).
10. Blotting membrane, e.g., Zeta-Probe GT (Bio-Rad Labs. Ltd.).
11. 80°C Incubator/oven.
12. 25×35-mm Radiation bags (Jencons Scientific Ltd., Leighton Buzzard, UK).
13. Bag sealer, artist's roller tool, and darkroom developing trays for gel and filter washings.
14. Prehybridization and hybridization mix: 0.25*M* Na$_2$HPO$_4$, pH 7.2, 7% SDS.
15. Shaking water bath or incubator with shaking tray.

16. Redivue [α³²P]dCTP at 3000 Ci/mmol (Amersham International plc, Little Chelfont, UK). **Caution** (*see* Note 22).
17. DNA probe PW71b (D15S63) *(5)*.
18. Labeling kit, e.g., High Prime (Amersham International).
19. Water bath at 37°C.
20. Wash buffer 1: 20 m*M* Na₂HPO₄, pH 7.2, and 5% SDS. Wash buffer 2: 20 m*M* Na₂HPO₄, pH 7.2, 1% SDS.
21. Sephadex G50-150 and a 0.7 × 20-cm glass column (Bio-Rad Labs. Ltd., Econo-Columns).
22. Autoradiography cassettes, screens, and films (as in Section 2.3.).

3. Methods
3.1. FISH Analysis
3.1.1. Slide Preparation and Denaturation

1. Clean a microscope slide by spraying with 70% IMS and wiping dry with tissue. Make sure that the surface is grease free.
2. Make chromosome preparations using conventional methods (3:1 methanol:acetic acid), but it is best to place one drop of suspension centrally on each slide. Mark the underside of the slide with a diamond pencil, thereby defining the outer limits of the cell suspension (*see* Note 4).
3. Immerse the slide in freshly prepared 3:1 methanol:acetic acid for 30 min (i.e., postfixation). Air-dry.
4. RNase slides using a working concentration of 100 μg/mL made up in 2X SSC (i.e., 100 μL of stock + 900 μL of 2X SSC). Add 60 μL/slide under a 24 × 50 mm coverslip, and incubate slides for 30 min at 37°C (*see* Note 2).
5. Remove coverslips gently and wash slides briefly in 2X SSC. Dehydrate by 2 min washes at room temperature in 70, 90, and 100% IMS series. Air-dry.
6. Make up and preheat to 70°C the denaturing solution, **take care and wear gloves**: 70% formamide, 30% 2X SSC (*see* Note 3).
7. Place the slides in a staining trough or coplin jar, and place at 72°C for 1–3 min to prewarm.
8. Pour the hot denaturing solution onto the slides and incubate for 2 min at 72°C.
9. Pour off the denaturing solution and immerse slides in ice-cold 70% IMS for 2 min.
10. Wash slides for 2 min in 90% and 2 min in 100% IMS. Air-dry.

3.1.2. Hybridization

1. Approximately 10 min prior to setting up the hybridization, remove the probe(s) from the –20°C freezer and place in a 37°C water bath to warm up. The commercial probes used in this protocol are supplied precompeted with human Cot-1 DNA, and so are ready for use (*see* Notes 5 and 6).
2. Place the required number of 22 × 22-mm coverslips on a flat surface, and aliquot 10 μL of probe mixture onto each trying to avoid bubbling.

3. Place the slide—denatured cell surface downward—gently onto the 22 × 22-mm coverslip using the diamond pencil mark to identify where the cells are located. Seal the edge of the coverslip with rubber solution.

4. Place the slide into a deep-sided slide rack (or some suitable container that will keep the slides horizontal and level during incubation). Position the slides/rack in a chamber, e.g., a plastic lunch box with a sealable lid, and pour 5 mL of 2X SSC into the bottom for humidifiication. Incubate overnight in a 37°C water bath (*see* Note 7).

3.1.3. Posthybridization Stringent Washing and Detection

1. Prior to beginning the next step (usually the morning after setting up the hybridization), make up the stringent wash solutions, and preheat them to 42°C in the water bath, i.e., 50% formamide, 50% 2X SSC. Make up sufficient volume for two 5-min washes.

2. Gently remove the hybridization coverslip, and place the slides immediately into 2X SSC at room temperature.

3. When all the slides have had their coverslips removed, pour off the 2X SSC, and immediately pour the preheated stringent wash onto them. Incubate for 5 min in the 42°C water bath.

4. Pour off the first solution, and replace with the second aliquot of preheated stringent wash solution. Incubate for 5 min in the 42°C water bath.

5. Pour off the second wash and replace with 2X SSC at room temperature. Incubate for 5 min.

6. Remove slides from 2X SSC, attach them to a disposable plastic coverplate (Shandon), and place them in a rack as shown in Fig. 1 (*see* Note 12).

7. Inject 100 µL of block solution into each slide well. Incubate for 15 min at room temperature (*see* Note 9).

8. Inject 100 µL of antidigoxigenin (mouse monoclonal) diluted 1:500 in 1% Boehringer block solution into each slide well. Incubate for 20 min at room temperature (*see* Note 10).

9. Inject 500 µL of 4X SSC/Tween-20 to each slide well. Incubate for 2 min at room temperature.

10. Repeat step 9.

11. Inject 100 µL antimouse-FITC (made in rabbit) diluted 1:500 in 1% Boehringer block solution into each slide well. Incubate for 20 min at room temperature (*see* Note 10).

12. Repeat washing steps 9 and 10.

13. Inject 100 µL antirabbit-FITC (made in goat) diluted 1:500 in 1% Boehringer block solution into each slide well. Incubate for 20 min at room temperature.

14. Repeat washing steps 9 and 10.

15. Remove slides from the coverplates, and immerse in 4X SSC/Tween-20 wash solution.

16. Place one small drop of antifade on 22 × 50 mm coverslip, and inject 1 µL of a 0.05 mg/mL solution of PI (*see* Note 11).

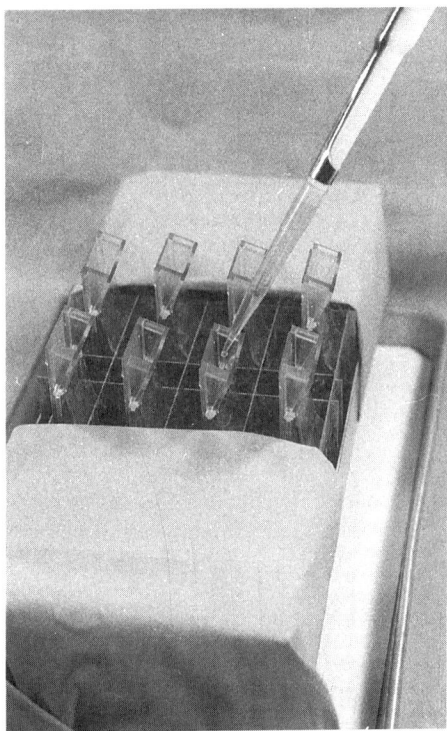

Fig. 1. Shandon coverplates and the posthybridization slides can be arranged in a "homemade" rack, made in the example from a Denley storage rack. One hundred microliters of each detection reagent are pipeted (arrow) into the well formed by the slide and coverplate. The fluid drains down the slide by gravity, but once the well is empty, a residue is trapped between the slide and coverplate by surface tension. Adding 0.5 mL of the wash buffer reagent displaces the detection reagent, washes the slide, and prepares the slide surface for the next 100 µL of detection reagent.

17. Drain slide briefly from 4X SSC/Tween-20, and place cell side downwards onto coverslip/antifade/stain mixture.
18. Blot the excess thoroughly with tissue paper, and seal the coverslip with rubber solution. The slides are now ready for examination under a fluorescent microscope using either Carl Zeiss filter combination 15 or Chroma Technology Filters. With these filter combinations, the chromosomes stain red and the FITC signal is green. A minimum of 10 metaphases should be scored, and the distribution of signal expected in normal and deleted patients.

3.2. DNA Extraction

Genomic DNA was prepared from whole blood taken in EDTA tubes from patients and parents and collected into EDTA tubes. The following procedure was designed for 10-mL blood samples but may be scaled down for smaller volumes (*see* Note 13).

1. Place blood on ice for 20 min in a 50-mL screw-cap tube (*see* Note 14).
2. Add cold sterile distilled water on ice to a final volume of 50 mL.
3. Centrifuge at 2000*g* at 4°C for 10 min.
4. Pour off supernatant and resuspend the pellet in 25 mL ice-cold sucrose lysis buffer (*see* Note 15).
5. Centrifuge at 2000*g* at 4°C for 10 min.
6. Pour off supernatant and resuspend pellet in 3 mL resuspension buffer. Add 150 µL of 10% SDS and 8 µL proteinase K (50 mg/mL, stored frozen as 20-µL aliquots) (*see* Note 15).
7. Incubate overnight at 37°C or for 2–3 h at 60°C until fluid.
8. Add 1.5 mL of 6*M* NaCl, and shake vigorously for 20 s.
9. Centrifuge at 2200*g* at room temperature for 30 min.
10. Collect supernatant in a 15-mL tube and fill with 100% ethanol at room temperature. Invert two to three times until the DNA "hair ball" forms.
11. Lift out the DNA with a sterile disposable syringe needle (carefully "hooked" by catching the tip against the inside of the needle case), and wash quickly in 70% ethanol.
12. Resuspend in 1 mL of TE.
13. Store short term (weeks) at 4°C, or long term (years) at –20 to –80°C.

3.3. CA Repeat Analysis

1. Prepare four hot kits. End-label each selected primer separately as in Table 2, adding 1 µL of T_4 kinase to each hot kit, followed by $[\gamma^{32}P]$ATP to give a total volume of 10 µL/reaction.
2. Incubate at 37°C for 1 h.
3. Prepare a multiplex 10X cold kit as in Table 3. This kit provides enough material for 9–10 PCR reactions and may be stored at –20°C for future use. After the hot kit 1-h incubation add the end-labeled primers to the cold kit as shown in Table 3 (*see* Note 16).
4. Add 1 µL *Taq* polymerase enzyme, and divide into 19-µL aliquots in PCR tubes.
5. Add 1 µL of DNA to each tube (*see* Note 16).
6. PCR for 24 cycles with an initial denaturation of 94°C for 4 min, followed by 24 cycles of 94°C for 1 min, 55°C for 2 min, 72°C for 2 min, and a final extension of 72°C for 10 min.
7. After PCR amplification, add 20 µL stop buffer/tube, and denature at 100°C for 5 min just before use.
8. Keep on ice and load onto a 5% polyacrylamide denaturing gel as soon as possible (*see* Note 17).
9. Run for 3–3.5 h at 120 W.
10. Dismantle the apparatus, remove siliconized top plate (*see* Note 18), and identify radioactive products by scanning the gel surface with a Geiger counter.

Table 2
Hot Kit Preparation

Primers 20 μM		Primer	T$_4$ × 10 buffer	H$_2$O	T$_4$ kinase	[γ^{32}P]ATP
				Reagent volumes, μL		
4-3RCA	F	3	1	4	1	1
GABRB3CA	R	5	1	1	1	2
AFM 200wb4	F	3	1	4	1	1
LS6-1CA	R	5	1	1	1	2

Table 3
Cold Kit Preparation

Reagents	Volumes, μL
10X PCR buffer	20
25 mM MgCl$_2$	12
2 mM dNTP mix	25
20 μM 4-3RCA	1
20 μM GABRB3CA	2.5
20 μM AFM 200wb4	1.5
20 μM LS6-1CA	2.5
H$_2$O	109.5
End-labeled primers[a]	
4-3RCA	2
GABRB3CA	5
AFM 200wb4	3
LS6-1CA	5

[a]*See* Table 2.

11. Roll on an appropriate sized sheet of Whatman 3MM paper.
12. Trim off surrounding gel with scalpel, and lift up gel on the Whatman paper, transfer to cassette with intensifying screens, cover the gel in polythene, and expose to an X-ray film at –80°C for 2 h to overnight (Fig. 2, Table 1) (*see* Note 19).

3.4. Methylation Analysis

1. Digest 5 μg of DNA with 30 U of *Hpa*II and 20 U of *Hin*dIII, 6 μL 10X 'M' buffer (Boehringer Mannheim), and 1 μL of the magnesium/spermidine mix in a total volume 60 μL made up with double-distilled water or equivalent.
2. Incubate overnight at 37°C.

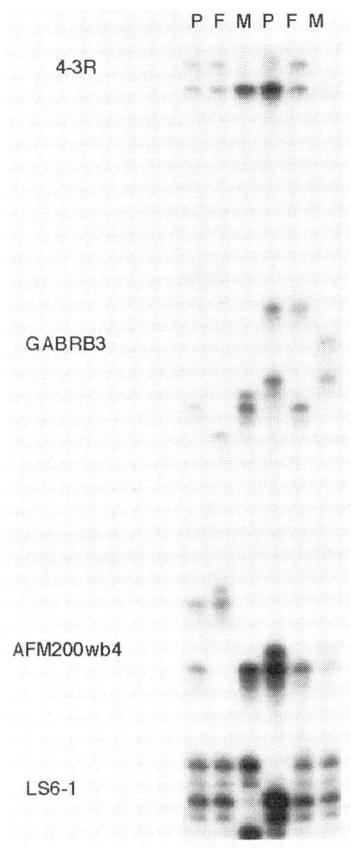

Fig. 2. Multiplex PCR of four CA repeats in the PWS/AS critical region in two normal families. P, proband; F, father; M, mother.

3. Pulse spin samples, and add 10 μL tracking dye to each digest.
4. Prepare a 20 × 20 cm horizontal 0.7% agarose gel, including 5 μL/100 mL of 5 mg/mL ethidium bromide into the molten agarose mix. **Caution** (*see* Note 20). Electrophorese the digests overnight at 80 V.
5. Wear disposable gloves while handling the gel and filters and using appropriate face and eye protective visor and goggles, transfer the gel to a UV transilluminator and photograph.
6. Transfer the gel to a tray, and cover with DN solution until the gel can move freely. Shake gently for 70 min (*see* Note 21).
7. Carefully pour off DN, holding gel down with gloved hand, rinse with distilled water, and then cover with N solution. Shake as before for 70 min.

8. Remove the gel, using a sheet of old X-ray film, and place onto the bottom surface of an inverted gel former, cover with a gel-sized perspex sheet (preferably with a block at one side to prevent gel slip), and with hands at each end, invert the gel.

9. For wet blotting, prepare a standard Southern blot apparatus with a 20X SSC reservoir and Whatman 3MM wick at least two layers thick folded across a glass or perspex platform. Add the inverted gel to the apparatus and follow the filter manufacturer's instructions (Zeta-Probe GT, Bio-Rad). Surround the gel with cut strips of polythene or used X-ray film to prevent filter/wick solution bypass effects.

   For dry blotting, line the bench with a sheet of polythene, cut four pieces of Whatman 3MM paper to the gel size, soak in 20X SSC, stack on the polythene, add the inverted gel, and then continue as for wet blotting.

10. Blot overnight, remove towels, and turn over gel and filter. Mark well positions, track 1 position, and unique filter number with pencil. Carefully peel away gel and rinse filter in 2X SSC. Air-dry between two sheets of Whatman 3MM paper and bake at 80°C for 1 h.

11. Prior to labeling PW71b, amplify the plasmid insert and flanking regions by PCR using the ScreenTest Recombinant Screening Kit (Stratagene) according to the manufacturer's instructions. Check the PCR product sizes on an agarose mini-gel, running 5 μL of the products against known size standards. Purify the remaining products using the Prep-A-Gene DNA Purification Kit (Bio-Rad). Check the final products as before for size and concentration against known markers.

   Label 25 ng of purified product with 50 μCi of Redivue [α^{32}P]dCTP, 3000 Ci/mmol (Amersham) using the High Prime Labeling Mix for Random Prime Labeling Kit (Boehringer Mannheim, UK) according to manufacturer's instructions. After a 30-min incubation at 37°C, run the labeled probe down a 12-cm Sephadex G50-150 (TE buffered) column to remove free nucleotides. Monitor the separation of free nucleotides from probe on the column with a hand-held Geiger counter. Collect the probe peak running ahead of the (red) free nucleotide peak, in a "screw-cap" Eppendorf tube held with a pair of forceps. Replace the Eppendorf cap, and denature the probe in a boiling water bath for 10 min. Cool rapidly on ice, and then add to the prehybridized filter as described in the following step (*see* Note 22).

12. Prehybridize for 5–30 min. Hybridize and wash the membrane using the standard aqueous protocol according to manufacturer's instructions (Zeta-Probe GT. Bio-Rad). Use about 40 mL prehybridization solution, and after squeezing out, add 5–10 mL of prewarmed hybridization solution and the labeled probe PW71b. Seal the bag and thoroughly treat with an artist's roller to ensure mixing. Incubate in a shaking water bath at 65°C or preferably on a shaking tray in a hot air oven (Hybaid, Teddington, UK). Hybridize for at least 18 h.

13. After washing twice for 30 min in wash buffer 1 and twice for 30 min in wash buffer 2, enclose the filter in clear plastic wrap, and transfer to a cassette beneath two facing intensifying screens with Kodak X-Omat AR5 X-ray film sandwiched in between. Expose at –80°C overnight up to 5 d and develop (Fig. 3) (*see* Note 23).

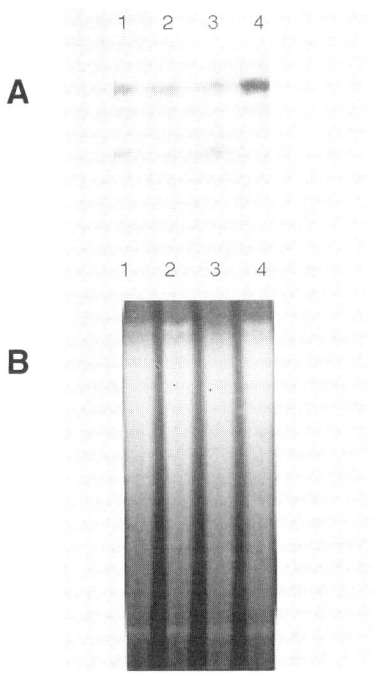

Fig. 3. (A) An autoradiograph of a Southern blot analysis of the methylation patterns at the locus D15S63(probe PW71b) in *Hin*dIII/*Hpa*II-digested DNA. The 6-kb band represents the maternal methylation imprint, and the 4.4-kb band represents the paternal methylation imprint. 1, Normal female; 2, PWS sample deleted for the unmethylated paternal allele; 3, normal male; 4, PWS sample with uniparental disomy. **(B)** A gel photograph of the ethidium bromide-stained *Hin*dIII/*Hpa*II-digested DNA corresponding to 1, 2, 3, and 4 in (A), demonstrating the equivalent DNA concentrations of the enzyme digest.

4. Notes

4.1. FISH Analysis

4.1.1. Slide Preparation and Denaturation

1. Dissolve the salts initially in 800 mL water and adjust volume to 1 L when fully dissolved. 2X SSC = 1:10 dilution of 20X SSC in ultra-pure water
2. RNase A stock solution of 10 mg/mL made up in RNase buffer: Boil for 30 min to destroy any contaminating DNase. Store this boiled stock at −20°C.
3. Formamide is a possible teratogen and must be handled with caution. *See* local control of substances hazardous to health (COSHH [UK]) assessments (or other mandatory regulations) for the correct handling and disposal of this chemical.

4. Slides for *in situ* hybridization can be used after the short pretreatment schedule noted here. However, older slides can be used if necessary, but the postfixation step can be omitted. If the only patient material available is older unstained slides, then the *in situ* technique should be attempted. The optimal way of storing material for future studies is as cells suspended in 3:1 methanol:acetic acid fixative at –20°C.

4.1.2. Hybridization

5. The current strategy for the use of commercially available cosmids from the PWS/AS regions is based on the observation that the vast majority of deletions involving this region will remove sequences detected by the probes D15S11 (at the centromeric end) and GABRB3 (at the telomere end of the region). However, very rare cases of PWS have been reported with deletions in the SNRPN region only. Since SNRPN lies proximal to GABRB3, it is advisable to use SNRPN together with D15S11 for PWS and D15S11 and GABRB3 for AS. However, this is an extremely active area of research, and developments should be carefully followed at all times

6. ONCOR catalog numbers: D15S11, P5150; SNRPN, P5152; GABRB3, P5151.

7. There are many ways in which slides can be placed in a humidified chamber for hybridization, but slides should be kept horizontal and humidified during this step.

4.1.3. Posthybridization Stringent Washing and Detection

8. 4X SSC/Tween-20: 20X SSC 200 mL, ultra-pure water 800 mL, and Tween-20 (Sigma, catalog #P1379), 500 μL.

9. Boehringer blocking reagent (catalog #1096176): Make a 1% solution in 4X SSC/Tween-20, and place on a magnetic stirrer for 1 h. Spin the solution in a microfuge for 5 min to remove the undissolved solids. The block solution can be stored at 4°C for several weeks.

10. Digoxigenin detection reagents:

a. Antidigoxigenin (mouse monoclonal) (Boehringer catalog #133062): Dilute 1:500 in 1% Boehringer block for use. If stored at 4°C, this reagent remains stable for several weeks.

b. Antimouse-FITC (made in rabbit) (Sigma catalog #F-9137): Dilute 1:500 in 1% Boehringer block for use. If stored at 4°C, this reagent remains stable for several weeks.

c. Antirabbit-FITC (made in goat) (Sigma catalog #F-0382): Dilute 1:500 in 1% Boehringer block for use. If stored at 4°C, this reagent remains stable for several weeks.

d. If the FITC signal appears weak after this protocol, an additional layer of FITC can be added by destaining the slides with two 5-min washes in 4X SSC/Tween-20, followed by incubation in antigoat-FITC (made in rabbit) diluted 1:500 in 1% Boehringer block. This reagent should be applied as described for previous antibodies, and the slide restained (*see* Section 3.1.3., steps 13–16).

11. Vector Vectashield Mounting Medium (Antifade) catalog #H-1000.

12. It is highly recommended that the FISH staining protocol should use Shandon coverplates for the delivery of the staining reagents to the slides. This is the method described in this protocol. Alternatively, the reagents can be delivered by adding 60 µL/slide using 24 × 50 mm glass or plastic coverslip. If this method is to be used, pipet the solution onto the coverslip, and invert the slide gently touching the slide onto the solution—this helps to disperse the reagent and eliminate air bubbles. Use a slide rack and humidified chamber for all the incubations. Shandon Coverplates catalog #7211013. *See* Fig. 1 for details of how a rack can be made for use with the coverplates.

4.2. DNA Extraction

13. Small tissue samples, such as chorionic villi, or cultured cells may be extracted in Eppendorf tubes. For 30 mg of tissue (*see* Section 3.2., step 6), add 500 µL of resuspension buffer, 5 µL of 10% SDS, and 2 µL of proteinase K (50 mg/mL). Incubate as before, add 150 µL of 6*M* NaCl, shake vigorously, and centrifuge at 2000*g* for 20 min. Collect the supernate, add 2 vol of ethanol, and continue as before. If no pellet is obtained, cool to –20°C for 20 min and recentrifuge at 4°C for 30 min.
14. When possible, execute operations 1, 2, 4, and 6 in a safety cabinet.
15. Pour off supernatant into a freshly prepared 2% Virkon solution (Antec International, UK) solution, and discard after a minimum of 15 min. Ensure the pellets are broken up.

4.3. CA Repeat Analysis

16. Possible cross-contamination effects may be avoided or at least reduced by designating three separate areas or rooms for PCR kit preparations, DNA additions, and PCR product manipulations, using only designated pipeters in each area. Aerosol-resistant tips (Northumbria Biologicals Ltd.) may be used as an additional precaution. It is often beneficial to incubate DNA samples at 37°C for at least 30 min before use, particularly after freezing, to ensure the solutions are homogeneous.

    The kits are usually prepared in the multiplex format as shown, but if problems arise, it may be easier to prepare and run each primer set as separate kits at least until the problems are resolved. Similarly, if the relative intensities of primer products in the multiplex reactions are consistently unsatisfactory, it may be necessary to alter the amounts of each primer added.
17. Resolution of alleles tends to deteriorate if there is a long gap between denaturing and gel loading. Gels are prerun for at least 1 h before use and loaded when hot (50°C).
18. To prevent sticking and possible tearing of the gel on dismantling, treat the plates before every run by cleaning twice with distilled water and then twice with ethanol. The top plate is then siliconized by wiping on the siliconizing fluid with a tissue, air-dried, wiped with distilled water, and then with alcohol.

19. Ideally samples from both parents should be run with the proband. Single-band, homozygous, or hemizygous allele patterns are difficult to distinguish, and lack of a paternal contribution (PWS) or maternal contribution (AS) may signify a deletion, isodisomy, or nonpaternity (in the absence of a paternal allele). Prior FISH analysis should at least distinguish the first two situations (*see* Note 5). Further microsatellite or fingerprint studies for loci outside the PWS/AS critical regions may be considered necessary if nonpaternity is suspected. Similarly for heterodisomy (the presence of both alleles from the mother) when there is no paternal contribution, nonpaternity may need to be excluded. Rare "null" alleles have been found by some laboratories using LS6-1CA. The detection of an apparent deletion with LS6-1CA should therefore be confirmed using other markers from this region.

4.4. Methylation Analysis

20. **Caution:** Ethidium bromide is a powerful mutagen. Handle with care. Do not boil with the agarose, but add and mix just prior to pouring into the gel former.
21. A depurination stage involving a preliminary wash in 0.25M HCl for 15 min may be included before denaturation. This will slightly improve transfer of larger fragments to the nylon membrane.
22. Follow national and local safety regulations when using radioisotopes. The probe may be labeled while the filter is prehybridizing (5 min to 1 h). Whole plasmid (vector + insert) labeling, although usually successful, gave poor results with PW71b. The Stratagene kit is useful because it will efficiently amplify from most pBR322-based vectors.

    The success of the labeling reaction can be easily monitored using a G50-150 Sephadex gravity column. Soak Sephadex in TE overnight, or boil for 5 min before use. A clear separation between labeled probe and the free nucleotide peak (migrating with the red isotope dye) should easily be detected. Ten microliters of Orange G (10 mg/mL) may be added to the probe mix just prior to column addition to highlight the free nucleotide peak. Spin columns may be used as a quick alternative to gravity columns. These are available commercially or may be simply made from a 1-mL syringe. Using the syringe plunger, plug the syringe with a small ball of glass wool. Fill with Sephadex G50, and centrifuge in a 15-mL centrifuge tube with syringe flanges resting on the tube neck, at 1000g for 1 min. Discard TE from the tube, add a collecting "screw-cap" Eppendorf tube (lid removed), and replace the syringe. Add 50 µL of TE to the labeled probe, and carefully add the mix onto the G50 bed followed by another 50 µL of TE. Centrifuge at 1000g for 1.5 min. Carefully remove the Eppendorf (this can be done by opening a pair of surgical long-handled tweezers against the inside of the tube, maintaining pressure and withdrawing), replace the screw-cap lid, and heat-denature as before.
23. Methylation analysis allows direct detection of deletions or disomy without recourse to parents. At least one positive (deleted) control for PWS and/or AS and one normal control should be included with the digests. A uniparental disomy,

positive control is also useful, if available, for demonstrating dosage differences between deleted and disomy patients (Fig. 4).

The single-allele deletion or disomy pattern in PWS (larger maternally methylated allele[s] present) or in AS (smaller paternally unmethylated allele present) as opposed to the normal two-allele pattern, is diagnostic. In PWS, approx 75% of cases have deletions and 25% have maternal disomy. In AS, the absence of these pertubations does not exclude the diagnosis, since they are not detected in approx 40% of AS patients (for AS, approx 60% have deletions and 4% have paternal disomy) *(1)*.

A fainter 5.5-kb band lying between the two normal alleles and an array of faint smaller bands below the normal pattern are sometimes seen on longer autoradiograph exposures. In PWS-deleted/disomy cases, long exposures sometimes reveal a faint unmethylated "paternal-like" band, suggesting that either maternal methylation is not complete, or that excess methyl-sensitive enzyme may overcome the methyl inhibition and cut the methylated site. A single allele at this stage combined with a normal FISH pattern is indicative of uniparental disomy. However, an unusually intense signal for the single allele on the autoradiograph, relative to the concentration of ethidium-bromide stained DNA on the gel photograph, may be compared with the DNA "concentration to signal ratios" of neighboring positive (deleted) and normal control tracts, and is a useful subjective diagnostic measure. Alternatively, the filter may be hybridized (together with, or separately from, PW71b) with a nonpolymorphic probe, chosen to give a product size close to, but outside, the PW71b product size range. This allows direct signal-to-DNA concentration measurements by densitometry, working within defined calibration limits. The speed of detection of the radioactive allele patterns can be substantially improved using phosphoimaging techniques, e.g., the imaging analyzer Fujix Bas 1000/Millipore in place of standard X-ray autoradiography. A 1–2 h imaging plate exposure is equivalent to an overnight autoradiograph. This has the advantage of allowing the rapid detection and repeat of failed tests, increasing the rate of overall throughput.

References

1. Cassidy, S. B. (1992) Conference report—first international scientific workshop on Prader-Willi Syndrome and other chromosome 15q deletion disorders. *Am. J. Med. Genet.* **42,** 220–230.
2. Delach, J. A., Rosengren, S. S., Kaplan, L., Greenstein, R. M, Cassidy, S. B., and Benn, P. A. (1994) Comparison of high resolution chromosome banding and fluorescence in situ hybridization (FISH) for the laboratory evaluation of Prader-Willi Syndrome and Angelman Syndrome. *Am. J. Med. Genet.* **52,** 85–91.
3. Mutirangura, A., Greenberg, F., Butler, M. G., Malcolm, S., Nicholls, R. D., Chakravarti, A., and Ledbetter, D. H. (1993) Multiplex PCR of 3 dinucleotide repeats in the Prader-Willi–Angelman critical region (15q11–q13)—molecular diagnosis and mechanism of uniparental disomy. *Hum. Mol. Genet.* **2,** 143–151.

4. Dittrich, B., Robinson, W. P., Knoblauch, H., Buiting, K., Schmidt, K., Gillessen-kaesbach, G., and Horsthemke, B. (1992) Molecular diagnosis of the Prader-Willi and Angelman Syndromes by detection of parent-of-origin specific DNA methylation in 15q11-13. *Hum. Genet.* **90**, 313–315.

5. Dittrich, B., Buiting, K., Gross, S., and Horsthemke, B. (1993) Characterization of a methylation imprint in the Prader-Willi Syndrome chromosome region. *Hum. Mol. Genet.* **2**, 1995–1999.

6. Ozcelik, T., Leff, S., Robinson, W., Donlon, T., Lalande, M., Sanjines, E., Schinzel, A., and Francke, U. (1992) Small nuclear ribonucleoprotein polypeptide N (SNRPN), an expressed gene in the Prader-Willi syndrome critical region. *Nature Genet.* **2**, 265–269.

7. Buiting, K., Dittrich, B., Robinson, W. P., Guitart, M., Abeliovich, D., Lerer, I., and Horsthemke, B. (1994) Detection of aberrant DNA methylation in unique Prader-Willi syndrome patients and its diagnostic implications. *Hum. Mol. Genet.* **3**, 893–895.

8. Mutirangura, A., Kuwano, A., Ledbetter, S. A., Chinault, A. C., and Ledbetter, D. H. (1992) Dinucleotide repeat polymorphism at the D15S11 locus in the Angelman/Prader-Willi region (AS/PWS) of chromosome 15. *Hum. Mol. Genet.* **1**, 139.

9. Malcolm, S. and Donlon, T. A. (1994) Report of the second international workshop on human chromosome 15 mapping 1994. *Cytogenet. Cell Genet.* **67**, 2–22.

10. Mutirangura, A., Ledbetter, S. A., Kuwano, A., Chinault, A. C., and Ledbetter, D. H. (1992) Dinucleotide repeat polymorphism at the GABAa receptor beta3 (GABRB3) locus in the Angelman/Prader-Willi region (AS/PWS) of chromosome 15. *Hum. Mol. Genet.* **1(1)**, 67.

13

Noninvasive Prenatal Diagnosis
Using Fetal Cells in Maternal Blood

Y. M. Dennis Lo

1. Introduction

It has been a long-sought goal of human genetics to develop safe and reliable prenatal diagnostic procedures that constitute no risk to the fetus. At present, the safety of available methods is limited by the need to obtain fetal tissues through invasive means, such as chorionic villus sampling (CVS) and amniocentesis, which constitute a risk to the fetus. One potential noninvasive approach for prenatal diagnosis is to use fetal cells that have entered into maternal circulation during pregnancy as a source of fetal material for analysis.

There are several reports suggesting the existence of fetal cells in maternal blood during pregnancy (reviewed in refs. *1* and *2*), but the first molecular evidence that fetal genetic materials can be detected in maternal circulation had to await the development of the polymerase chain reaction (PCR) *(3)*. In 1989, Lo et al. *(4)* used a nested PCR system to detect a Y repeat from peripheral blood DNA from 19 pregnant women. All 12 pregnant women whose samples gave rise to a positive Y signal later gave birth to boys, whereas all 7 whose samples were negative gave birth to girls. This provided the first molecular proof that fetal nucleated cells do indeed circulate in maternal blood and that genetic information regarding the fetus can be obtained from analyzing maternal peripheral blood. Since then a number of groups have confirmed these observations using a number of Y-specific sequences as targets for amplification *(5,6)* (for review, *see* ref. *1*).

Following the success using Y-specific PCR, investigators then turned their attention to the possibility of diagnosing autosomal disorders using a similar approach. Since the fetal cells in maternal circulation are surrounded by a great excess of maternal cells, the use of the PCR for autosomal fetal gene detection

From: *Methods in Molecular Medicine: Molecular Diagnosis of Genetic Diseases*
Edited by: R. Elles Humana Press Inc., Totowa, NJ

is limited to the detection of fetal-derived, paternally inherited sequences. Because of the limits in the specificity of the PCR (for review, *see* ref. *7*), the most successful systems to date are from clinical scenarios where there exists a unique paternally inherited DNA sequence, which is possessed by the fetus but not by the mother.

The first example is the detection of a paternally inherited hemoglobin Lepore-Boston gene from maternal peripheral blood *(8)*. The Lepore-Boston gene is caused by the fusion of the 5' half of the δ-globin gene and the 3' half of the β-globin gene, together with a 7-kb deletion between these two fusion partners. This constitutes a good target for PCR amplification.

The second example is the detection of fetal-derived rhesus D gene from the peripheral blood of rhesus D negative pregnant women *(9,10)*. This approach is possible because the rhesus negative mother does not possess the rhesus D gene *(11,12)*, and thus, the system is directly analogous to that of the Y chromosome system. The noninvasive prenatal determination of fetal rhesus D status has potential clinical implications in the management of previously sensitized rhesus negative women with a partner heterozygous for the rhesus D gene. Hence, if the fetus can be shown to be rhesus D negative, then no further prenatal diagnostic and therapeutic procedure is necessary.

The further extension of this noninvasive approach to detect paternally inherited DNA polymorphisms that differ from those of the mother by one or several nucleotides is much more demanding on the specificity of the PCR. This can, however, be implemented by the use of systems based on the amplification refractory mutation system (ARMS) *(13)*. ARMS enables the PCR to be discriminatory down to a single-nucleotide level. It is based on the principle that the specificity of the PCR is conferred by the 3' end of the primers. Thus, if there is a 3'-terminal mismatch between a PCR primer and the DNA target, then the amplification efficiency will be greatly reduced. When using ARMS to detect paternally inherited polymorphisms of the fetus from maternal peripheral blood, ARMS primers are designed such that the last base of the primer matches the paternal allele, but has a 3'-terminal mismatch with the maternal alleles. It is important to realize that ARMS only confers relative selectivity for the detection of fetal-specific sequence. In other words, the mismatched allele will also be amplified, although with reduced efficiency compared with the matched one. Hence, one is faced with a dilemma when applying ARMS to the detection of an extremely small amount of fetal genetic materials from maternal blood: The small quantities of fetal material require the use of a large number of PCR cycles; however, this high degree of cycling means that the extent to which this mismatched reaction will take place is also increased. With further development in ARMS technology, such as the double ARMS *(14)*, one is able to achieve the goal of detecting a minority DNA population at a level of

1 in 10^5 or below. Using double ARMS, it has recently been shown that a paternally inherited polymorphism in the β -globin locus can be detected from maternal blood *(15)*. This latter system may potentially be used for the diagnosis of β-thalassemia.

It can be seen that the PCR has been instrumental in proving that fetal cells do indeed circulate in maternal blood during pregnancy and that certain prenatal genetic analysis may be possible using PCR alone. However, the precision of noninvasive prenatal diagnosis using this approach has not reached the level sufficient for clinical use. This has prompted a number of investigators to pursue approaches for enriching for circulating fetal cells prior to genetic analysis.

At present, three populations of fetal cells are thought to be candidates for enrichment from maternal blood, namely nucleated red blood cells (NRBC), trophoblasts, and lymphocytes *(1,2)*. Current data suggest that NRBCs are the most promising candidate cell type. This approach was first pioneered by Bianchi et al. *(16)*, who used the fluorescence-activated cell sorter (FACS) and antitransferrin receptor antibody to enrich NRBCs prior to genetic analysis using the PCR. Since then, variations of this theme have been adopted by many investigators using other markers or combinations of markers *(17,18)*, or other enrichment techniques, such as the magnetic activated cell sorter (MACS) *(19,20)*. Using these techniques encouraging data on fetal sex diagnosis *(16,17)*, diagnosis of chromosomal aneuploidies *(17,21,22)* and detection of fetal-derived autosomal sequences *(23)* have been reported. Further developments in fetal cell enrichment techniques will be expected to complement techniques based on the PCR and *in situ* hybridization to improve the diagnostic accuracy of this approach.

In the following sections, the use of the PCR to detect fetal-derived DNA sequences using a Y-specific sequence and the rhesus D gene as examples is outlined. Technical problems are then discussed. Similar methodological considerations can be applied to the use of the PCR for detecting other minority nucleic acid populations.

2. Materials

1. A thermal cycler is necessary for the PCR. The author uses either a Biometra (Göttingen, Germany) TRIO thermoblock or a Perkin-Elmer Cetus DNA Thermal Cycler.
2. Reagents for the PCR, including the *Thermus aquaticus (Taq)* DNA polymerase, deoxynucleotides (dNTPs), Ampliwax for Hot Start PCR *(24)*, and PCR buffer are obtained from a GeneAmp DNA Amplification Reagent Kit (Perkin-Elmer, Emeryville, CA).
3. Oligonucleotide primers for the PCR were obtained from Genosys (Cambridge, UK). Two PCR systems are described as examples, namely the amplification of the DYS14 locus (a Y-specific sequence) *(25)* and the amplification of the rhesus

Fig. 1. Schematic diagram showing the location of the primers for the DYS14 amplification system.

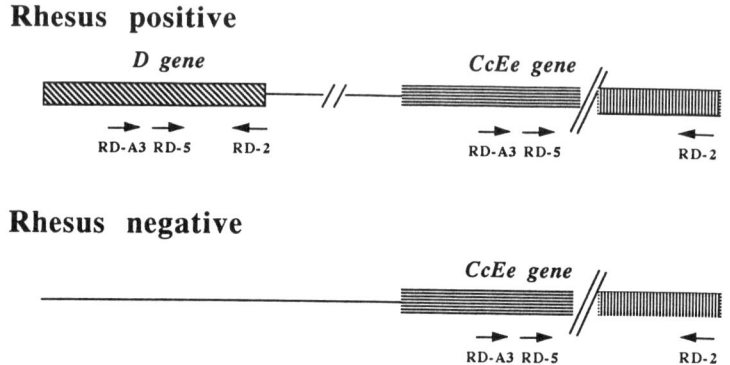

Fig. 2. Schematic representation showing the difference in the structure of the rhesus locus in RhD-positive and RhD-negative individuals. Primer locations are marked in the diagram.

D gene *(12)*. Primer sequences are listed here, and primer locations are shown in Figs. 1 and 2. The primer combinations Y1.5/Y1.6 (product size 239 bp) and Y1.7/Y1.8 (product size 198 bp) are nested with respect to one another, being the external and internal pair, respectively. The primer combinations RD-A3/RD2 (product size 291 bp) and RD-5/RD-2 (product size 262 bp) are both specific for the RhD gene and are heminested with respect to each other, with the latter primer combination being the internal set.

Primer sequences:

Y1.5: 5'CTA GAC CGC AGA GGC GCC AT3'
Y1.6: 5'TAG TAC CCA CGC CTG CTC CGG3'
Y1.7: 5'CAT CCA GAG CGT CCC TGG CTT3'
Y1.8: 5'CTT TCC ACA GCC ACA TTT GTC3'
RD-A3: 5'GGA TTT TAA GCA AAA GCA TCC AAG AA3'
RD-2: 5'ACT GGA TGA CCA CCA TCA TAT3'
RD-5: 5'CAA GGC CTG TTC AAA AAC AAG3'

3. Methods

1. Collect peripheral blood samples from pregnant women either into EDTA or lithium heparin tubes. Perform DNA extraction by the standard proteinase K, phenol-chloroform method (*see* Note 1) *(26)*. Carry all extraction, and set up procedures in a laminar flow cabinet (*see* Notes 2–8).
2. Set up PCR in 100-μL reaction volumes with 5 U of *Taq* DNA-polymerase in each tube. $MgCl_2$ concentration for the DYS14 and RhD systems has been optimized at 1.5 m*M*. Use 1–5 μg of genomic DNA extracted from pregnant women/reaction (*see* Note 9). For Y-specific PCR using primer combinations Y1.5/Y1.6 and Y1.7/Y1.8, first-round PCR consists of 40 cycles of 94°C 1 min, 55°C 1 min, and 72°C 1 min using the primer pair Y1.5 and Y1.6. Transfer 2 μL of the first-round PCR product into fresh reagents, and reamplify for 25 cycles using the same thermal profile with the internal primer pair Y1.7 and Y1.8. For RhD amplification from maternal peripheral blood, 50 cycles of Ampliwax-mediated Hot Start PCR (*see* Note 10) are carried out using RD-A3 and RD-2. Reamplify 2 μL of this first-round reaction using RD-5 and RD-2 for a further 10 cycles using the same cycling parameters.
3. Electrophorese 10 μL of PCR products using a 1.5% ethidium bromide-stained agarose gel. Visualize PCR products under UV transillumination.

4. Notes

1. Great care should be taken during DNA extraction, since the labor-intensive nature of conventional DNA extraction protocols provides many opportunities for the introduction of contaminants. We have tested a number of commercially available DNA extraction kits and have found the Nucleon system from Scotlabs (Strathclyde, Scotland) to be fast, efficient, and to involve a smaller number of steps than the conventional proteinase K/phenol-chloroform extraction method.
2. The main strength of the PCR, namely its sensitivity, is also its chief weakness, since it is extremely prone to false-positive results owing to contamination *(27,28)*. This disadvantage is especially obvious in applications requiring the highest sensitivity, such as in the detection of fetal cells in maternal blood. Thus, for the performance of noninvasive prenatal diagnosis using PCR, a lot of effort should be directed toward avoiding and detecting contamination.
3. Negative controls should be included in every PCR experiment. In many situations, multiple controls are preferred. Negative controls should include water blanks to test for reagent contamination as well as appropriate genomic DNA controls, e.g., female cord blood DNA for the DYS14 system and rhesus negative male DNA for the RhD system.
4. Physical separation of the pre- and post-PCR areas should be instituted. The use of a laminar flow cabinet is recommended for setting up the PCR.
5. All PCR reagents should be aliquoted, and reagents that could be autoclaved should be so treated.
6. Gloves, face, and head masks are recommended.

7. Separate pipet sets should be allocated to the DNA extraction phase, PCR setting up phase, and post-PCR phase. Pipet tips with filters should be used.

8. When multiple reactions are needed, a master mix should be set up to reduce the number of maneuvers and thus reduce the chance of possible contamination. One method that has been found to be useful for destroying contaminating sequence is restriction enzyme treatment. Restriction enzymes that cleave within the target sequence for PCR may be used to restrict any contaminating sequence prior to the addition of the target *(4)*. Following decontamination, the enzyme should be destroyed by thermal denaturation (e.g., 94°C for 10 min) before addition of the template DNA.

9. The amount of DNA used for PCR is important, since this quantity is a reflection of the number of maternal cells (and hence the volume of maternal blood) among which one is searching for the minority fetal cells. Thus, if the amount of DNA is reduced, then one is effectively reducing the chance of finding the rare fetal cells. Since 1 μg of genomic DNA corresponds to approx 150,000 diploid cells, at single molecule sensitivity, this corresponds to a sensitivity of 1 in 150,000. This consideration, however, has to be balanced against the fact that increasing the amount of DNA will lead to the increase in the number of nonspecific amplification bands and to the increase in PCR inhibition owing to inhibitors existing in genomic DNA. As a guide, maternal DNA from 1–5 μg provides satisfactory results.

10. An alternative to the nested PCR strategy is the use of hot start PCR *(24)*. In this technique, the PCR reagents are separated by a plug of wax that melts in the PCR block at an elevated temperature, preventing the formation of nonspecific PCR products. This enables the achievement of single molecule sensitivity in the RhD system following just one round of 50 PCR cycles. Note that although a second round of hemi-nested PCR is also used in the RhD system, this second amplification reaction is only used for confirmatory purposes, to prove that the signal obtained after the first-round PCR is indeed owing to the amplification of the RhD gene. The use of hot start PCR for prenatal sex determination has also been described *(29)*. In general, hot start PCR can be regarded as equivalent in sensitivity and specificity to nested PCR, except that the former is more sensitive to slight change in amplification conditions. Thus, a hot start system may take more time to optimize than the more tolerant nested system.

Acknowledgment

The author is supported by a Career Development Fellowship by the Wellcome Trust.

References

1. Lo, Y. M. D. (1994) Noninvasive prenatal diagnosis using fetal cells in maternal blood. *J. Clin. Pathol.* **47,** 1060–1065.

2. Simpson, J. L. and Elias, S. (1993) Isolating fetal cells from maternal blood: advances in prenatal diagnosis through molecular technology. *JAMA* **270,** 2357–2361.

3. Saiki, R. K., Gelfand, D. H., Stoffel, S., Scharf, S. J., Higuchi, R., Horn, G. T., et al. (1988) Primer-directed enzymatic amplification of DNA with a thermostable DNA polymerase. *Science* **239,** 487–491.

4. Lo, Y. M. D., Patel, P., Wainscoat, J. S., Sampietro, M., Gillmer, M. D. G., and Fleming, K. A. (1989) Prenatal sex determination by DNA amplification from maternal peripheral blood. *Lancet* **2**, 1363–1365.

5. Kao, S. M., Tang, G. C., Hsieh, T. T., Young, K. C., Wang, H. C., and Pao, C. C. (1992) Analysis of peripheral blood of pregnant women for the presence of fetal Y chromosome-specific ZFY gene deoxyribonucleic acid sequences. *Am. J. Obstet. Gynecol.* **166**, 1013–1019.

6. Hamada, H., Arinami, T., Kubo, T., Hamaguchi, H., and Iwasaki, H. (1993) Fetal nucleated cells in maternal peripheral blood: frequency and relationship to gestational age. *Hum. Genet.* **91**, 427–432.

7. Lo, Y. M. D. (1994) Detection of minority nucleic acid populations by PCR—a review. *J. Pathol.* **174**, 1–6.

8. Camaschella, C., Alfarano, A., Gottardi, E., Travi, M., Primignani, P., Caligaris, C. F., and Saglio, G. (1990) Prenatal diagnosis of fetal hemoglobin Lepore-Boston disease on maternal peripheral blood. *Blood* **75**, 2102–2106.

9. Lo, Y. M. D., Bowell, P. J., Selinger, M., MacKenzie, I. Z., Chamberlain, P., Gillmer, et al. (1993) Prenatal determination of fetal RhD status by analysis of peripheral blood of rhesus negative mothers. *Lancet* **341**, 1147,1148.

10. Lo, Y. M. D., Noakes, L., Bowell, P. J., Fleming, K. A., and Wainscoat, J. S. (1994) Detection of fetal RhD sequence from peripheral blood of sensitised RhD-negative pregnant women. *Br. J. Haematol.* **87**, 658–660.

11. Colin, Y., Chérif-Zahar, B., Le Van Kim, C., Raynal, V., van Huffel, V., and Cartron, J.-P. (1991) Genetic basis of the RhD-positive and RhD-negative blood group polymorphism as determined by Southern analysis. *Blood* **78**, 2747–2752.

12. Le Van Kim, C., Mouro, I., Chérif-Zahar, B., Raynal, V., Cherrier, C., Cartron, J.-P., and Colin, Y. (1992) Molecular cloning and primary structure of the human blood group RhD polypeptide. *Proc. Natl. Acad. Sci. USA* **89**, 10,925–10,929.

13. Newton, C. R., Graham, A., Heptinstall, L. E., Powell, S. J., Summers, C., Kalsheker, N., et al. (1989) Analysis of any point mutation in DNA. The amplification refractory mutation system (ARMS). *Nucleic Acids Res.* **17**, 2503–2516.

14. Lo, Y. M. D., Patel, P., Newton, C. R., Markham, A. F., Fleming, K. A., and Wainscoat, J. S. (1991) Direct haplotype determination by double ARMS: specificity, sensitivity and genetic applications. *Nucleic Acids Res.* **19**, 3561–3567.

15. Lo, Y. M. D., Fleming, K. A., and Wainscoat, J. S. (1994) Strategies for the detection of autosomal fetal DNA sequence from maternal peripheral blood. *Ann. NY Acad. Sci.* **731**, 204–213.

16. Bianchi, D. W., Flint, A. F., Pizzimenti, M. F., Knoll, J. H., and Latt, S. A. (1990) Isolation of fetal DNA from nucleated erythrocytes in maternal blood. *Proc. Natl. Acad. Sci. USA* **87**, 3279–3283.

17. Price, J. O., Elias, S., Wachtel, S. S., Klinger, K., Dockter, M., Tharapel, A., et al. (1991) Prenatal diagnosis with fetal cells isolated from maternal blood by multi-parameter flow cytometry. *Am. J. Obstet. Gynecol.* **165**, 1731–1737.

18. Bianchi, D. W., Zickwolf, G. K., Yih, M. C., Flint, A. F., Geifman, O. H., Erikson, M. S., and Williams, J. M. (1993) Erythroid-specific antibodies enhance detection of fetal nucleated erythrocytes in maternal blood. *Prenat. Diagn.* **13,** 293–300.

19. Gänshirt-Ahlert, D., Börjesson-Stoll, R., Burschyk, M., Dohr, A., Garritsen, H. S. P., Helmer, E., et al. (1993) Detection of fetal trisomies 21 and 18 from maternal blood using triple gradient and magnetic cell sorting. *AJRI* **30,** 193–200.

20. Zheng, Y. L., Carter, N. P., Price, C. M., Colman, S. M., Milton, P. J., Hackett, G. A., et al. (1993) Prenatal diagnosis from maternal blood: simultaneous immuno-phenotyping and FISH of fetal nucleated erythrocytes isolated by negative magnetic cell sorting. *J. Med. Genet.* **30,** 1051–1056.

21. Bianchi, D. W., Mahr, A., Zickwolf, G. K., Houseal, T. W., Flint, A. F., and Klinger, K. W. (1992) Detection of fetal cells with 47,XY,+21 karyotype in maternal peripheral blood. *Hum. Genet.* **90,** 368–370.

22. Elias, S., Price, J., Dockter, M., Wachtel, S., Tharapel, A., and Simpson, J. L. (1992) First trimester prenatal diagnosis of trisomy 21 in fetal cells from maternal blood. *Lancet* **340,** 1033.

23. Geifman-Holtzman, O., Holtzman, E. J., Vadnais, T. J., Phillips, V. E., Capeless, E. L., and Bianchi, D. W. (1995) Detection of fetal HLA-DQ-alpha sequences in maternal blood—a gender-independent technique of fetal cell identification. *Prenat. Diagn.* **15,** 261–268.

24. Chou, Q., Russell, M., Birch, D. E., Raymond, J., and Bloch, W. (1992) Prevention of pre-PCR mis-priming and primer dimerization improves low-copy-number amplifications. *Nucleic Acids Res.* **20,** 1717–1723.

25. Arnemann, J., Epplen, J. T., Cooke, H. J., Sauermann, U., Engel, W., and Schmidtke, J. (1987) A human Y-chromosomal DNA sequence expressed in testicular tissue. *Nucleic Acids Res.* **15,** 8713–8724.

26. Maniatis, T., Fritsch, E. F., and Sambrook, J. (1982) *Molecular Cloning: A Laboratory Manual.* Cold Spring Harbor Laboratory, Cold Spring Harbor, NY.

27. Lo, Y. M. D., Mehal, W. Z., and Fleming, K. A. (1988) False-positive results and the polymerase chain reaction. *Lancet* **2,** 679.

28. Kwok, S. and Higuchi, R. (1989) Avoiding false positives with PCR. *Nature* **339,** 237,238.

29. Lo, Y. M. D., Schmidtke, J., Wainscoat, J. S., and Fleming, K. A. (1994) An improved PCR-based system for prenatal sex determination from maternal peripheral blood. *Ann. NY Acad. Sci.* **731,** 214–216.

14

PCR from Single Cells
for Preimplantation Diagnosis

Pierre F. Ray and Alan H. Handyside

1. Introduction

The detection of genetic defects in human embryos following in vitro fertilization (IVF) or preimplantation genetic diagnosis (PGD) allows the selection and transfer of unaffected embryos in couples known to be at risk of transmitting an inherited disorder. This avoids the need to terminate an affected pregnancy, following prenatal diagnosis at later stages *(1)*. Diagnosis of a single gene defect is usually performed on one or two single cells (blastomeres) biopsied from 8- to 10-cell embryos on the 3rd d postinsemination using nested polymerase chain reaction (PCR) to amplify informative fragments. Nested PCR allows amplification from a limited number of target sequences *(2)*, and under carefully optimized conditions, amplification of as few as one or two target copies present in a single haploid or diploid cell is possible *(3–5)*. PGD was first achieved for X-linked diseases by determining the sex of the embryos using a Y chromosome-specific repetitive sequence and selective transfer of only female embryos *(6)*. More recently, specific diagnosis has been achieved for cystic fibrosis (CF), by amplifying across the cystic fibrosis transmembrane regulator (CFTR) gene ΔF508 locus *(7)* and for Lesch-Nyhan syndrome by amplifying across a familial base substitution nullifying a natural *Xho*I restriction site in the hypoxanthine phophoribosyl transferase (HPRT) gene *(8)*. In both instances, nested PCR strategies were chosen to amplify the mutated sequence allowing sufficient amplification for detection on ethidium bromide-stained gels. The limited cycling with the outer primers (20 cycles) reduces nonspecific amplification, and only specific fragments that contain the complementary sequence to the internal primers are amplified to a detectable level in the second round of PCR. Although extra handling is involved, any

From: *Methods in Molecular Medicine: Molecular Diagnosis of Genetic Diseases*
Edited by: R. Elles Humana Press Inc., Totowa, NJ

245

genomic contaminant introduced after the first round of amplification would not be amplified to a detectable level by the inner primers alone. The efficiency of the second amplification is improved because the denaturation of the first amplification product (amplicon) is easier. Also, the great excess of these amplicons compared with nonspecific sequences eliminates competition, thereby enhancing specificity and yield.

Lesch-Nyhan syndrome is caused by heterogeneous mutations in the HPRT gene on the X-chromosome. In one family, sequencing revealed a basepair substitution in exon 3 of the HPRT gene, which deleted a natural *Xho*I restriction site (Hughes, personal communication). After nested amplification of a 158-bp fragment surrounding the mutation and restriction with *Xho*I, a diagnosis could be made by analyzing the pattern of digestion. Fully digested and undigested products corresponded, respectively, to homozygous unaffected and affected (male), whereas partial digestion was characteristic of heterozygous female cells. The test was applied successfully, and PGD resulted in the birth of a healthy unaffected baby girl *(8)*. The described primers could be used for other mutations located in exon 3 of the HPRT gene that are encompassed by the inner primers. In that case, only the detection system would have to be modified, and single-stranded conformational polymorphism (SSCP) could be used for mutations that do not affect restriction sites.

To date, we have performed PGD for 12 couples in which both partners carry the ΔF508 mutation in a total of 18 cycles. This resulted in five singleton births confirmed to be homozygous normal *(9)*. Single blastomeres from disaggregated embryos that had not been transferred were analyzed to confirm the original diagnosis and assess reliability in clinical practice. Amplification efficiency and accuracy were high with blastomeres from embryos diagnosed as homozygous normal or affected. In a proportion of blastomeres from presumed carrier embryos, one of the parental alleles failed to amplify, apparently at random (allele dropout [ADO]), despite preliminary results with single-cell analysis of the ΔF508 locus, which indicated high efficiency and 100% accuracy *(10)*. Further investigation of single lymphocytes confirmed the occurrence of ADO, and showed that it can be reduced using stringent cell lysis conditions and by increasing the denaturation temperature to 96°C during the first few cycles of amplification *(11)*. This stresses the importance of control experiments on heterozygous cells and optimization with individual thermocyclers, especially if single-cell diagnosis is to be applied to dominant disorders since this kind of error could lead to serious misdiagnosis. Although good amplification rates were obtained, with both thermal and chemical lysis protocols on blastomeres and lymphocytes, the use of lysis buffer appeared to reduce the occurrence of ADO. We therefore recommend its use, especially for clinical applications of single-cell PCR.

For diseases caused by heterogeneous mutations, analysis of several loci would be an advantage. However, multiplex PCR has not proven reliable at the single-cell level because of the difficulties involved in optimizing the reaction conditions for more than one pair of primers. Zhang and colleagues *(12)*, using random 15 mers in a modified PCR reaction, primer extension preamplification (PEP), demonstrated that at least 30 copies of any specific DNA fragment from >78% of the genome can be produced from a single cell. Small aliquots from the PEP reaction can then be reamplified with specific primers, thus allowing analysis, for example, of two independent mutations or flanking linked informative markers. The latter would be particularly useful for patients with uncharacterized mutations, but with an informative pedigree. Closely linked markers, such as variable copy number tandem repeats (VNTR) *(13,14)* are multiallelic polymorphisms with a polymorphic information content (PIC) often >0.7, which make them ideal candidates for linkage analysis. Unfortunately, their amplification and the identification of the different alleles are often difficult because of amplification of extra bands (stutter bands) possibly generated by the slippage of the *Taq* polymerase while copying the repeats. We amplified two CA repeats located at the 3' and 5' ends of the dystrophin gene, as an approach to the diagnosis of Duchenne muscular dystrophy (DMD) *(15)*. Although good amplification efficiency could be obtained after PEP, separation of the alleles could not be achieved reliably. By contrast, Kristjansson and colleagues *(16)* amplified five commonly deleted exons in the dystrophin gene as well as the X/Y-linked genes, *ZFX* and *ZFY*, to provide a test informative for most of the DMD carriers. In conclusion, although the use of VNTRs is very promising, the amplification of such repeated sequences (and especially that of dinucleotide repeats) from a single cell is technically very difficult. When possible, it might be safer to perform a direct analysis (such as those described for CF or Lesch-Nyhan) or to use a combination of less informative, but more reliable longer repeats or restriction fragment length polymorphisms (RFLPs).

The use of a more sensitive detection system, like DNA fluorescent analysis using labeled primers, could be of great advantage for single-cell PCR. It precludes the need for nesting, and the reduced number of cycles could allow for reliable multiplex PCR even from a single cell. Findlay et al. *(17,18)* suggested its use for DNA fingerprinting as a control for contamination, and described a single-cell protocol for the detection of ΔF508 and the determination of sex.

At present, only 14 centers have attempted PGD, and clinical experience is therefore limited *(19)*. Overall, 197 PGD cycles have resulted in 50 (25%) clinical pregnancies. Most of these were for X-linked diseases, and involved identification of sex either by PCR or fluorescent *in situ* hybridization (FISH). Among these, one misdiagnosis resulted from amplification failure of the Y-repeat. Subsequently, this has been avoided using other protocols that simultaneously amplify X and Y sequences. Two misdiagnoses of CF have also been reported. In these cases, only one partner carried the ΔF508 deletion; the other partner carried a different mutation. The reason for these errors is not clear, but may have included ADO or contamination possibly by sperm DNA. Any attempt to detect compound heterozygotes should therefore be extensively tested on appropriate single cells.

2. Materials
2.1. Single-Cell Preparation
2.1.1. Lymphocyte Preparation

1. Ficoll-Paque (Pharmacia, St. Albans, Hertsfordshire, UK).
2. Phosphate-buffered saline (PBS) (Gibco BRL, Glasgow, UK).
3. Crystallized bovine serum albumin (BSA) (ICN Immuno Biologicals, Thame, Oxfordshire, UK).

2.1.2. Blastomere Preparation and Biopsy

1. Silicone fluid (Dow Corning 299/50 cs, BDH Chemicals Ltd, Poole, Dorset, UK)
2. Acid Tyrode's solution: 2 g NaCl, 0.05 g KCl, 0.06 g $CaCl_2 \cdot 2H_2O$, 0.025 g $MgCl_2 \cdot 6H_2O$, 0.25 g glucose (all from BDH Chemicals, Poole, Dorset, UK), and 1 g polyvinylpyrrolidone (PVP; Calbiochem, Nottingham, UK), dialyzed against PBS and lyophilized in <250 mL of H_2O. Note that the PVP should be sprinkled and allowed to dissolve. Adjust to pH 2.2 by adding a very small amount of $5M$ HCl and make up the volume to 250 mL by adding more H_2O (high-quality water; FL (manufacturing) Ltd., Fresenius Health Care Group, Basingstoke, UK). The solution should be aliquoted and stored at −20°C.

2.2. PCR

"In-house" buffers and water are filtered using a 0.22-μm filter (Millipore, Molsheim, France) and autoclaved. All of the following are aliquoted and stored at −20°C:

1. Ampli-*Taq* DNA-polymerase 5 U/μL (Applied Biosystems, Warrington, Cheshire, UK).
2. 10X PCR buffer II: 500 m*M* KCl, 100 m*M* Tris HCl, pH 8.3 (Applied Biosystems).
3. 25 m*M* $MgCl_2$ (Applied Biosystems)
4. Lysis buffer (LB): 200 m*M* KOH, 50 m*M* dithiothreitol (DTT) *(20)*.
5. Neutralizing buffer (NB): 900 m*M* Tris HCl, pH 8.3, 300 m*M* KCl, 200 m*M* HCl *(20)*.
6. 10X PCR [K⁺] free: 25 m*M* $MgCl_2$, gelatine 1 mg/mL, 100 m*M* Tris HCl, pH 8.3 *(12)*, used in conjunction with LB and NB.
7. dNTP Mixture (Pharmacia): 10 m*M* stock (100-fold dilution).
8. Mineral oil (Applied Biosystems).
9. Thin-wall PCR tubes (Sorenson Bioscience, Inc., Salt Lake City, UT).
10. Oligonucleotide primers were synthesized by Pharmacia. The nucleotide sequence of the different primer sets is shown in Table 1. They were diluted and stored at a concentration of 40 μ*M*.

Table 1
Nucleotide Sequence and Cycling Conditions of the Different Primer Sets[a]

Primer	Sequence, 5'→3'	Expected size, bp	Cycling conditions	No. of cycles
CF ΔF508[b]				
Outer	GAC TTC ACT TCT AAT GAT GAT CTC TTC TAG TTG GCA TGC	193	96°/94°C for 45 s 40°C for 45 s 72°C for 90 s	10 then 12
Inner	TGG GAG AAC TGGAGC CTT GCT TTG ATG ACG CTT CTG TAT	154/151	94°C for 45 s 50°C for 45 s 72°C for 90 s	30
HPRT exon 3				
Outer	GCA GGC ATG GGG TCT CAC GCC CCC CTT GAG CAC ACA	199	94°C for 30 s 52°C for 45 s 72°C for 90 s	20
Inner	TTG CCC AGG TTG GTG TGG AA AGG GCT ACA ATG TGA TGG CC	158	93°C for 30 s 52°C for 45 s 72°C for 90 s	30
Amelogenin[c]				
Outer	CTG ATG GTT GGC CTC AAG CCT GTG TAA AGA GAT TCA TTA ACT TGA CTG	X Band: 927 Y Band: 738	94°C for 30 s 58°C for 60 s 72°C for 60 s	28
Inner	TGA CCA GCT TGG TTC TA(A/T) CCC CA(A/G) ATG AG(A/G) AAA CCA GGG TTC CA	X Band: 290 Y Band: 105	94°C for 30 s 68°C for 90 s 72°C for 30 s	35

[a]All the cycling parameters indicated in the table for the different primer sets were preceded by an initial 3-s denaturation step at 94°C and included a final extension step of 5 s at 72°C.
[b]Described in ref. 7.
[c]The outer primers were described in ref. 21, and the inner primers were a gift from Roger Mountford (St. Mary's Hospital, Manchester, UK).

11. Random 15 mers for whole genome amplification by PEP were synthesized using a Cyclon Milligene synthesizer. Because the synthesis reaction is initiated by one specific nucleotide bound to the column, and no column coated with all four nucleotides is available, the last nucleotide at the 3' end of the oligonucleotide could not be random. Therefore, for all 15 nucleotides to be completely random, where N is any nucleotide, the following four oligonucleotides, $[N]_{14}$-A, $[N]_{14}$-C $[N]_{14}$-T, and $[N]_{14}$-G were mixed in equimolar amounts to obtain a 400 μM stock.

12. Temperature cycling was performed on a Perkin Elmer/Cetus DNA Thermal cycler model.

2.3. Gel Electrophoresis

2.3.1. Polyacrylamide Gel Electrophoresis

1. Acrylamide–bis-acrylamide 29:1 (v/v) (Bio-Rad, Hemel Hempstead, Hertfordshire, UK).
2. *N,N,N',N'*-tetramethylethylenediamine (TEMED) (Sigma, UK), store at 4°C.
3. 10% (w/v) Ammonium persulfate (Sigma), store at 4°C for no more than 1 wk.
4. 10X TBE (Tris base, boric acid, EDTA from Sigma), store at room temperature.
5. Loading buffer: 0.25% (w/v) bromophenol blue, 0.25% (w/v) xylene cyanole, 40% (w/v) sucrose (Sigma).

2.3.2. Heteroduplex Formation for Δ F508

Preamplified DNA from homozygous normal and ΔF508 cells, premixed with loading buffer.

2.4. Restriction Digestion (Lesch-Nyhan Syndrome)

*Xho*I enzyme and 10X buffer (Promega, Southampton, UK).

3. Methods

3.1. Single-Cell Preparation

3.1.1. General Code of Practice for Single-Cell Preparation

Single cells or blastomeres are handled in a clean laboratory (overshoes and gown are worn at all times) with restricted access, and no DNA work is performed in this room (*see* Notes 1 and 2).

3.1.2. Blastomere Preparation

Blastomeres are either obtained by micromanipulation of cleavage-stage embryos *(22)* or for research purposes by disaggregating the whole embryo under a binocular microscope with a mouth tube and pulled Pasteur pipet as follows:

1. Remove the zona pellucida from cleavage-stage embryos with acid Tyrode's solution, pH 2.2, for 10–30 s at room temperature, and return the embryo immediately to an excess of HEPES-buffered embryo culture medium.

2. Separate the blastomeres by gentle pipeting using a pulled, flamed polished glass capillary.
3. Rinse the pipet thoroughly by pipeting PBS in and out.
4. Introduce the blastomeres into individual microcentrifuge tubes containing 5 μL of lysis buffer with minimal medium. Rinse the pipet as before between each blastomere manipulation.
5. After tubing blastomeres from individual embryos, prepare one or two control blanks by introducing a small volume of the medium that had contained the blastomeres into the control tubes.
6. Add 50 μL of mineral oil, and complete the lysis by heating the samples for 10 min at 65°C.
7. If not used immediately, cells may be kept at –20°C for up to 3 mo.
8. Alternatively, the lymphocytes are placed in 10 μL of ddH$_2$O; 50 μL of mineral oil are added and the samples are denatured at 95°C for 5 min (*see* Note 3).

3.1.3. Lymphocyte Isolation

1. Separate lymphocytes from unclotted blood collected in EDTA-treated tubes by centrifugation through Ficoll-Paque: Layer 4 mL of a 1:1 dilution of blood and PBS onto 3 mL of Ficoll-Paque. Centrifuge for 30 min at 1600 rpm, remove the supernatant, and rinse three times with an excess of PBS (*see* Note 3).
2. Dilute the lymphocytes in filtered PBS containing 10 mg/mL of BSA.
3. Under visual control, using a binocular microscope and a mouth-controlled, finely pulled glass pipet, distribute two to five lymphocytes into microdrops (volume of about 1 μL) of the same medium under silicone oil.
4. Transfer single lymphocytes into 0.5-mL thin-wall microcentrifuge tubes containing 10 μL ddH$_2$O or 5 μL of lysis buffer.
5. Transfer a sample of medium from each drop (every two to five lymphocytes) into control blank tubes
6. Add 50 μL of mineral oil, and for the cells in water, heat the tubes to 95°C for 5 min, or to 65°C for 10 min for cells in lysis buffer, to assure complete cell lysis (*see* Note 4).
7. If not used immediately, cells may be kept at –20°C for up to 3 mo.
8. Alternatively, the lymphocytes are placed in 10 μL of ddH$_2$O; 50 μL of mineral oil are added and the samples are denatured at 95°C for 5 min (*see* Note 3).

3.2. PCR

3.2.1. PCR Setup

1. Prepare PCR reaction mixtures for the number of tubes to be analyzed plus one to allow for inaccuracy of pipeting (Tables 2 and 3). Both outer and inner amplification mix can be prepared at the same time and the inner mix kept at 4°C during the outer amplification.
2. Dispense the outer mix into the sample tubes, and perform the first PCR amplification.
3. In a separate laboratory with different pipetor, transfer 2-μL aliquots of each sample into a fresh tube containing all the reagents for the inner amplification.

Table 2
Concentration of the PCR Reagents for Diagnosis of Lesch-Nyhan Syndrome and ΔF508 Deletion for the Diagnosis of CF Using the ΔF508 Deletion

Outer amplification				Inner amplification	
Lysis buffer protocol	Vol, μL	Lysis with ddH$_2$O	Vol, μL	Reagents	Vol, μL
LB-containing cell	5	H$_2$O with cell	10	Amplified product	2
NB	5	MgCl$_2$ (25 mM)	3	MgCl$_2$	3
10X [K+]-free	5	10 X (buffer II)	5	10X (buffer II)	5
Nucleotides (10 mM)	0.5	Nucleotides	0.5	Nucleotides	0.5
Forward primer (40 μM)	1	Forward primer	1	Forward primer	1
Reverse primer (40 μM)	1	Reverse primer	1	Reverse primer	1
AmpliTaq (5 U/μL)	0.2	Taq polymerase	0.2	Taq polymerase	1
ddH$_2$O	32.3	ddH$_2$O	29.3	ddH$_2$O	36.5
Total	50	Total	50	Total	50

Table 3
Concentration of the PCR Reagents for the Determination of Sex
Using the Amelogenin Primers

Outer amplification		Inner amplification	
Reagents	Vol, µL	Reagents	Vol, µL
ddH$_2$O containing cell	10	Amplified product of the first reaction	2
MgCl$_2$ (25 mM)	3	MgCl$_2$	1.8
10X (buffer II)	5	10X (buffer II)	3
Nucleotides (10 mM)	0.5	Nucleotides	0.3
Forward primer (40 µM)	1	Forward primer	0.6
Reverse primer (40 µM)	1	Reverse primer	0.6
Ampli*Taq* (5 U/µL)	0.2	Ampli*Taq*	0.2
ddH$_2$O	29.3	ddH$_2$O	21.5
Total	50	Total	30

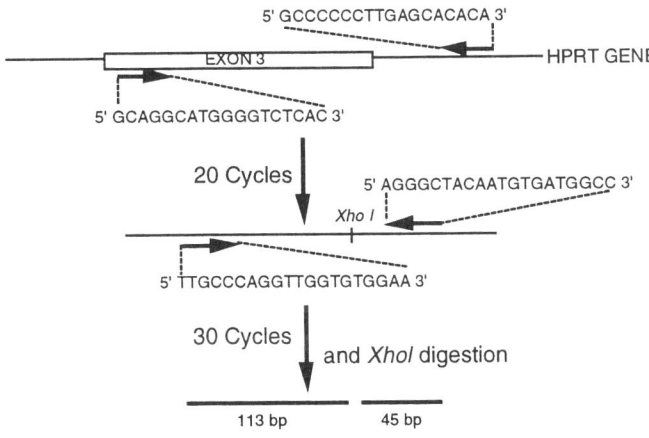

Fig. 1. Schematic representation of the nested PCR protocol for Lesch-Nyhan diagnosis.

Refer to Note 1 for contamination containment precautions during the setup. A diagram of the nested protocol for amplification of part of the HPRT gene is shown in Fig. 1.

3.2.2. PEP

1. The PEP protocol is almost identical to the original protocol described in ref. *12*. The reaction volume is 50 µL instead of the described 60 µL. Each reaction tube contains 5 µL of LB, NB, and 10X [K$^+$]-free buffer, 5 µL of random primers, 1 µL of dNTPs and *Taq* polymerase, and 28 µL of ddH$_2$O.

2. Perform 50 of the following cycles: 1 min at 92°C, 2 min at 37°C, a ramping step of 10°/s to 55°C and a 4-min incubation at 55°C.
3. Aliquot 3–5 μL of the PEP product for subsequent amplification with specific primers.

3.3. Electrophoresis and Mutation Detection

All the detection techniques described here were chosen (at least in part) for their speed and simplicity (*see* Note 5).

3.3.1. Polyacrylamide Gel Electrophoresis

1. Mix 8 μL of the amplified product with 2 μL of loading buffer.
2. Load the samples onto a 10% polyacrylamide minigel (10 × 8 × 0.1 cm), and run for 30 min at 200 V in a Bio-Rad Mini Protean II minigel apparatus.
3. After electrophoresis, stain the gel for 10 min in 0.5 μg/mL ethidium bromide solution, view, and photograph under UV illumination.

3.3.2. Heteroduplex Formation for DF508

1. Since there is only a 3-bp size difference between the normal and the affected allele, heteroduplex formation is used to obtain a fast, unambiguous diagnosis by conventional gel electrophoresis.
2. After completion of amplification, dispense two 5-μL aliquots of each amplification product into two fresh microcentrifuge tubes.
3. Add 5 μL of previously amplified DNA product from a homozygous unaffected and affected individual to the aliquots of test DNA.
4. Heat the mixtures of DNA to 95°C for 2 min to separate all the DNA strands, and cool to room temperature to allow the random reannealing of the single-stranded DNA fragments.
5. Run the mixed products on a polyacrylamide gel.
6. Diagnosis is obtained from the pattern of heteroduplex formation given by the two mixtures (Fig. 2). Heteroduplex bands, i.e., hybrid double-stranded DNA made from the hybridization of the amplification product of one normal and one ΔF508 allele are retarded on the gel compared to homoduplex bands made of the perfect match of either two normal or ΔF508 alleles. For homozygous samples, one band (homoduplex) is visible when adding DNA of the same genotype, whereas there are two bands (homo- and heteroduplex) when adding DNA of a different genotype. With amplified product, homo- and heteroduplex bands are detected in both mixtures. In the case of amplification failure, there are no heteroduplex bands in either of the two tracks. Polyacrylamide gel showing the amplification of single blastomeres of different genotypes is shown in Fig. 2.

3.3.3. Restriction Digestion (Lesch-Nyhan Syndrome)

The pattern of digestion after the *Xho*I digest is indicative of the cell genotype. Fully digested samples with two shorter fragments are characteristic of homozygous unaffected cells; undigested samples with only one full-length

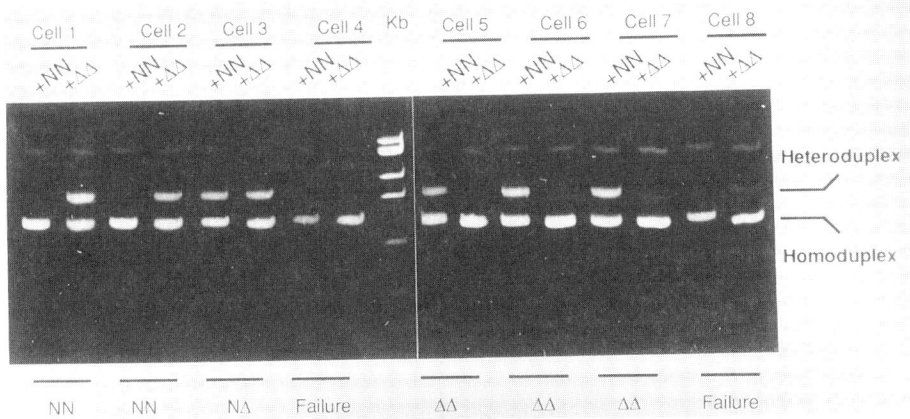

Fig. 2. ΔF508 PCR amplification from single blastomeres.

fragment indicate a homozygous affected (male) cell. A partial digest with three DNA fragments indicates a heterozygous carrier (female) cell.

1. Incubate 17 μL of PCR product with 10 U of enzyme (*Xho*I) and 2 μL of the supplied 10X buffer for 1 h at 37°C.
2. As a control for complete digestion, an aliquot of amplified homozygous unaffected product should be digested with each batch of samples.

3.3.4. Sexing With the Amelogenin Primers

Direct visualization of the X band only (290 bp) or of both X and Y (105 bp) bands allows easy sex determination after gel electrophoresis (*see* Note 6).

4. Notes

1. The handling of all the reagents and the preparation of the PCR mix are carried out in a laminar downflow cabinet with the worker wearing a clean gown and gloves. No extracted DNA or amplified PCR product is ever brought into this protected environment. Dedicated Gilson pipets and sterile filtered tips are used to prevent contamination. All of the reagents are filtered (0.22-μm Millipore filters) and aliquoted into sterile tubes. Numerous control blanks containing only an aliquot of the cell containing media are also prepared.
2. As previously emphasized, extreme caution should be exercised to avoid contamination. Despite stringent precautions, we occasionally observe false positives in 0–10% of our control blanks. This level of contamination may be acceptable if the amplification efficiency is high and transfer of heterozygotes is avoided, since it is only the combination of amplification failure and contamination that potentially leads to the most serious risk of misdiagnosis (i.e., misdiagnosis of an affected embryo as unaffected). Contamination seems to build up after periods

of extensive use of one set of primers in the lab. This suggest that contamination from previous PCR is the most prevalent source, despite the measures for containment taken during the different steps of the PCR. Amplified PCR products must accumulate either in the laminar flow cabinet despite UV decontamination or in the room where single-cell tubing is performed. This stresses the need for regular quality control with numerous control blanks (at least 50) to test the reagents, and the procedures involved in blastomere handling and PCR preparation.

3. There are three critical steps to achieve a clean separation devoid of red cells, which could be confused with lymphocytes during the selection, and excessive impurities:

   a. Be very gentle when layering the diluted blood onto the Ficoll, so as not to mix the two phases.

   b. Start the first centrifugation as slowly as possible, and increase the speed very slowly up to 1600 rpm.

   c. The rinses are important to remove cell debris and platelets that might later introduce contamination

4. A freezing step might be incorporated to assure complete cell lysis. Although not necessary with the use of lysis buffer, freezing seems to improve amplification efficiency slightly.

5. Presently, because of IVF imperatives, it is preferable that embryos are transferred on d 3 postinsemination, the same day as embryo biopsy. Hence the genetic analysis has to be rapid, if possible no more than 8 h to avoid late transfers. For the CF and Lesch-Nyhan tests described here, the outer amplification takes about 2 h, the inner about 3 h, and the gel loading, running, and staining about 1 h. Allowing for some breathing space, the whole procedure takes about 7 h, when testing a typical number of samples and controls.

6. We have used the amelogenin primers both directly on single cells and on PEP product. Amplification rate is relatively low (~75%). Also on a number of occasions, we observed a failure of amplification of either the X or the Y fragment, i.e., ADO *(11)*. The amelogenin primers are not used for clinical cases. Sexing by FISH is more informative, allowing the detection of aneuploidy or abnormal numbers of sex chromosomes and also is not susceptible to contamination *(23)*. Other sexing primers amplifying sequences common to the X and the Y chromosome have been described for single-cell amplification, including hemi-nested primers amplifying the steroid sulfatase gene on the X chromosome and pseudogene on the Y *(12)*. We obtained good amplification with them, but found the ratio of X and Y specific primers to be critical to obtaining good amplification of both chromosomes when amplifying male cells. Primers have also been described that amplify the *ZFX* and *ZFY* sequences with high efficiency and accuracy *(24)*. Their main advantage is that the amplified sequences on the X and the Y chromosomes are of equal size, but are distinguishable by restriction digestion because of an additional site in the Y fragment. This feature therefore decreases the risks of preferential amplification.

References

1. Handyside, A. H. (1993) Diagnosis of inherited disease before implantation. *Reprod. Med. Rev.* **2,** 51–61.
2. Mullis, K. and Faloona, F. (1987) Specific synthesis of DNA in vitro via a polymerase-catalysed chain reaction. *Methods Enzymol.* **155,** 335–350.
3. Li, A., Gyllenstein, U. B., Cui, X., Saiki, R. K., Erlich, H. A., and Arnheim, N. (1988) Amplification and analysis of DNA sequences in single human sperm and diploid cells. *Nature* **335,** 414–419.
4. Cui, X. F., Li, H. H., Goradia, T. M., Lange, K., Kazazian, H. H. J., Galas, D., and Arnheim, N. (1989) Single-sperm typing: determination of genetic distance between the G gamma-globin and parathyroid hormone loci by using the polymerase chain reaction and allele-specific oligomers. *Proc. Natl. Acad. Sci. USA* **86,** 9389–9393.
5. Coutelle, C., Williams, C., Handyside, A., Hardy, K., Winston, R., and Williamson, R. (1989) Genetic analysis of DNA from single human oocytes: a model for preimplantation diagnosis of cystic fibrosis. *Br. Med. J.* **299,** 22–24.
6. Handyside, A. H., Kontogianni, E. H., Hardy, K., and Winston, R. M. (1990) Pregnancies from biopsied human preimplantation embryos sexed by Y-specific DNA amplification. *Nature* **344,** 768–770.
7. Handyside, A. H., Lesko, J. G., Tarin, J. J., Winston, R. M., and Hughes, M. R. (1992) Birth of a normal girl after in vitro fertilization and preimplantation diagnostic testing for cystic fibrosis. *N. Engl. J. Med.* **327,** 905–909.
8. Ray, P. F., Winston, R. M. L., and Handyside, A. H. (1994) Single cell analysis for diagnosis of cystic fibrosis and Lesch-Nyhan syndrome in human embryos before implantation. *Miami Bio/Technol.* **5,** 46. (abstract)
9. Ao, A., Ray, P., Lesko, J., Harper, J. C., Handyside, A. H., Hughes, M. R., and Winston, R. M. L. (1996) Clinical experience with preimplantation diagnosis of the ΔF508 deletion causing cystic fibrosis. *Prenat. Diagn.* (in press).
10. Lesko, J., Snabes, M., Handyside, A. H., and Hughes, M. (1991) Amplification of the cystic fibrosis Δ F508 mutation from single cells: applications toward genetic diagnosis of the preimplantation embryo. *Am. J. Hum. Genet.* **49(4),** 223 (abstract).
11. Ray, P. F. (1996) Increasing the denaturation temperature during the first cycles of nested amplification reduces allele dropout from single cells for preimplantation genetic diagnosis. *Mol. Hum. Reprod.* (in press).
12. Zhang, L., Cui, X., Schmitt, K., Hubert, R., Navidi, W., and Arnheim, N. (1992) Whole genome amplification from a single cell: implications for genetic analysis. *Proc. Natl. Acad. Sci. USA* **89,** 5847–5851.
13. Jeffreys, A. J., Wilson, V., and Thein, S. L. (1985) Hypervariable "minisatellite" regions in human DNA. *Nature* **314,** 67–73.
14. Nakamura, Y., Leppert, M., O'Connell, P., Wolff, R., Holm, T., Culver, M., et al. (1987) Variable number of tandem repeat (VNTR) markers for human gene mapping. *Science* **235,** 1616–1622.
15. Ray, P. F., Harper, J., Mountford, R., Elles, R., and Handyside, A. H. (1992) Analysis of simple tandem repeats following whole genome amplification from

single cells for preimplantation diagnosis of Duchenne muscular dystrophy. *J. Reprod. Fert.* **Abstr. Series No. 10,** 52.

16. Kristjansson, K., Chong, S. S., Van den Veyver, I. B., Subramanian, S., Snabes, M. C., and Hughes, M. R. (1994) Preimplantation single cell analyses of dystrophin gene deletions using whole genome amplification. *Nature Genet.* **6,** 19–23.

17. Findlay, I., Ray, P., Quirque, P., Rutherford, A., and Lilford, R. (1995) Allelic drop-out and preferential amplification in single cells and human blastomeres: implications for preimplantation diagnosis of sex and cystic fibrosis. *Hum. Reprod.* **10,** 1609–1618.

18. Findlay, I., Urquart, A., Quirque, P., Sullivan, K. M., Rutherford, A., and Lilford, R. (1995) Simultaneous DNA "fingerprinting", diagnosis of sex and single-gene defect status from a single cell. *Hum. Reprod.* **10,** 1005–1013.

19. Harper, J. C. (1996) Preimplantation diagnosis of inherited disease. An update of world figures. *J. Assoc. Reprod. Genet.* (in press).

20. Li, H., Cui, X., and Arnheim, N. (1991) *A Companion to Methods in Enzymology*, Academic, New York.

21. Nakahori, Y., Hamanao, K., Iwaya, M., and Nakagome, Y. (1991) Sex identification by polymerase chain reaction using X-Y homologous primer. *Am. J. Med. Genet.* **39,** 472,473.

22. Handyside, A. H., Pattinson, J. K., Penketh, R. J., Delhanty, J. D., Winston, R. M., and Tuddenham, E. G. (1989) Biopsy of human preimplantation embryos and sexing by DNA amplification. *Lancet* **1,** 347–349.

23. Delhanty, J. D. A., Griffin, D. K., Handyside, A. H., Harper, J., Atkinson, G. H. G., Pieters, M. H. E. C., and Winston, R. M. L. (1993) Detection of aneuploidy and chromosomal mosaicism in human embryos during preimplantation sex determination by fluorescent in situ hybridization (FISH). *Hum. Mol. Genet.* **2(8),** 1183-1185.

24. Chong, S. S., Kristjansson, K., Cota, J., Handyside, A. H., and Hughes, M. R. (1993) Preimplantation diagnosis of X-linked disease: reliable and rapid sex determination of single human cells by restriction site analysis of simultaneously amplified ZFX and ZFY sequences. *Hum. Mol. Genet.* **8,** 1187–1191.

15

FISH in Preimplantation Diagnosis

Joyce C. Harper and Joy D. A. Delhanty

1. Introduction

Analysis of chromosomes in human embryonic nuclei would ideally be achieved by karyotyping. Several studies have used this technique to examine human embryonic chromosomes *(1–4)*, but information is limited, since it is difficult to obtain bandable metaphase spreads. For preimplantation genetic diagnosis (PGD) where only one or maybe two cells are available, karyotyping is not a viable option because of its low success rate per single cell. However, in certain cases, fluorescent *in situ* hybridization (FISH) can be used, for instance, for sexing embryos for couples at risk of passing on X-linked disorders for which there is, as yet, no specific molecular diagnosis. In addition FISH is useful for couples who are subfertile owing to chromosomal disorders (translocations or gonadal mosaicism). Since these are among the most common reasons for requesting PGD, a laboratory contemplating providing this service should include FISH in its repertoire.

Although it is now possible to amplify simultaneously X and Y sequences for sexing embryos using the polymerase chain reaction (PCR) *(5,6)*, there are several drawbacks that apply when amplifying DNA from single blastomeres, and FISH is preferable. The first is the risk of selective amplification failure. The second is the risk of amplifying contaminating material; this applies to any reaction involving PCR. The third is that the presence of an amplified band only indicates that an X or Y chromosome is present and gives no information on copy number. Because we have accumulated data from preimplantation diagnosis cases by FISH analysis, the importance of the copy number has become apparent. It is our experience that in about one-third of embryos, the biopsied cell contains an abnormal number of X signals making the embryo unsuitable for transfer despite the absence of a Y-specific signal *(7,* Harper and

From: *Methods in Molecular Medicine: Molecular Diagnosis of Genetic Diseases*
Edited by: R. Elles Humana Press Inc., Totowa, NJ

Delhanty, unpublished observations). From apparently normal embryos, blastomere nuclei with a single X chromosome and those with three, four, or more signals are frequently observed *(8–10)*. The former is potentially the most disastrous when the aim is to avoid X-linked disease from the carrier mother, since in the majority of fully X-monosomic embryos, it is the paternal sex chromosome that is lacking. Since 45,X conceptuses are considered to occur with a frequency approaching 1%, such a finding will not be rare when carrying out PGD and has been reported *(7)*.

Information on chromosome copy number has enabled us to avoid the transfer of abnormal or chromosomally mosaic embryos. This facility is enhanced by the use of an autosomal probe in addition to probes for the sex chromosomes, since this gives extra information and allows a more exact analysis. We routinely perform PGD of sex using triple-color FISH with probes for chromosomes X, Y, and 1 (Fig. 1).

Since we first reported the use of FISH for PGD *(11)*, several improvements to the technique have been made. The initial method used to spread interphase human blastomeres was a modification of Tarkowski *(12)*, which used 3:1 methanol acetic acid as the fixative *(11)*. For spreading single human blastomeres, this method is problematic since a large amount of cytoplasm cannot be effectively removed and the blastomeres are easily lost during the procedure.

More recently, we have used a spreading method developed in mouse embryos *(13)*, which can be successfully applied to human blastomeres *(9)* or whole embryos *(10,14,15)*. The spreading solution used is HCl and Tween-20, which dissolves the cell membrane and allows direct visualization of the blastomere, so that the cytoplasm can be totally washed away leaving a clear nucleus. Second, the original method described used a long RNase and proteinase K digestion to make the nuclei accessible to the probes. With the improved spreading method, we have been able to reduce this digestion to 20 min using pepsin. Finally, using DNA probes labeled with biotin or digoxygenin requires long detection procedures. We now use probes directly labeled with the fluorochromes, which greatly reduces the overall procedure time. Our original FISH method took approx 7 h, but with the improvements outlined here, the whole procedure now takes just 2 h *(9)*. Since the biopsy, diagnosis, and transfer all take place on the same day (d 3 postinsemination), the diagnosis is completed at an earlier time, allowing the embryo transfer to take place within normal working hours.

There have to date been no misdiagnoses following the identification of sex by FISH, and the number of deliveries per cycle is slightly higher with FISH than with PCR *(16,17)*. However, interestingly, an excess of male-to-female embryos has been observed when performing sexing for X-linked disease *(18,* Harper and Delhanty, unpublished observations). The use of cosmid and YAC

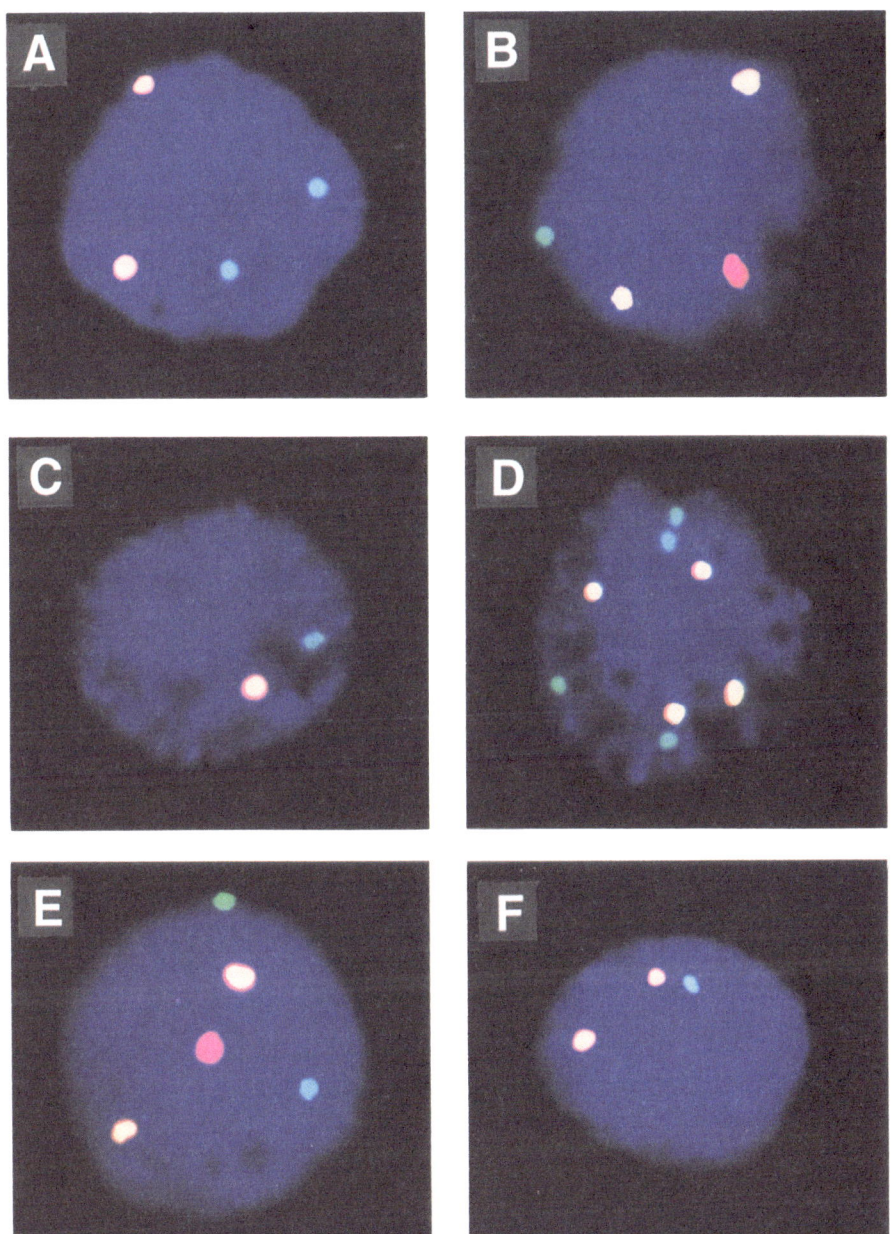

Fig. 1. Triple-color FISH in human embryonic nuclei: X probe labeled green, Y probe labeled red, and chromosome 1 probe labeled orange. **(A)** Normal male, XY11; **(B)** normal female, XX11; **(C)** haploid, X1; **(D)** tetraploid, XXXX1111; **(E)** aneuploid, XXY11; **(F)** X11. All images were captured on a cooled CCD camera using Smart Capture Software (software from Digital Scientific, Cambridge, UK).

DNA probes carrying large inserts has been successfully applied to embryonic nuclei and could be used in specific cases. However, FISH for the diagnosis of chromosomal disorders (translocations or gonadal mosaicism) is still in the research stage (Harper and Delhanty, unpublished observations). Therefore, in this chapter, we concentrate on the use of FISH using α-satellite probes for sexing human embryos.

2. Materials

2.1. Nick Translation of DNA Probes

2.1.1. DNA Probes

The DNA probes used for sexing human embryos are:

1. X chromosome: pBam X5 *(19)*.
2. Y chromosome: cY98 (Wolfe, personal communication).
3. 1 chromosome: pUC1.77 *(20)*.

2.1.2. Nick Translation

1. 1 μg DNA probe.
2. 10X Nick translation buffer: $0.5M$ Tris-HCl, pH 7.5, $0.1M$ magnesium sulfate, 1 mM dithiothreitol (DTT, Sigma [St. Louis, MO], D0632). Store stock at –20°C.
3. $0.1M$ DTT.
4. Nucleotide mix consisting of:
    a. 0.5 mM 2'deoxyguanosine 5'-triphosphate (100 mM, pH 7.5, Pharmacia [Uppsala, Sweden], 27-2070-01).
    b. 0.5 mM 2'deoxyadenosine 5'-triphosphate (100 mM, pH 7.5, Pharmacia, 27-2050-01).
    c. 0.5 mM 2'deoxycytidine 5'-triphosphate (100 mM, pH 7.5, Pharmacia, 27-2060-01).
    d. 0.1 mM 2'deoxythymidine 5'-triphosphate (100 mM, pH 7.5, Pharmacia, 27-2080-01).
5. 1 mM Label: either FITC-12-dUTP (Boehringer Mannheim [Mannheim, Germany], 1373242) or Fluorored (Amersham [Amersham, UK], RPN 2122).
6. DNA polymerase I (Promega [Madison, WI], 3642302).
7. DNase I (Boehringer Mannheim, 104159), from bovine pancrease, grade II. Make 1 mg/mL stock in 20 mM Tris-HCl, pH 7.6, 50 mM NaCl, 1 mM DTT, 50% glycerol. Store at –20°C. When required, dilute 1 in 1,000 with distilled water, store on ice, and discard when nick translation is complete.
8. $0.5M$ EDTA, disodium salt (BDH [Poole, UK], 10093).
9. Herring sperm DNA (Sigma, D-7290).
10. $3M$ Sodium acetate.
11. TE (10 mM Tris-HCl, 1 mM EDTA, pH 7.6).
12. Hybridization buffer: 2X SSC, 60% deionized formamide (BDH, product 103264R).

2.2. Preparation of Cells

2.2.1. Spreading Single Blastomeres

1. Poly-L-lysine coated slides stored at 4°C (Poly-L-lysine, Sigma, P8920).
2. Spreading solution: 0.01M HCl, 0.1% Tween-20. Stocks are made of 1% Tween-20 and 1M HCl, and the final solution made fresh on day of use.

2.2.2. Preparation of Control Lymphocyte Slides

Standard cytogenetic preparations of male control lymphocytes are stored in 3:1 methanol:acetic acid at –20°C.

2.3. FISH

1. 100 µg/mL Pepsin (Sigma, P6887) in 0.01M HCl. Pepsin is stored as 10 mg/mL stock (500-µL aliquots) and is stable at –20°C for up to 2 mo. Do not refreeze.
2. 1% Paraformaldehyde in phosphate-buffered saline (PBS, 0.01M phosphate buffer, 0.0027M potassium chloride, and 0.137M sodium chloride, pH 7.4).
3. 2X SSC stored as stock of 20X SSC (3M sodium chloride, 0.3M trisodium citrate, pH 7.2).
4. 60% Deionized formamide in 2X SSC.
5. 4X SSC, 0.05% Tween-20.
6. Mounting medium: 1 mL Vectarshield (Vector Laboratories, Burlingame, CA) mixed with 6 µL 0.2 mg/mL 4',6-diaminidino-2-phenyolindole (DAPI) stored at 4°C in the dark.

3. Methods

3.1. Nick Translation of DNA Probes

The method described here is slightly modified from Rigby et al. *(21)* (*see* Note 1).

1. On ice, mix: 5 µL 10X nick translation buffer, 5 µL 0.1M DTT, 4 µL nucleotide mix, 2 µL 1 mM label, *xx* µL probe DNA (1 µg), *xx* µL filtered bidistilled water, 2 µL DNA polymerase I, 5 µL DNase I. The volume of the probe required for 1 µg will depend on the stock, and the volume of filtered bidistilled water should be adjusted to give a final volume of 50 µL.
2. Incubate at 15°C for 1 h, and add an additional 5 µL of DNase I.
3. Incubate for a further hour.
4. Stop the reaction by adding 5 µL of 0.5M EDTA, and keep on ice.
5. Ethanol-precipitate the DNA by adding 5 µL herring sperm DNA, 1/10 vol 3M sodium acetate (6 µL) and 1 µL ice-cold ethanol. Invert several times, and leave for 1 h at –70°C or overnight at –20°C.
6. Spin on a microcentrifuge at top speed for 15 min, remove ethanol, and allow pellet to dry. Resuspend probe in either TE (store at –20°C) or hybridization buffer (store at 4°C) in the dark.

3.2. Preparation of Cells

3.2.1. Spreading Single Blastomeres

Single embryonic cells are obtained from embryo biopsy or by disaggregation of whole embryos as detailed in Chapter 14. For blastomere handling, a fine, flame-polished glass capillary tube is used. A video of this procedure has been produced *(22)*.

1. Make a circle on the underside of a poly-L-lysine slide using a diamond marker.
2. Under a dissecting microscope, wash the cell in PBS to remove serum proteins, and other contaminating material.
3. Prime the capillary with spreading solution, and transfer the blastomere to a small drop of spreading solution within the circle, ensuring minimum transfer of PBS.
4. Under an inverted microscope, gently remove and replace the spreading solution. The shape of the blastomere may distort and form "buds." At this stage, the nucleus should be visible.
5. With constant observation, keep removing and replacing the solution until the cell membrane lyses and the cytoplasm washes away from the nucleus (*see* Note 2).
6. Once the nucleus is clear, leave the slide to air-dry, and incubate in PBS for 5 min.
7. Dehydrate the slides for 5 min in 70, 90, and 100% ethanol, and store for up to 2 wk at room temperature (*see* Note 3).

3.2.2. Preparation of Control Lymphocyte Slides

1. Centrifuge the fixed cell suspension at 400g for 5 min, and resuspend cells in fresh fixative (3:1 methanol:acetic acid).
2. Drop the suspension onto a clean slide; leave to air-dry.
3. Flood with fixative for 10 s, and leave to air-dry.
4. Flood the slide with 70% acetic acid for 10 s, leave to air-dry, and dehydrate through a 70, 90, and 100% ethanol series.

3.3. FISH

1. Incubate the slides for 20 min at 37°C in 100 µg/mL pepsin in 0.01M HCl to remove any remaining protein, and make the nuclei accessible to the probes.
2. Briefly wash the slides in bidistilled water and PBS, and incubate for 10 min at 4°C in 1% paraformaldehyde in PBS to refix the nuclei.
3. Briefly wash in PBS and a further two washes in water, and dehydrate slides through a 70, 90, and 100% ethanol series. The nuclei are now ready for denaturation and hybridization to the probes. The probes are used in a concentration of 5–10 ng/µL of hybridization mix (60% formamide, 2X SSC, 10% dextran sulfate). For triple-color FISH, we use the X probe labeled with FITC, the Y with rhodamine, and the probe for chromosome 1 in a 50:50 mix of FITC:rhodamine, which will give an orange fluorescence *(23,24)*.
4. Add the probes to the nuclei under a coverslip (*see* Note 4), and denature the probe and nuclear DNA simultaneously at 75°C for 3 min.

5. Leave to hybridize in a moist chamber at 37°C for 45 min.
6. To remove unbound probe, wash the slides for 5 min at 42°C in 60% formamide, 2X SSC, 5 min at 42°C in 2X SSC, and two 5-min washes at room temperature in 4X SSC/0.05% Tween-20. All posthybridization washes should be performed in the dark.
7. Dehydrate the slides through a 70, 90, and 100% ethanol series, mount in Vectarshield mounting medium containing DAPI, and analyze (*see* Note 5).
8. Slides should be stored in the dark at 4°C.

3.3.1. Interpretation and Artifacts

FISH signals are analyzed according to Hopman et al. *(25)*. For two signals lying close together to be considered as separate signals, they must be more than one signal diameter apart. Since the DNA of interphase nuclei is decondensed compared to chromosomes in metaphase, there is a much greater likelihood of the signals from homologous chromosomes overlying one another with the result that only one signal is scored. For this reason, it is advantageous to have two independently biopsied cells, so that if a reduced signal number is seen for one chromosome pair in one nucleus only and the other is normal female, the embryo can still be considered for transfer. In this situation, the additional information provided by an autosomal probe provides valuable reassurance. Diagnosis of a normal female embryo is only made when two X signals are present in the absence of a Y signal, with two autosomal signals.

3.3.2. Mosaicism

Mosaicism in a basically normal diploid embryo is of four types: diploid/haploid (Fig. 1C), diploid/tetraploid (Fig. 1D), diploid/aneuploid (owing to mitotic nondisjunction) (Fig. 1E,F), and completely chaotic division. Diploid/haploid mosaicism is common, and has important implications for the diagnosis of both dominant single gene disorders and chromosomal trisomies, should a haploid cell be biopsied *(10,16)*.

It is important not to disregard abnormal signal numbers, particularly when only a single cell is available for analysis. In our experience, it is indicative of a full or mosaic abnormality in the remainder of an embryo in 9 of 10 cases (Harper and Delhanty, unpublished observations). Human cleavage-stage embryos seem to constitute a special case with regard to genetic instability, both at the chromosomal and DNA levels, and the criteria are not the same as when dealing with cells from somatic sources *(26)*.

4. Notes

1. α-Satellite probes can be obtained as plasmids or already transformed into bacteria, which can be grown up and the DNA purified to give large quantities of unlabeled probe. The probes can be directly labeled by nick translation using first

principle methods or using commercial kits for biotin or digoxygenin labeling. Some methods purify the labeled probe through Sephadex columns, but we have experienced loss of our directly labeled probes using these columns. We have found that an ethanol precipitation is sufficient and the probe can then be stored in either TE or hybridization buffer (60% formamide, 2X SSC). Directly labeled α-satellite probes can also be obtained commercially. The reliability of any probe used must be confirmed on male control lymphocytes, ensuring that the majority of the nuclei show the expected number of signals.

2. It is important to observe constantly the cell/nucleus throughout the procedure. The spreading solution must not be allowed to dry out before the cell lyses. Nuclei can be obscured by the addition of too much spreading solution and lost owing to inconsistent observation, especially after cell lysis. If too much cytoplasm is left around the nucleus during spreading, the nucleus may be lost from the slide during the pepsin digestion. It should take no longer than 5 min to spread a nucleus.

3. For easy location of the nucleus after spreading, coordinates can be recorded either from the microscope stage or using an England finder.

4. Since each slide only contains one nucleus, we use 5 μL of the final hybridization mix under a 13-mm coverslip. The hybridization time is only 45 min, so sealing the coverslips with glue is not required.

5. Using triple-color FISH, it is best to use a double band pass filter, which detects FITC and rhodamine, allowing the three colors to be detected simultaneously.

References

1. Angell, R. R., Templeton, A. A., and Messinis, I. E. (1986) Consequences of polyspermy in man. *Cytogenet. Cell Genet.* **42,** 1–7.

2. Plachot, M., Mandelbaum, J., Junca, A.-M., Grouchy, J., de Salat-Baroux, J., and Cohen, J. (1989) Cytogenetic analysis and developmental capacity of normal and abnormal embryos after IVF. *Hum. Reprod.* **4,** 99–103.

3. Zenzes, M. T. and Casper, R. F. (1992) Cytogenetics of human oocytes, zygotes and embryos after in vitro fertilisation. *Hum. Genet.* **88,** 367–375.

4. Jamieson, M. E., Coutts, J. R. T., and Connor, J. M. (1994) The chromosome constitution of human preimplantation embryos fertilised in vitro. *Hum. Reprod.* **9,** 709–715.

5. Chong, S. S., Kristjansson, K., Cota, J., Handyside, A. H., and Hughes, M. R. (1993) Preimplantation prevention of X-linked disease: reliable and rapid sex determination of single human cells by restriction analysis of simultaneously amplified ZFX and ZFY sequences. *Hum. Mol. Genet.* **2,** 1187–1191.

6. Liu, J., Lissens, W., Devroy, P., Van Steirteghem, A., and Liebers, I. (1994) Amplification of X- and Y-specific regions from single human blastomeres by polymerase chain reaction for sexing of preimplantation embryos. *Hum. Reprod.* **9,** 716–729.

7. Delhanty, J. D. A., Griffin, D. K., Handyside, A. H., Harper, J., Atkinson, G. H. G., Pieters, M. H. E. C., and Winston, R. M. L. (1993) Detection of aneuploidy and chromosomal mosaicism in human embryos during preimplantation sex determination by fluorescent *in-situ* hybridisation. *Hum. Mol. Genet.* **2,** 1183–1185.

8. Munne, S., Lee, A., Rosenwaks, Z., Grifo, J., and Cohen, J. (1993) Diagnosis of major chromosome aneuploidies in human preimplantation embryos. *Hum. Reprod.* **8,** 2185–2191.

9. Harper, J. C., Coonen, E., Ramaekers, F. C. S., Delhanty, J. D. A., Handyside, A. H., Winston, R. M. L., and Hopman, A. H. N. (1994) Identification of the sex of human preimplantation embryos, in two hours using an improved spreading method and fluorescent in situ hybridisation using directly labelled probes. *Hum. Reprod.* **9,** 721–724.

10. Harper, J. C., Coonen, E., Handyside, A. H., Winston, R. M. L., Hopman, A. H. N., and Delhanty, J. D. A. (1995) Mosaicism of autosomes and sex chromosomes in morphologically normal, monospermic, preimplantation human embryos. *Prenat. Diagn.* **15,** 41–49.

11. Griffin, D. K., Wilton, L. J., Handyside, A. H., Winston, R. M. L., and Delhanty, J. D. A. (1992) Dual fluorescent in-situ hybridisation for the simultaneous detection of X and Y chromosome specific probes for the sexing of human preimplantation embryonic nuclei. *Hum. Genet.* **89,** 18–22.

12. Tarkowski, A. K. (1990) An air drying method for chromosome preparations from mouse eggs. *Cytogenetics* **5,** 394–400.

13. Coonen, E., Dumoulin, J. C. M., Ramaekers, F. C. S., and Hopman, A. H. N. (1994) Optimal preparation of preimplantation embryo interphase nuclei by fluorescent in situ hybridisation. *Hum. Reprod.* **9,** 533–537.

14. Harper, J. C., Robinson, F., Duffy, S., Griffin, D. K., Handyside, A .H., Delhanty, J. D. A., and Winston, R. M. L. (1994) Detection of fertilisation in embryos with accelerated cleavage by fluorescent in situ hybridisation (FISH). *Hum. Reprod.* **9,** 1733–1737.

15. Coonen, E., Harper, J. C., Ramaekers, F. C. S., Delhanty, J. D. A., Hopman, A. H. N., Garaedts, J. P. M., and Handyside, A. H. (1994) Presence of chromosomal mosaicism in abnormal preimplantation embryos detected by fluorescent in situ hybridisation. *Hum. Genet.* **54,** 609–615.

16. Delhanty, J. D. A. (1994) Preimplantation diagnosis. *Prenat. Diagn.* **14,** 1217–1227.

17. Harper, J. C. and Handyside, A. H. (1994) The current status of preimplantation diagnosis. *Curr. Obstet. Gynaecol.* **4,** 143–149.

18. Griffin, D. K., Handyside, A. H., Harper, J. C., Wilton, L. J., Atkinson, G. H. G., Soussis, I., et al. (1994) Clinical experience with preimplantation diagnosis of sex by dual fluorescent in-situ hybridisation. *J. Assist. Reprod. Genet.* **11,** 132–143.

19. Willard, H. F., Smith, K. D., and Sutherland, J. (1983) Isolation and characterisation of a major tandem repeat family from the human X chromosome. *Nucleic Acids Res.* **19,** 3237–3241.

20. Cooke, H. J. and Hindley, J. (1979) Cloning of the human satellite III DNA: different components are on different chromosomes. *Nucleic Acids Res.* **6,** S3177–S3179.

21. Rigby, P. W. J., Dieckmann, M., Rhodes, C., and Berg, P. (1977) Labelling deoxyribonucleic acid to high specific activity in vitro by nick translation with DNA polymerase I. *J. Mol. Biol.* **113,** 237–241.

22. Harper, J. C. and Delhanty, J. D. A. (1995) Spreading single human blastomeres and multicolour fluorescent in situ hybridisation (FISH). *Hum. Reprod.* Update. CD-ROM, 1, No 6, item 28, video.

23. Dauwerse, J. G., Wiegant, J., Raap, A. K., Breuning, M. H., and van Ommen, G. J. B. (1992) Multiple colors by fluorescence in situ hybridisation using ratio-labelling DNA probes create a molecular karyotype. *Hum. Mol. Genet.* **1(8),** 593–598.

24. Reid, T., Baldini, A., Rand, T., and Ward, D. C. (1992) Simultaneous visualization of seven different DNA probes by in situ hybridization using combinational fluorescence and digital imaging microscopy. *Proc. Natl. Acad. Sci. USA* **89,** 1388–1392.

25. Hopman, A. H. N., Ramaekers, F. C. S., Raap, A. K., Beck, J. L. M., Devilee, P., Ploeg van der, M., and Vooijis, G. P. (1988) *In situ* hybridisation as a tool to study numerical chromosome aberrations in solid bladder tumours. *Histochemistry* **89,** 307–316.

26. Delhanty, J. D. A. and Handyside, A. H. (1995) The origin of genetic defects in man and their detection in the preimplantation embryo. *Hum. Reprod. Update* **1,** 201–215.

16

Microtiter Array Diagonal Gel Electrophoresis (MADGE) for Population Scale Genotype Analyses

Ian N. M. Day, Manjeet Bolla, Lema Haddad, Sandra O'Dell, and Steve E. Humphries

1. Introduction

Human populations display enormous genetic variation, evident both at the phenotypic level and at the DNA level. These variations include both single "mutations" causative of profound disease and variations that contribute to susceptibility to particular "polygenic" diseases. To date, genetic diagnostics have been applied mainly in the context of isolated diagnoses for individuals or families for single gene disorders. Population screening, for example, for carrier status for recessive disorders such as cystic fibrosis, has not yet advanced beyond feasibility studies. Such studies require satisfaction of the criteria of Wilson and Jungner (1), in that there must be the knowledge and resources (counseling, treatment, and so on) to confer benefit, and that there must be a viable and affordable means to undertake screening. For research into the genetic epidemiology of common disorders, such as cardiovascular disease and cancers, some of the feasibility shortfalls correspond with those for population screening for single gene mutations. First, tests for genetic variation are still very expensive, both in staff time and in reagents. Second, the combination of informed consent, collection of appropriate clinical detail, and collection of samples is expensive on a population scale. For these reasons, many associations, such as those between apolipoprotein E (APOE) genotype, hypercholesterolaemia and premature vascular disease (2), APOE genotype and late-onset Alzheimer disease (3), and angiotensinogen-converting enzyme (ACE) genotype and cardiovascular disease (4), have mainly been researched on groups of a few hundred individuals. However, larger studies of more genetic markers

From: *Methods in Molecular Medicine: Molecular Diagnosis of Genetic Diseases*
Edited by: R. Elles Humana Press Inc., Totowa, NJ

would demonstrate more convincing confidence intervals, with respect to candidate genes tested, and to look at the effects of multiple genes in combination. By contrast, traditional epidemiological studies of biochemical phenotype have involved tens or hundreds of thousands of individuals *(5)* and the biochemical risk factors identified have led on to functional studies and therapeutic strategies. By analogy, it should be possible eventually to achieve similar goals in genetic epidemiology. Not all gene variations can be identified from a biochemical phenotype, for example where the biochemical phenotype is a continuous trait, where the biochemical assays are more difficult than the genetic assays, or where the biochemical phenotype varies so much with time that there is essentially no intermediate trait that can be measured usefully. In these instances at a minimum, and in all epidemiological studies at a maximum, it would be valuable to examine genotypic markers and variations in genes that could conceivably be involved in the intermediate traits or overt clinical phenotypes under study. These research arguments pertain equally to population screening for single gene disorders.

One goal in molecular genetics at present is to establish screening programs for whole populations. For example, for cystic fibrosis, knowledge of carrier status would be helpful to identify at-risk couples. Unfortunately, this demands testing for one of a large number of point mutations known to cause cystic fibrosis *(6)*. Invariably, the first step is polymerase chain reaction (PCR) amplification of the regions of interest; the second step often is either a capture-binding assay (in which labeled allele-specific oligonucleotides [ASOs] are used in high stringency binding assays to test for the presence of particular mutations); or an electrophoretic assay (with the PCR arranged to generate fragments of a particular size according to presence/absence of a particular mutation. Capture-binding assays are similar in principle to two site immunometric assays *(7)*, but instead use a capturable group such as biotin incorporated into one PCR primer and a detectable label such as a fluorescent group attached to the ASO. (The configuration can be reversed and some liquid phase automation is possible.) Analytical electrophoresis is widely recognized as being manual and time-consuming and therefore also expensive. It would seem obvious, therefore, to aim to avoid electrophoresis for all mutation analysis. Unfortunately, many variations and mutations involve changes in *length* of sequence rather than composition of sequence. This is true for the many small deletions and insertions that occur *(8)*, in variable number dinucleotide *(9)* and tetranuceotide repeats that are very useful for linkage analysis, and in the triplet repeat slippage disorders. Among the latter, population screening for premutation expansion of repeat number is being considered as a possibility to identify carrier mothers for risk of fragile X mutation *(10)*. The determination of size of PCR products is almost unavoidable in these situations.

There are several categories of analysis for which it would be advantageous to have systems for high throughput electrophoresis, but in which the eventual pattern recognition commonly will hinge on mobility differences greater than 5%. These include PCR checking gels, sizing of PCR products, and analysis of restriction digests of PCR products. In addition, digests of PCR products for direct haplotyping (haplotyping of an individual without recourse to family studies), would often be useful. In this case two markers on the same strand must be analyzed in conjunction. This is impossible using ASOs, which do not allow determination of the phase between markers.

Many procedures in research and diagnostic laboratories are undertaken using 96-well microtiter plates as devised by Dynatech 30 yr ago. The rigid 8 × 12 arrays (rows A–H and columns 1–12, with 9-mm center-to-center spacing between adjacent wells), have been established for a wide range of disposable plastic plates that may be suitable for biological cultures, as a solid-phase coated plastic, for reading in spectrophotometric and fluorescence plate readers, or for PCR. For example, we have devised a very rapid DNA preparation method from blood, suitable for many PCRs, which manipulates the samples entirely in the 96-well array in which they are originally placed *(11)*. Subsequent PCRs are set up from pre-PCR dried DNA template 96-well replicas that are stored at room temperature and can be posted to other laboratories *(12)*. The configuration offers several advantages:

1. Information storage is on a "master grid" and there is no need for any labeling of tubes and storage of tubes in racks.
2. A wide range of purpose-made manual and automated multichannel pipeting and other devices are available for subsequent replications or other manipulations. For example, it becomes very easy to set up several different PCRs from the same set of samples.
3. The compact nature of the arrays is convenient for storage in large numbers in standard laboratories.

History and the test of time have established the 96-well plate as an industry standard for the foreseeable future. However, electrophoresis still is inconvenient because slots for loading gels traditionally are placed closely adjacent in row(s) for ready alignment of bands. These are not conveniently compatible with 96-well arrays (i.e., sample redistribution and recoding becomes necessary, and most arrangements preclude the use of multichannel devices). In addition, polyacrylamide is a better resolving matrix for PCR products and digests of PCR products than agarose. However, acrylamide does not polymerize in the presence of air, so most laboratories prepare polyacrylamide gels between two glass plates, with a "well-former" inserted at one end. This has three consequences:

1. Inconvenient setup;
2. Inability to "access" the whole area of the gel in the way that is commonly used to prepare multiple rows of wells in horizontal agarose gels; and
3. An obligation to load the gel with the glass plates vertical so that the samples do not leak out of the wells.

In this chapter, we describe a very simple device and method to prepare and manipulate horizontal polyacrylamide gels *(13,14)*. In addition, the open-faced horizontal arrangement enables loading of arrays of wells. Therefore, we have designed a device which preserves the exact configuration of the 8 × 12 array, and enables electrophoresis along a 71.6° diagonal line-of-sight between wells (MADGE, microtiter array diagonal gel electrophoresis), using either acrylamide or agarose. This eliminates almost all of the staff time taken in set up, loading, and record keeping and offers high resolution for genotyping pattern recognition. The nature and size of the gels allows direct stacking of gels in one tank, so that a tank used typically to analyze 30–60 samples can be used readily to analyze 1000–2000 samples with no increase in operator time. This system opens a wide variety of possibilities for diagnostic and research genotyping centered around existing microtiter plate technology, and is in essence an electrophoretic counterpart to the microtiter plate. Our interests have been in the development of tools suitable for research into the genetic epidemiology of cardiovascular disease on a population scale, but the utility for genotyping markers in the diagnostic context should be apparent.

2. Materials

The approach described here reflects the initial development of the technique and will be superceded by the commercial availability of ready made gels, gel formers, and a range of ancillary apparatus.

2.1. Preparation of Prototype Devices for Making Horizontal Polyacrylamide Gels (H-PAGE) and MADGE

Perspex blocks, 200 × 100 × 8 mm were machined away at one face using a computer controlled CNC machining center (Mazak, Worcester, UK) to leave either conventional rows of teeth (for H-PAGE) or teeth in a microtiter array format, i.e., 8 columns, 12 rows, 9-mm center to center between adjacent teeth. For MADGE format, the teeth were cut at an angle of 71.6° to the row axis of the array but perpendicular to the long edge of the perspex.

Various teeth were tried and 2 × 2 × 2 mm was selected as the "standard" size. This type of tooth enables loading of 5–7 microliter samples, the wells are open enough to take account of the imprecision of alignment of standard tips on standard multichannel devices, and the gel is of a convenient thickness. A plan view of the resultant gel is shown in Fig. 1. Approaches to making gel formers are described in Note 1. Other possible formats of gel are considered in Notes 4 and 5. Precast gels are available commercially (*see* Note 8).

—————————————————————————————cathode

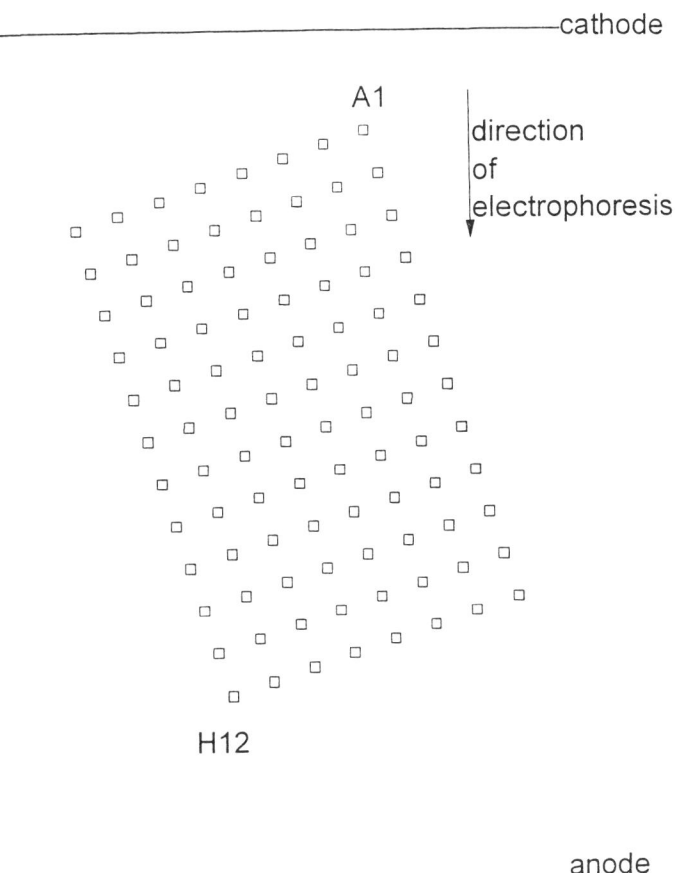

direction
of
electrophoresis

Fig. 1. Plan and gel former (two dimensional "comb") for MADGE. Schematic plan view of the wells of a MADGE gel in which the electrophoretic line-of-sight is diagonally across a 2 × 4 rectangle of wells. The distance between adjacent wells is 9 mm, as standard for 96-well microtiter plates. In the plan shown, the wells are 2 mm square, the angle between the direction of electrophoresis and the 12-well rows of the array is 71.6°, and the track length per well is 26.5 mm. Relative to standard designation on 96-well plates (rows A–H, columns 1–12), the orientation places well A1 nearest the cathode.

2.2. Reagents

Gamma-methacryloxypropyltrimethoxysilane is available from Sigma (Poole, Dorset, UK), Hydrolink from J. T. Baker (Swallowfield, Nr Reading, Berkshire, UK), hydrophilic electrophoresis film from Sigma, and Plasticard from Slater's Plastikard (Matlock Bath, Derbyshire, UK).

3. Methods

3.1. Preparing an H-PAGE or Polyacrylamide MADGE Gel

1. Tape around the edges of the H-PAGE or MADGE comb, leaving approx 3 mm of tape jutting up on the side where the (2 mm) teeth are. Sequencing gel (Scotch 3MM electrical) tape works well. The tape does not need removal after polymerization and rarely needs to be changed at all.
2. Lay the MADGE comb flat on paper towel or in a tray, with the teeth and jutting edge of the tape facing upward.
3. Silanize a suitably sized piece (e.g., 160 × 100 × 2 mm) of standard soda lime float glass (new or reused, *see* Note 2) with 0.5% gamma-methacryloxy-propyltrimethoxysilane, 0.5% glacial acetic acid, ethanol (v/v).
4. Prepare a volume of acrylamide gel mix (a few milliliters more than necessary to fill the volume bounded by the tape and the glass plate that will be pressed directly onto the ends of the teeth). Polymerization is by TEMED and ammonium persulfate as for any acrylamide gel *(8,9)*. A volume of 150 µL of TEMED and 150 µL of 10% ammonium persulphate are used for 50 mL of gel mix (*see* Note 6).
5. Pour the gel mix onto the comb, then lay the glass plate, silanized side down, onto the comb. The glass plate is rested in the gel at one end, then the other end smoothly lowered until the gel/air front is driven out and the plate contacts all the teeth. A 250-g weight is then placed on the plate to maintain pressure between plate and teeth. Note that it is critical not to release pressure from the glass plate once it is in contact with the teeth, otherwise some air bubbles will seep in under the glass.
6. Once polymerized, the glass plate with gel attached is prized off the comb by inserting a broad flat spatula at one end and rotating firmly until the glass can be grasped and lifted. Robustness of gel slots is considered in Note 6.

   Gels on glass can be stored in piles of 5–10 in buffer at 4°C for many weeks (*see* Note 7).

3.1.1. Variation I. Hydrolink

Gels were set up as for acrylamide.

3.1.2. Variation II. Agarose

Hydrophilic electrophoresis film can be used to form wells whose bases are formed by the plastic support, using the setup principle described for acrylamide. A rigid surface such as a glass plate should be placed above the electrophoresis film to ensure even distribution of a 250-g weight used to press the film firmly against the teeth. It is also possible to prepare polyacrylamide MADGE gels on such a plastic, rather than glass support, but the gel does not adhere as strongly as it does to glass (*see* Note 3) and also must be removed from the plastic prior to viewing on a transilluminator.

3.2. Loading and Electrophoresis of Samples on H-PAGE and MADGE Gels

1. Immerse the gel horizontally in the electrophoresis tank. Polyacrylamide or Hydrolink gels are anchored on their glass plate and the bases of the wells are formed by the glass.
2. Prepare samples for loading. They will probably have come from a microtiter plate PCR, or some subsequent or other procedure undertaken in a microtiter plate. For 2-mm cubic wells, 5 μL is an appropriate volume to load.
3. Load using a multichannel pipet, preferably one designed for pipeting in the 1–10 μL range, so that thumb travel is long and smooth during loading. It is easy to feel the glass or plastic base of each well when the pipet is correctly positioned. A reflective white surface such as plasticard under the gel and a light source (ideally parallel light from a parabolic reflector or a light placed approx 1 m above the gel) are very helpful to facilitate visualization of wells.
4. Electrophorese at 1–10 V/cm. As for any other type of gel, if power supplied exceeds heat dissipation, then temperature and hence conductivity inequalities across the gel will lead to "smiling." Indeed, the general properties of these gels are no different from standard gels for which detailed reviews are available *(15)*. Optionally, a glass plate can be laid on top of the gel to ensure symmetry of conditions between the top and the bottom of the gel. An important corollary to this is that a set of MADGE gels on glass plates can be stacked directly on top of each other in one tank. Thus, the same tanks previously used to electrophorese 32 samples on a small agarose gel on a special tray can be used to electrophorese 480 samples on five horizontal acrylamide MADGE gels anchored on 2-mm float glass plates.

3.3. DNA Detection on MADGE Gels: Different Methods

1. Incorporate ethidium bromide in the gel. For agarose, remove carefully from the plastic support and view on a transilluminator as for traditional agarose gels. For polyacrylamide gels anchored on glass, little UV would pass through the glass; therefore, place the gel side down on the transilluminator and view the orange fluorescence through the glass.
2. Stain postelectrophoresis with ethidium bromide. For a 2-mm thick polyacrylamide gel anchored on glass, this takes approx 30 min.
3. Silver staining of polyacrylamide gels. For 2-mm thick gels the 30–60 min period for each step for gel on glass may be inconvenient. However, the gel can be detached from the plate (*see* step 4).
4. Gels can be detached from the plate if they are not to be reused. The gel can be cut off the glass by pushing a 200 × 10 × 0.1-mm strip of overhead transparency film, a long straight-edged razor blade, or a cheesewire on a handle between gel and glass. If the thin glass plates are to be reused, they can be cleaned using household liquid detergent, ethanol, and water. (Acetone or 1*M* sodium hydroxide are other well known releasing/cleaning agents for silanized plates. However, tanks of either are inconvenient in the laboratory and the former can introduce background fluorescence, *see* Note 2.)

5. Detached gels can be dried down after silver staining or for autoradiography.

6. Detached polyacrylamide gels would be amenable to other procedures, such as electroblotting, and so on.

3.4. Record Keeping

For MADGE gels, the most cathodal well corresponds in our arrangement with well A1 of a microtiter plate. For photography, a transparency of a microtiter grid is overlaid on the gel or glass plate, with its letters and numbers suitably oriented to identify sample wells or bands of interest, and with the lines of the grid arranged to assist interpretation of patterns.

3.5. Examples

A range of checking gels, resolving gels for PCRs informative from the size of products, and resolving gels of post-PCR restriction digests are shown in Figs. 2 and 3. The specific genotypic markers are explained in the figure legends.

4. Notes

1. Three possible ways to obtain the gel formers described are first to glue suitable slot formers to a smooth-faced piece of plastic (difficult in our experience); second to machine away from one face of a piece of plastic to leave slot formers, using specialist computerized cutters of limited availability (expensive in our experience); or third, to mold plastics (a commercial process). The latter eventually should be the simplest and cheapest option for those requiring such apparatus and has the advantage that associated items such as suitable transparent photographic grids, glass plates, and other reagents and equipment will be simultaneously available. However, "unique" machining runs will be most appropriate for users with special needs, for example slots greater or less than 2 mm in length between cathode and anode, gels of different thickness, different diagonal angles, and so on.

2. We have been reusing our glass plates. However, if the glass were to be treated as a disposable and the gel used once only, the cost of the glass per sample would be approx 0.0032 \$US; for comparison, we estimate the cost of one (10 µL) sample PCR to be 0.026 \$US. The simplest way to clean the glass is to "shave" the gel off the plate with a long straight-edged razor blade, then to clean the plate with Fairy Liquid Excel (Proctor and Gamble Ltd, Newcastle, UK), ethanol then water. Several reagents, either singly or in combination with each other and ethidium bromide, introduce background fluorescence that can be problematic: Traces of acetone (which is well known to remove silane) cause smeared and speckled orange fluorescence; Jeybrite (Jeyes, Bucks, UK) liquid cleaner causes heavily smeared orange fluorescence; and excess residual nonvolatile component of the silanizing mix also induces a heavy background fluorescence with ethidium bromide. The latter background problem never occurs with the first use of glass plates and presumably reflects combination with some trace from cleaning procedures; however, wiping of the (dried) silanized plate with tissue and water prevents this cause of background.

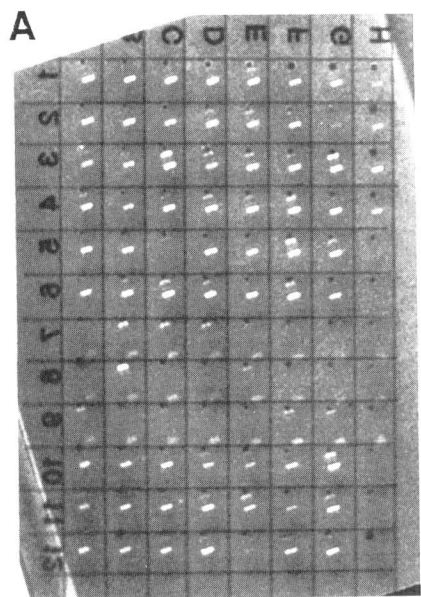 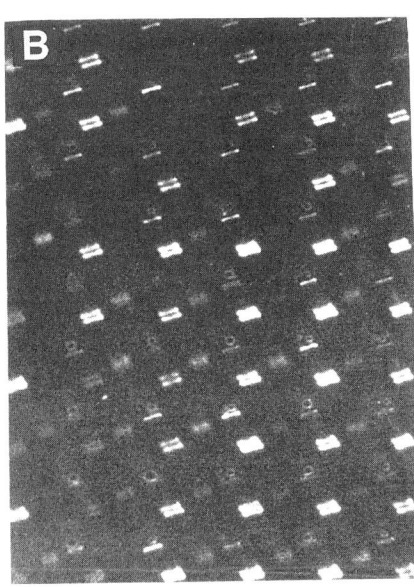

Fig. 2. Examples of MADGE gels for checking of PCR products. **(A)** 7.5% poly-acrylamide/1X TBE checking gel for presence of PCR products from a 96-well plate PCR. The bands in the centers of the grid boxes represent the PCR product. Their wells of origin are (for the wells that contain an air bubble) visible within their respective grid boxes. In some cases high-mol-wt DNA, representing an excess of genomic DNA template put into the PCR reaction, is visible at the leading edges of some wells. Columns 7, 8, and 9 contain no PCR product, but the unincorporated oligonucleotide is recognizable as a smear of high mobility. Primers of higher mobility are visible. **(B)** 7.5% polyacrylamide/1X TBE checking gel of a duplex PCR. The 174 and 202 bp products are clearly resolved after a migration of less than 1 cm. The leading edges of their wells of origin are in some tracks marked by genomic DNA PCR template that cannot migrate a significant distance into the gel.

It should be noted that the mirror images of the array codes are intentional and used in the laboratory as part of a mnemonic aid system when gels are viewed "upside-down" relative to orientation during loading and electrophoresis: This ensures that only one set of transparency grids are in circulation in the laboratory, which must themselves be inverted if the gel is inverted. If there were two orientations of transparency grid available in the laboratory, there would be high potential for use of the inappropriate grid (e.g., the one for a detached gel in usual orientation rather than gel anchored on glass and viewed inverted) and consequent misidentification of all positions in the array.

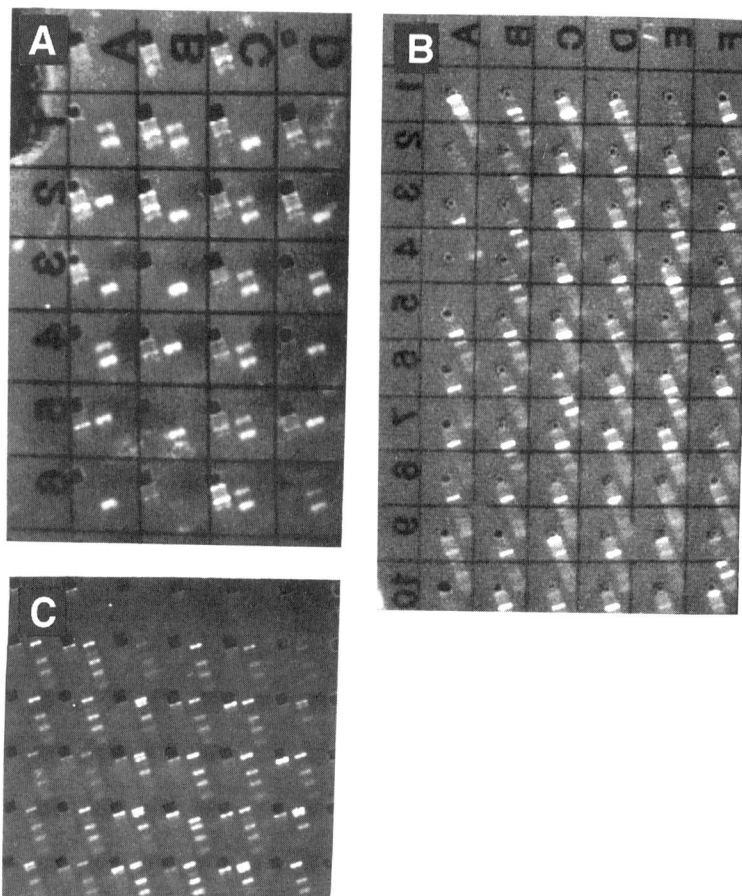

Fig. 3. Examples of MADGE gels for genotyping either by resolution of size products of an informative PCR or resolution of fragments from a post-PCR restriction enzyme digestion. **(A)** PCR products from a three oligonucleotide PCR designed to distinguish an *Alu* insertion/deletion polymorphism in intron 16 of the human ACE gene *(4)*. Homozygotes and heterozygotes are distinguishable on the size of the PCR products, 84 and 65 bp. Heteroduplex and/or long PCR product are also observed near the wells in samples generating the smaller (65 bp) fragment, which is arranged (paradoxically) to represent the *presence* of the *Alu* insertion sequence. Tracks D2, D3, and D4, respectively, represent insertion homozygote, heterozygote, and deletion homozygote. **(B)** PCR of exon 13 of the low density lipoprotein receptor gene was followed by drying of PCR product (a simple means of DNA concentration for large scale studies), then *Ava*II digestion for typing of a restriction fragment length polymorphism. For example, tracks 6A, 6C, and 6E represent a homozygote lacking the restriction site, a homozygote for the presence of the site, and a heterozygote. Although drying is a convenient means of concentrating arrays of DNA so that smaller bands of low yield

3. Hydrophilic GelBond plastic can be used instead of glass for polyacrylamide as well as agarose MADGE, but H-PAGE is more difficult because the closely spaced teeth do not permit much adherence of gel to plastic in the critical region around the slots. The hydrophilic nature of the adherence also means that MADGEs on GelBond (unlike polyacrylamide MADGEs on glass) cannot be stored submerged in TBE in the refrigerator long-term, because the gel peels off the backing.

4. Other formats of MADGE may be useful for different applications. For example, if it is necessary to visualize faint bands of small fragments from digests, then slots that are longer (e.g., 4 mm) between cathode and anode would be helpful with less than a 10% compromise of the total track length possible. If gels are to be dried, for example for autoradiography, then a thinner gel (e.g., 1 mm rather than 2 mm) will give sharper resolution and will enable the drying of high percentage (e.g., 20%) polyacrylamide gels.

5. As an alternative to longer slots, more sample can be loaded by concentration/drying prior to loading, if faint bands are to be visualized. When there is significant salt in the sample, its concentration may cause a salt gradient from bottom (salty sample) to top (TBE buffer) of the well. This will cause tilted bands, DNA at the base of the wells migrating more slowly: Prior flushing of slots with high salt buffer should minimize this effect. However, for PCR amplifications tending toward low yield, we prefer to increase the concentration of *Taq* polymerase—economy is achieved by maintaining the total PCR volume at the minimum necessary, for example 10 μL.

6. We prefer our gels to set rapidly (2–5 min) so that the device can immediately be reused to prepare another gel. The use of higher concentrations of ammonium persulfate and TEMED, as listed, expedites this and does not cause any problems.

Fig. 3. *(continued)* PCR products can be visualized on MADGE (where, unlike vertical gels, the slots cannot be "overloaded"), the process tends to cause some smearing. For high throughput applications, it is preferable to avoid secondary procedures post-PCR if possible, and to optimize PCR conditions for high yield. More sensitive detection systems will also be advantageous. **(C)** PCR of the APOE gene *(2,3)* followed directly by restriction digestion (addition of a master mix of restriction enzyme/salt buffer to PCR product). The digest simultaneously analyzes two restriction sites in one PCR product, distinguishing three alleles (E2/3/4) and hence six genotypes. The various patterns observed represent different combinations of fragments of 90 (present for E3 and E2), 84 (present for E2 only), 72 (present for E4 only), 60 (constant), 48 (present for E3 and E4), 36 (present for E3 and E4) bp, and some very small fragments not visible. The 90-bp fragment has been electrophoresed so that it is level with the anodal edge of the well of an adjacent track and it can be noted that the 90/84 doublets are readily recognized in E2/E3 and E2/E2 samples as a closely spaced but clearly resolved doublet. Thus resolution on MADGE of 6.7% relative mobility is readily possible—ultimately, the resolution possible with MADGE will be determined by the gel thickness, the imaging system used, and the quality of the gel matrix, so considerable improvements will be possible.

7. Polyacrylamide gels on glass anchors can readily be stored piled on top of each other in electrophoresis buffer in the refrigerator. The convenience of storage, robustness, and reuse has one drawback: Ethidium bromide incorporated into the gel decays in TBE buffer. Gels stored for a few weeks are best stained post-electrophoresis, or soaked in intercalating dye (10 min on a shaker) prior to electrophoresis. The bands in 2-mm gels appear very fine and sharp compared with agarose if ethidium bromide is incorporated in the gel. The sharpness of these bands means that even the limited diffusion occurring during poststaining gives a surprising thickening of the band and often also substantial apparent gain in quantity of fluorescence present in the band.

8. Ready-made gels are now available from *genetiX*, (Wimborne, Dorset, UK) and extend to pattern recognition electrophoretic analyses all of the conveniences associated with the use of disposable microtiter plates. Disposable ready-made gels may turn out to be the most convenient and popular option for many laboratories, in view of the safety objective to avoid handling unpolymerized acrylamide, coupled with time saving. This "use-and-dispose" strategy is common in laboratories using microtiter plates to achieve high throughput and save staff time, usually the most expensive component of progress in the laboratory.

Acknowledgments

I. N. M. Day, L. Haddad, and S. E. Humphries have been supported, respectively, by Intermediate Fellowship, PhD studentship and Chair Award from the British Heart Foundation. I. N. M. Day is currently the recipient of a Lister Institute Research Fellowship. Support for M. Bolla was kindly provided by L. G. Fine and S. O'Dell was supported, respectively, by an award to S. E. Humphries from Merck Sharpe and Dohme MEDPED program and a ROPA award from the MRC to I. N. M. Day. The staff of *genetiX* (Dorset, UK) are thanked for assistance and loan of equipment.

References

1. Wilson, J. M. G. and Jungner, G. (1968) *Principles and Practice of Screening for Disease* (Public Health Paper No. 34), WHO, Geneva.

2. Davignon, J., Gregg, R. E., and Sing, C. F. (1988) Apolipoprotein E polymorphism and atherosclerosis. *Arteriosclerosis* **8**, 1–21.

3. Corder, E. H., Saunders, A. M., Strittmatter, W. J., Schmechel, D. E., Gaskell, P. C., Small, G. W., et al. (1993) Gene dose of apolipoprotein E type 4 allele and the risk of Alzheimer's disease in late onset families. *Science* **261**, 921–923.

4. Cambien, F., Poirier, O., Lecerf, L., Evans, A., Cambou, J. P., Arvelier, D., et al. (1992) Deletion polymorphism in the gene for angiotensin-converting enzyme is a potent risk factor for myocardial infarction. *Nature* **359**, 641–644.

5. Kannel, W. B., Neaton, J. D., Wentworth, D., Thomas, H. E., Stamler, J., Hulley, S. B., et al. (1986) Overall and coronary heart disease mortality rates in relation to major risk factors in 325,348 men screened for the MRFIT. *Am. Heart J.* **112**, 825–836.

6. Gille, C., Grade, K., and Coutelle, C. (1991) A pooling strategy for heterozygote screening of the ΔF508 cystic fibrosis mutation. *Hum. Genet.* **86,** 289–291.

7. Hales, C. N. and Woodhead, J. S. (1980) Labelled antibodies and their use in the immunoradiometric assay. *Meth. Enzymol.* **70,** 334–355.

8. Cooper, D. N. and Krawczak, M. (1991) Mechanisms of insertional mutagenesis in human genes causing genetic disease. *Hum. Genet.* **87,** 409–415.

9. Weissenbach, J., Gyapay, G., Dib, C., Vignal, A., Morissette, J., Millasseau, P., et al. (1992) A second-generation linkage map of the human genome. *Nature* **359,** 794–801.

10. Snow, K., Doud, L. K., Hagerman, R., Pergolizzi, R. G., Erster, S. H., and Thibodeau, S. N. (1993) Analysis of a CGG sequence at the FMR-1 locus in fragile X families and in the general population. *Am. J. Hum. Genet.* **53,** 1217–1228.

11. O'Dell, S., Humphries, S. E., and Day, I. N. M. (1995) A rapid approach to genotyping of the insertion/deletion polymorphism in intron 16 of the angiotensin converting enzyme gene using simplified DNA preparation and microtitre array diagonal gel electrophoresis. *Br. Heart J.* **73,** 368–371.

12. Day, I. N. M., Whittall, R., Gudnason, V., and Humphries, S. E. (1995) Dried template DNA, dried PCR oligonucleotides and mailing in 96-well plates: LDL receptor gene mutation screening. *BioTechniques* **18,** 981–984.

13. Day, I. N. M. and Humphries, S. E. (1994) Electrophoresis for genotyping: devices for high throughput using horizontal acrylamide gels (H-PAGE) and microtitre array diagonal gel electrophoresis (MADGE). *Nature* (product review) 36,37.

14. Day, I. N. M. and Humphries, S. E. (1994) Electrophoresis for genotyping: microtitre array diagonal gel electrophoresis (MADGE) on horizontal polyacrylamide (H-PAGE) gels, Hydrolink or agarose. *Anal. Biochem.* **222,** 389–395.

15. Rickwood, D. and Hames, B. D. (eds.) (1982) *Gel Electrophoresis of Nucleic Acids: A Practical Approach.* IRL Press, Oxford, UK.

17

Pulsed Field Gel Electrophoresis for Detection of Gene Rearrangements in Duchenne Muscular Dystrophy

David J. Cockburn and Anneke Seller

1. Introduction

In diseases with a high new mutation rate, such as Duchenne and Becker muscular dystrophy (DMD, BMD), linkage analysis often produces highly unsatisfactory results for carrier diagnosis compared to methods that rely on the direct detection of the mutation. The size of the dystrophin gene and the nature of mutations at this locus that give rise to DMD/BMD make pulsed field gel electrophoresis (PFGE) an appropriate and powerful technique for detection of mutations and hence accurate carrier diagnosis in these diseases.

The basis of PFGE analysis is to digest high-mol-wt DNA using a rare-cutting restriction enzyme, such as *Sfi*I, and to analyze the sizes of fragments produced using an electrophoresis system capable of resolving DNA fragments several hundred kilobases in size. These restriction fragments may be detected by standard Southern blotting and probe hybridization procedures. A physical map of the dystrophin gene, including *Sfi*I sites is illustrated in Fig. 1. The presence of rearrangements within the 2300 kb dystrophin locus may result in the production of abnormally sized *Sfi*I restriction fragments and since the majority of mutations responsible for DMD/BMD are large scale deletions or duplications (approx 60 and 7%, respectively) the majority of DMD/BMD mutations are potentially detectable by PFGE analysis *(2–7)*. Once an abnormally sized fragment has been detected, a qualitative test is available to female relatives for the presence or absence of the mutation.

In order to extract DNA of a size suitable for PFGE analysis, cells are immobilized in agarose blocks and all subsequent steps of DNA extraction, washing, and restriction enzyme digestion are performed by allowing diffu-

From: *Methods in Molecular Medicine: Molecular Diagnosis of Genetic Diseases*
Edited by: R. Elles Humana Press Inc., Totowa, NJ

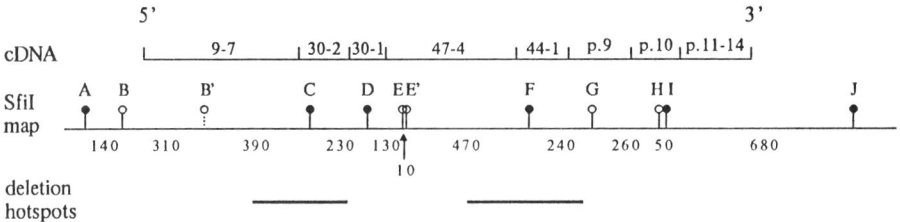

Fig. 1. Physical map surrounding the dystrophin locus, illustrating the positions of *Sfi*I restriction sites (A–J) and the sizes of restriction fragments (in kilobases; data based on ref. *1*). Unfilled circles indicate sites which are partially digestible. The presence/absence of site B' is polymorphic in the normal population (present on approx 11% of chromosomes; referred to as site S in ref. *1*). The approximate positions of exons to which cDNA probes hybridize is indicated above the map and positions of deletion hotspots is indicated below (corresponding to exons 3–19 and 44–55).

sion of solutions into the blocks. High-mol-wt DNA remains trapped within the agarose matrix and the blocks themselves are loaded into the wells of the gel. Electrophoretic separation of large DNA fragments is achieved by the PFGE technique, where the basis for resolution is thought to be the reorientation in direction of migration of the DNA with respect to the gel. The technical challenge of producing two uniform electric fields within a single tank is responsible for the unusual shapes and designs of PFGE gel tanks.

The methods described here are those used in our laboratory and employ the rotating gel "Waltzer" system, built in a workshop according to the design of Southern et al. *(8)*. Many commercial PFGE systems are available that give results of similar quality, however the conditions for optimal resolution vary between these systems. Since it would be inappropriate here only to describe the conditions used with our gel system, we have indicated the factors that individual operators should consider when selecting appropriate conditions for use with their own equipment.

Generally, investigations are performed in two types of family, first, those where a mutation has already been identified (usually a deletion) and accurate carrier diagnosis is requested, second, those where no mutation has yet been identified, either because no affected male is available from the family or because of the possibility of a duplication. Although duplications are readily detectable by PFGE analysis, they are not often detected using strategies currently employed in the majority of diagnostic laboratories. In the second type of investigation a full mutation screen must be performed using probes from throughout the dystrophin locus. If an abnormality is identified, it is often possible by use of further probes to characterize the mutation, i.e., determine whether it is a deletion or duplication, its size, and approximate location. Such information is especially valuable should any member of the family request a prenatal diagnosis.

PFGE is just one of several techniques available to diagnostic laboratories for mutation detection and carrier identification in dystrophinopathies. The power of the technique is demonstrated in its capacity for unambiguous carrier diagnosis and detection of duplications or more complex rearrangements. Therefore, we believe that the technique deserves to be more widely used and that this would improve the overall quality of service to patients.

2. Materials
2.1. Preparation of High-Mol-Wt DNA in Agarose Blocks

1. Lysis buffer: 155 mM NH$_4$Cl, 10 mM KHCO$_3$, 0.1 mM Na$_2$-EDTA. This solution may be autoclaved and stored at 4°C.
2. PBS: 0.8% NaCl, 0.23% Na$_2$HPO$_4$, 0.04% KH$_2$PO$_4$, 0.04% KCl. This solution may be autoclaved and stored at 4°C.
3. Block mold: The block mold should produce blocks which are compatible with the sizes of wells in the pulsed field gel, and may be supplied by the manufacturer of the pulsed field gel equipment. We use a perspex mold that produces blocks 11 × 6 × 1.5 mm in size (approx 100 μL in volume; these blocks are later cut into slices of approx 6 × 3.7 × 1.5 mm, *see the following*). The wells are formed by securing a strip of plastic sticky tape to one side of the block mold. Once the blocks have solidified, the tape is removed, allowing the blocks to be blown out of the mold using a rubber teat. The block mold must be kept clean by washing in a solution of 20% ethanol, 1% SDS for 16 h after use, rinsing in water, and thoroughly drying.
4. NDS: 30 g NaOH, 186 g EDTA, and 1.25 g Tris are dissolved in 700 mL H$_2$O; lauryl sarcosine (10 g sodium salt) is dissolved in 50 mL H$_2$O; the solutions are mixed, the pH is adjusted to 9.5 using 5M NaOH, and the volume is made up to 1000 mL. NDS may be stored at 4°C for up to 1 yr.
5. A plastic mesh strainer, marketed as a tea strainer and obtainable from a domestic hardware store, is suitable for draining wash solutions from PFGE blocks.

2.2. Restriction Enzyme Digestion

1. TE: 10 mM Tris-HCl, pH 8.0, 1 mM EDTA. This solution may be autoclaved and stored at 4°C.
2. *Sfi*I restriction buffer: 50 mM NaCl, 10 mM Tris-HCl, pH 7.9, 10 mM MgCl$_2$, 1 mM dithiothreitol, and 100 μg/mL bovine serum albumin. This solution is made up as a 10X stock and stored at –20°C.

2.3. Gel Electrophoresis

1. We use a "Waltzer" apparatus built in a university department workshop, as described by Southern et al. *(8)*. It is so called because the alternating electric

field is produced by rotating the gel with respect to the apparatus (the angle of rotation is fixed at 117°). The gel tank is square (260 × 260 mm) and the electrodes are straight, but the gel itself is circular (diameter 220 mm) to ensure a uniform electric field. This equipment produces consistently high quality DNA resolution in straight tracks.

2. 0.5X TAE: 0.24% Tris, 0.057% glacial acetic acid, 0.5 mM EDTA. A 50X TAE stock solution is stable at room temperature for up to 6 mo.

2.4. Southern Blotting

1. The blotting apparatus consists of a glass plate supported on a platform over a reservoir of alkali blotting solution (approx 1000 mL) with four sheets of 3MM chromatography paper (Whatman, Maidstone, UK) placed over the glass plate, their edges immersed in the reservoir. The gel is placed on top, a sheet of transfer membrane (Hybond N+; Amersham, Arlington Heights, IL) is laid over the gel followed by two sheets of 3MM paper, a 50-mm stack of paper towels, and finally a 500-g weight.

2. Alkali blotting solution: 0.4M NaOH and 1.6M NaCl.

3. 2X SSC: 1.75% NaCl and 0.88% trisodium citrate . This solution is made up as a 20X SSC stock which is stored at room temperature for 6 mo and is diluted as required.

2.5. Probe Hybridization

1. Hybridization solution: 300 mL 20X SSC and 100 mL 50X Denhardt's are mixed thoroughly with 550 mL H$_2$O at 37°C. Fifty milliliters 10% SDS is added with continuous stirring and the hybridization solution is aliquoted and stored at –20°C for up to 1 yr. Before use, dextran sulfate (sodium salt) is dissolved in hybridization solution warmed to 65°C to a final concentration of 5%. 50X Denhardt's solution is prepared by dissolving 10 g ficoll, 10 g bovine serum albumin, and 10 g polyvinyl pyrollidone in 900 mL H$_2$O. The solution is made up to 1 L and stored at –20°C.

2. cDNA clones, which were kindly provided by L. Kunkel, hybridize to the following dystrophin exons: 9–7 (probe 0–2a) to exons 1–11; 30–2 (probe 2b–3a) to exons 11–20; 30–1 (probe 3b–5a) to exons 20–30; 47–4 (probe 5b–7) to exons 31–47; 44–1 (probe 8) to exons 47–52 and 63–1 (probe 9–14) to exons 53–79 *(9)*. The insert of clone 63–1 may be restricted using *Bam*HI, generating three smaller probes. Probe 9 hybridizes to exons 53–59, probe 10 to exons 59–66 and probe 11–14 to exons 66–79. The approximate sites of hybridization of cDNA probes to the physical *Sfi*I map are illustrated in Fig. 1.

3. Methods

3.1. Preparation of High-Mol-Wt DNA in Agarose Blocks

The standard tissue for analysis is fresh blood, however, cultured cells (e.g., fibroblasts and chorionic villus samples [CVS]) or frozen blood are alternative starting materials (*see* Notes 1 and 2). It is not possible to obtain the clearest results unless the blocks themselves are of high quality. The DNA must be of high molecular weight (not degraded), the DNA must be evenly dispersed within the blocks at the correct concentration, and the blocks themselves must be firm so that they do not disintegrate during subsequent manipulations.

The DNA concentration within blocks is determined by counting the white cells and adjusting the number of blocks made accordingly. It is imperative that cells are evenly dispersed within the agarose block since clumps of cells produce localized high DNA concentrations that migrate more slowly in the gel, resulting in a smeared hybridization signal on the autoradiograph. Therefore, if cell clumps appear during the preparation of blocks they must be removed.

If the DNA from any sample is found not to have fully digested when the gel is run, the remaining blocks from the sample may be subjected to further pronase treatment followed by NDS washes (repeating steps 8–12 that follow).

1. Mix 5–10 mL of blood gently with 30 mL lysis buffer and stand on ice until the red cells have lysed (approx 15–30 min), mixing occasionally (*see* Notes 3 and 4).
2. Centrifuge at 200g for 10 min and resuspend the pellet evenly in 30 mL PBS.
3. Remove a sample and perform a white cell count (a Coulter counter or hemocytometer may be used).
4. Centrifuge at 200g for 10 min and resuspend the cell pellet evenly in PBS giving a cell concentration of 3×10^7/mL.
5. Warm the cell suspension briefly at 37°C and mix with an equal volume of molten 1.2% low melting point (LMP) agarose (UltraPure, Life Technologies, Bethesda, MD) at 37°C in PBS giving a final cell concentration of 1.5×10^7/mL.
6. Dispense the cell suspension into wells of a block mold that has been precooled on ice and leave to set for 10 min. Precooling the block mold ensures that the agarose sets before white cells begin to settle.
7. Blow the agarose blocks gently from the mold using a rubber teat into 10–20 mL NDS containing 1 mg/mL pronase (Sigma, St. Louis, MO) and incubate overnight at 50°C. Ten milliliters of solution is used for up to 15 blocks and 20 mL for 16–30 blocks.
8. Stand the tube on ice for 30 min to harden the blocks and drain the NDS/pronase solution using the plastic mesh strainer.
9. Replace with 10–20 mL fresh NDS containing 1 mg/mL pronase and incubate overnight at 50°C.
10. Harden blocks by standing on ice as described, drain NDS/pronase solution, and replace with 10–20 mL fresh NDS (without pronase).
11. Stand on ice for 30 min and replace NDS solution as described.
12. After a further 30 min repeat step 11 so that three NDS washes are performed in total. The blocks may be stored in the final NDS wash at 4°C indefinitely.

3.2. Restriction Enzyme Digestion

The following procedures must be performed on ice unless otherwise indicated to preserve the integrity of agarose blocks.

1. Transfer PFGE blocks individually to a glass microscope slide using a glass scoop (a glass Pasteur pipet may be modified in a flame for this purpose). Cut the blocks into slices corresponding to 0.5×10^6 cells using a glass coverslip and transfer slices to individual 2 mL screwcapped polypropylene tubes. These tubes are convenient since they permit rapid addition and removal of wash solutions, and are suitable for immersion of the block slice in a minimum volume of enzyme solution (100 µL).
2. Add 1 mL TE to each tube and incubate for 30 min (*see* Notes 5 and 6).
3. Remove TE wash taking care not to damage agarose slice, replace with 1 mL fresh TE, and incubate for a further 30 min. A disposable plastic Pasteur pipet has been found to be suitable for performing these washes.
4. Repeat step 3 so that three TE washes are performed in total.
5. Remove TE wash as in step 3 and replace with 1 mL *Sfi*I restriction buffer, incubating for 30 min.
6. Remove restriction buffer wash and add 100 µL *Sfi*I restriction buffer, including 10 U *Sfi*I (New England Biolabs, Beverly, MA). Incubate overnight at 50°C (*see* Notes 7 and 8).
7. If samples are to be loaded on gels within 24 h, add 1 mL gel-loading buffer to each tube and equilibrate for at least 15 min. Otherwise, add 1 mL NDS to each tube and store at 4°C, replacing the NDS with 1 mL gel-loading buffer within 24 h of loading the gel (*see* Note 9).

3.3. Gel Electrophoresis

The optimal procedures for loading, running, and blotting pulsed field gels are particularly dependent on the gel system being used, therefore we stress the overriding considerations that should be made. Conditions of electrophoresis that may be varied include voltage, agarose type and concentration, buffer type, temperature, and reorientation angle. Further information on selection of suitable conditions may be found in the excellent guide of Birren and Lai *(10)*.

The conditions described here give satisfactory resolution of DNA fragments over the range of 100–1000 kb using our equipment, a size range appropriate for the majority of DMD family investigations.

1. Cast the gel on a horizontal surface (230 mL of 1.5% agarose, Sigma type II, medium EEO; in 0.5X TAE) and leave to set.
2. Fill the wells with 0.5X TAE and carefully insert the agarose block slices. The slices may be manipulated using two small spatulas (approx 4 mm wide). A *Saccharomyces cerevisiae* chromosome size marker should be included (commercially available from a variety of sources, e.g., New England Biolabs). The block slices are sealed into the gel by covering the wells with molten 1% LMP agarose in 0.5X TAE at 37°C that is left for 5 min to solidify.

3. Ensure the gel tank is horizontal using a spirit level, wash out the heat exchanger with 70% ethanol, then the whole apparatus with distilled water. Refill with 0.5X TAE electrophoresis buffer and adjust temperature to 15°C (*see* Note 10).
4. Set the switching time. To give satisfactory resolution over a wide size range, we increase the switch time during electrophoresis. Standard conditions are a 30-s switch time for 16 h, 60 s for 8 h, and 80 s for 16 h (total run time 40 h). A constant voltage of 150 V is applied (starting current 250 mA). Many modern appliances employ microprocessors that permit the switch time to be ramped continuously during electrophoresis.

3.4. Southern Blotting

There is essentially no difference in blotting a pulsed field gel from blotting a conventional gel apart from the important consideration that high-mol-wt DNA will not transfer efficiently unless it is fragmented prior to blotting. The conditions of the fragmentation process are critical since if treatment is too severe, a poor hybridization signal will be obtained. It is therefore important to optimize this step and rigorously maintain conditions (*see* Note 11). The following method is for alkali transfer of DNA to positively charged nylon membranes.

1. Remove gel from tank and stain in 2 µg/mL ethidium bromide in 0.5X TAE for 15 min with gentle shaking. Destain in 0.5X TAE for 15 min and photograph over a UV transilluminator, taking care to expose gel to UV light for the shortest possible time to minimize DNA nicking.
2. Depurinate by transferring the gel to 700 mL 0.25M HCl and gently shaking for 20 min. The conditions of this step are critical and should be calibrated in individual laboratories to give maximum hybridization signal (*see* Note 11).
3. Transfer the gel to alkali blotting solution and leave to shake gently for 30 min.
4. Southern transfer DNA to a Hybond N+ membrane (Amersham) for 24 h using a reservoir of alkali blotting solution.
5. Rinse membrane briefly in 2X SSC and air dry.

3.5. Probe Hybridization

1. cDNA or genomic probes from throughout the dystrophin locus are labeled by the random hexanucleotide priming method (multiprime kit, Amersham). Label 50 ng of cDNA or genomic probe to a specific activity of 1×10^7 dps/µg with α-^{32}PdCTP (Amersham).
2. Prehybridize membranes for 30 min in sufficient hybridization solution to soak them plus 10 mL excess per bottle, add the labeled probe, and hybridize at 65°C overnight.
3. Wash membranes to a stringency of approx 0.5X SSC (with 0.1% SDS) at 65°C, air dry, and autoradiograph using X-ray film for 1–10 d at –70°C.
4. Before reprobing membranes, the old probe may be stripped by pouring boiling 0.1% SDS over the membrane and shaking gently for 10 min. Membranes are often reprobed successfully in our laboratory up to five times.

3.6. Interpretation of Results

Accurate interpretation of results from pulsed field gel investigations of the dystrophin locus requires care and skill. It is essential to recognize normal hybridization signals that may be produced by partial DNA digestion or polymorphism so that they are not confused with abnormally sized restriction fragments resulting from mutations. Careful evaluation of results is therefore essential and experience plays an important part in this aspect of PFGE analysis. The approach to analysis in any family depends on whether any other form of mutation screen has already been performed and on whether a mutation has been identified in such an analysis.

3.6.1. Mutation in Family Known

When the mutation responsible for disease in a particular family has already been identified using techniques other than PFGE analysis, it is generally possible to predict the approximate size of altered *Sfi*I restriction fragment that will be produced and to select probes appropriate for its detection (Fig. 1). Sometimes, however, this is not possible. The breakpoint positions of a deletion/duplication may not be precisely known, owing to incomplete characterization or because the intron in which the breakpoint lies is large. Alternatively, it may be uncertain whether the deletion/duplication includes a particular *Sfi*I site. Therefore, it is important to obtain a sample from an affected individual or known carrier and analyze this alongside the sample from the individual for whom carrier diagnosis is required whenever possible.

cDNA probes are usually suitable for detecting an abnormal *Sfi*I fragment, however, they may produce a faint hybridization signal from the abnormal fragment if this fragment contains only a small number of exons. In these circumstances, a genomic probe that hybridizes to the abnormal fragment may be used since this will be expected to give a stronger hybridization signal.

Occasionally an abnormal *Sfi*I fragment may be insufficiently resolved from the normal fragment to permit unambiguous carrier diagnosis. It is necessary in these cases to run another gel employing conditions that give optimal resolution in the required size range.

3.6.2. Mutation in Family Unknown

3.6.2.1. ANALYSIS OF BOYS IN WHOM NO DELETION HAS BEEN FOUND

If no deletion can be detected in an affected DMD/BMD boy by multiplex PCR analysis, there is still a chance that a deletion is present that does not include exons tested by this approach *(11)*. Such deletions are potentially detectable by PFGE analysis. There is a greater chance, however, that the mutation responsible for the disease is a duplication. Assuming frequencies of 60, 7, and 33% for deletions, duplications, and point mutations, respectively, one would expect 7/40 (17.5%) of nondeleted boys to show duplications. In our laboratory we have detected duplications in 7/25 (28%) nondeleted DMD boys by PFGE analysis, suggesting that the frequency of duplications may be higher than 7%, and that screening for duplications is a worthwhile test when no deletion has been detected (Cockburn et al., in preparation).

The distribution of duplications causing DMD/BMD is nonrandom and differs from that of deletions. The majority of duplications occur in the proximal region of the dystrophin gene, close to the more proximal of the two deletion hotspots *(2,7)*. The list of probes recommended for a mutation screen in this case therefore includes both 30–2 and 30–1 that are from this region, since some duplications may be detected using only one of these probes. The recommended list of probes used in a standard mutation screen for this type of investigation is: 9–7, 30–2, 30–1, 47–4, 44–1, probe 9, and probe 11–14.

An altered sized *Sfi*I restriction fragment from a DMD boy in whom no deletion had been found is illustrated in Fig. 2 (track 2). An explanation consistent with this result would be the presence of a 170-kb duplication within the 700-kb *Sfi*I fragment BC (Fig. 1). This interpretation could be tested by dosage examination of an orthodox Southern blot of *Hin*dIII digested DNA from the patient probed with cDNA 9–7 (exons 1–11).

3.6.2.2. ANALYSIS IN FAMILIES WHERE NO AFFECTED MALE IS AVAILABLE

The detection of a mutation by PFGE analysis in a family where no affected male is available for any type of molecular genetic analysis has a dramatic effect on carrier diagnosis. In such cases, carrier diagnosis is transformed from a situation relying on linkage analysis to one where highly accurate diagnosis can be made.

There is a very good prospect of identifying a mutation by PFGE analysis if an obligate carrier is available since most deletions and duplications are as straightforward to identify in a female sample as in a male. When no obligate carrier is available, however, the female relative who is closest in relationship to the affected boy should be analyzed. If an altered *Sfi*I restriction fragment is identified, the presence or absence of this fragment may be used as the basis of carrier diagnosis in other female relatives. If no altered fragment is identified, then this result reduces the risk that a deletion or duplication is present. A conservative figure of 50% sensitivity is probably appropriate for use in Baysian risk calculations, however (*see* Chapter 8), this figure depends on the quality of results and the rigor of the investigation. The recommended list of probes used in a standard mutation screen for this type of investigation is: 9–7, 30–2 or 30–1, 47–4, 44–1, probe 9, and probe 11–14.

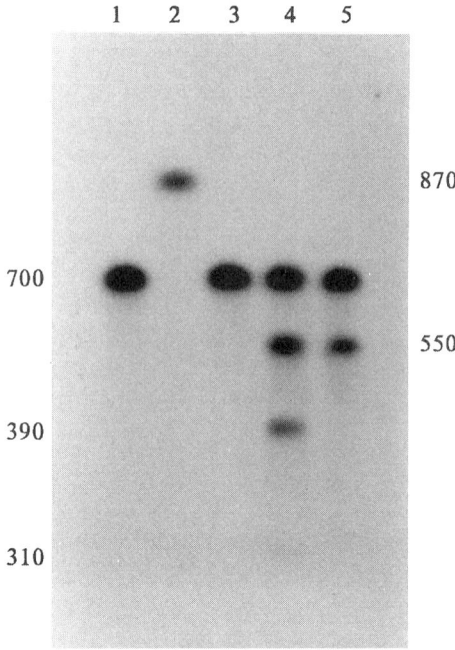

Fig. 2. Hybridization of cDNA clone 9–7 (exons 1–11) to Southern blot of *Sfi*I digested DNA resolved on a pulsed field gel. Fragment sizes (in kilobases) that represent normal results are shown on the left of the figure and the sizes of abnormal fragments that are caused by mutations are shown on the right. Tracks 1 and 3 show individuals with normal results. The sample in track 2 is from an affected boy in whom no deletion had been identified by multiplex PCR analysis. The altered 870-kb fragment may represent a 170-kb duplication within the *Sfi*I fragment BC (*see* Fig. 1). The sample in track 4 is from the mother of an affected boy who had died before any DNA was stored. An abnormal 550-kb fragment is present both in this sample and in that from her niece (track 5). Characterization of this mutation using other cDNA and genomic probes suggested that these individuals are carriers of a duplication of 550 kb that includes *Sfi*I site C. The 390- and 310-kb fragments additionally present in track 4 are owing to the presence of the partially digestible polymorphic site B' on the normal chromosome of this individual (*see* Fig. 1). The hybridization signal from the 390-kb fragment is significantly stronger than from the 310-kb fragment since probe 9–7 hybridizes to exons 2–11 on the 390-kb fragment but only to exon 1 on the 310-kb fragment.

An altered sized *Sfi*I restriction fragment in female relatives of a DMD boy who died without any DNA sample being obtained is illustrated in Fig. 2 (tracks 4 and 5). Additional PFGE results suggested that the mutation is a 550-kb duplication including *Sfi*I site C.

3.6.3. Mutation Characterization

The identification of a deletion in a sample from an affected boy is important since it allows accurate prenatal diagnosis to be offered to female relatives on the basis of a rapid PCR test. Therefore it is often helpful to characterize a mutation that has been identified in a female sample in case it can be demonstrated that the mutation is a deletion and some of the exons involved may be identified. It is simplest when characterizing a mutation to assume that it is a two-breakpoint deletion or duplication but to remember to consider the possibility that other gross rearrangements are capable of generating abnormally sized *Sfi*I fragments (translocations, inversions, complex rearrangements, and so on). Characteristic results from PFGE analysis of deletions and duplications are illustrated in Fig. 3 and Table 1. Information relating to the size of abnormal fragment, the positions of probes that detect or fail to detect the abnormal fragment, and the relative dosage of hybridization signal from normal and abnormal fragments helps to discriminate between the possible mutation types and positions.

The identification of a deletion should allow accurate prenatal diagnosis to be performed if required. If any doubt remains as to the nature or location of the mutation, then linkage analysis may also be performed. Linkage analysis is probably the course of action chosen for prenatal diagnosis should a duplication be identified. The accuracy of linkage analysis is improved in these cases once the duplication has been identified since markers closely surrounding the duplicated segment can be analyzed, reducing the chance of a recombination. It is also possible to perform PFGE analysis on cultured CVS cells, and this would be recommended if there is any difficulty in the interpretation of linkage results, for instance if the phase of the mutation cannot be established, if a recombination is detected, or for confirmation of linkage results.

4. Notes

1. The normal hybridization signals obtained from *Sfi*I-digested DNA from blood, cultured fibroblasts, and cultured CVS cells have been found to be identical, indicating that any methylation differences between these tissues do not affect *Sfi*I digestion at the dystrophin locus. Therefore, results derived from these tissues using *Sfi*I may be compared directly on pulsed field gels. The method described here for harvesting fibroblast or CVS cultures and preparing PFGE blocks gives the quantities required for each 25-cm^2 flask and should be scaled up as required. A yield of approx 1.5×10^6 cells is expected from each confluent 25 cm^2 culture flask, sufficient for three tracks on a gel, however, it is technically easier to prepare PFGE blocks from at least two to three times this quantity of cells.

   Growth medium should be drained from culture flasks and cells washed by adding 10 mL PBS and leaving for 5 min. The PBS solution is discarded and the cells are briefly rinsed (for approx 10 s) in 2 mL trypsin-EDTA solution (0.25%

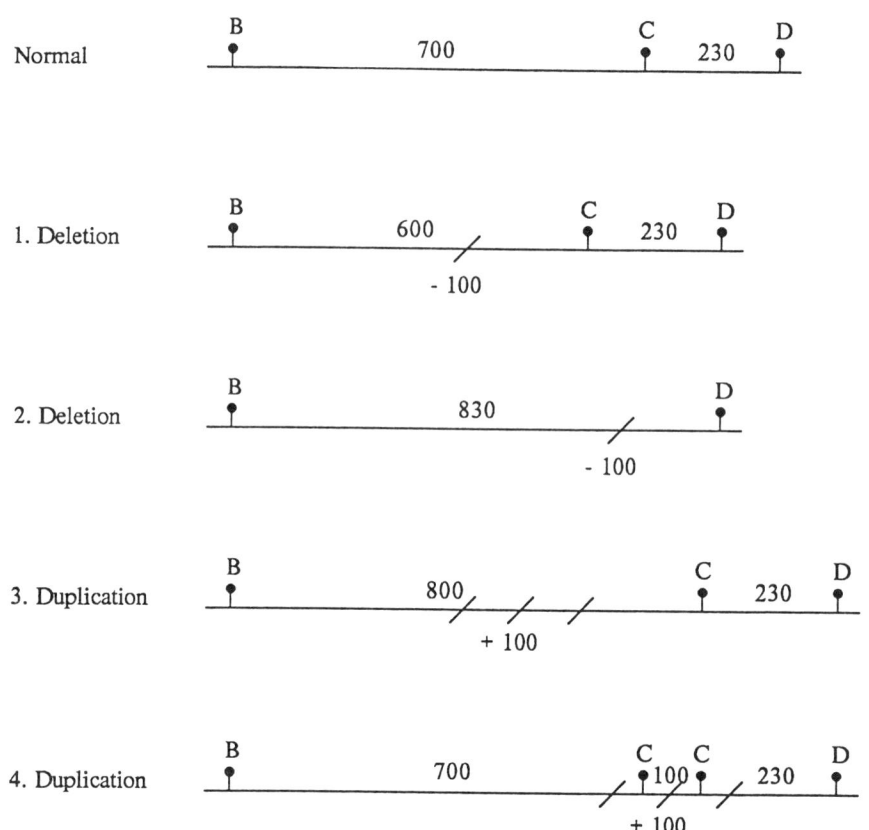

Fig. 3. Schematic effect of deletions and duplications on the sizes of *Sfi*I restriction fragments. Restriction sites (B, C, and D) and fragment sizes (in kilobases) are illustrated above the maps. Deletions or duplications are indicated below the maps and slashes indicate deletion sites or boundaries of duplicated segments. The numbered mutation types (1–4) correspond to those in Table 1.

trypsin; 0.02% EDTA), which is then also discarded. Fresh trypsin-EDTA solution is added (2 mL) and cells are incubated at 37°C for approx 2 min. The culture flask should be sharply banged on the palm of one hand two to three times to promote cell dissociation, which may be assessed using an inverted microscope, then an equal volume of growth medium is added to inhibit further trypsin activity. The cell suspension is transferred to a fresh tube and centrifuged at 200*g* for 10 min. The supernatant is discarded, the pellet is resuspended in 5 mL PBS, and a cell count may be performed using a hemocytometer. The block preparation is completed by proceeding from step 4 (*see* Section 3.1.).

Table 1
Characteristic Results of PFGE Analysis of Deletions and Duplications

Type of mutation[a]	Abnormal fragment size[b]	Detection of abnormal fragment using probe within the mutation[c]	Detection of abnormal fragment using probe not within the mutation[c]	Results using probe from adjacent SfiI fragment
Deletion, not including an SfiI site	Always smaller	–	+	Always normal
Deletion, including an SfiI site	May be smaller or larger	–	+	May show same abnormal fragment[d]
Duplication, not including an SfiI site	Always larger	+[e]	+[f]	Always normal
Duplication, including an SfiI site	May be smaller or larger[g]	+[h]	–	May show same abnormal fragment[i]

[a]See also Fig. 3.

[b]In relation to the normal fragment size detected by the same probe.

[c]Presence (+) or absence (–) of hybridization to the abnormal fragment using probe from the same SfiI fragment as another probe that detects the abnormal fragment.

[d]Unless probe is within the deleted segment.

[e]1:2 dosage (normal:abnormal) in female carriers.

[f]1:1 dosage (normal:abnormal) in female carriers.

[g]If the duplicated segment contains only 1 SfiI site, the size of the altered fragment will equal the size of the duplication.

[h]A normal sized fragment is additionally detected in males; 2:1 dosage (normal:abnormal) in female carriers.

[i]Unless probe is not within the duplicated segment.

295

2. A method for preparing high-mol-wt DNA from frozen blood has been described by Nguyen et al. *(12)*. It is not recommended as a routine procedure since it does not allow the white cell concentration to be measured. A yield of approx 4×10^7 white cells from 10 mL of blood should be assumed. We have used the method only occasionally but have achieved satisfactory results. The blood (10 mL) is thawed slowly on ice, and is mixed gently with 40 mL ice-cold TE. The tube is centrifuged for 5 min at 2000g and the supernatant is discarded. The pellet, which is red in color, is gently resuspended in 1.3 mL TE and the preparation of agarose blocks is completed by proceeding from step 5 (*see* Section 3.1.).

3. We recommend that blood samples should be collected in EDTA tubes and processed promptly. Although satisfactory results are often obtained from samples in lithium heparin tubes, we experienced a large number of failures at one time derived from a single batch of lithium heparin tubes. We are unsure whether this was a defect of the batch of tubes or a general problem of samples collected in these tubes. Good quality blocks are often prepared from blood samples several days old, however, samples that are not fresh appear to be more prone to producing cell clumps during block preparation, which can be a serious problem. We always try to obtain blood specimens within 24 h and prepare blocks on the day of receipt.

4. Red cell lysis is determined by observing an increase in translucency of the sample. Occasionally, lysis of some samples is slow, especially if they are fresh. If red cell lysis has not occurred after 30 min, the tube may be centrifuged, the supernatant discarded, and the pellet resuspended in 30 mL fresh lysis buffer. The red cells generally lyse within a few minutes and agarose block preparation can continue from step 2 (*see* Section 3.1.). If lysis is incomplete, a number of red cells will be present in the pellet but small numbers do not seem to interfere with the quality of the blocks.

5. Many protocols for restriction enzyme digestion of DNA in pulsed field blocks recommend treatment with phenylmethylsulfonylfluoride (PMSF), a protease inhibitor that is extremely toxic. We have found that PMSF treatment is unnecessary (at least for *Sfi*I digestion) providing that thorough TE washes are performed. PMSF may however be incorporated in the first TE wash if desired at a concentration of 0.1 mM. A 1M stock of PMSF dissolved in isopropanol or dimethyl sulfoxide (DMSO) is stable at $-20°C$ for up to 5 yr.

6. In order to ensure that washes are thorough, it is important to invert tubes before removal of wash solutions. Residual NDS solution adhering to the tube cap might otherwise be carried over and inhibit restriction enzyme digestion.

7. The volume of restriction enzyme solution should be sufficient to completely immerse the block slice. Ideally this volume should be kept to a minimum and will be determined partly by the shape and size of the block slice as well as the shape of the tube.

8. Covering the caps of the tubes with a layer of heat insulation during restriction enzyme digestion reduces condensation formation inside the caps and helps to maintain the optimal buffer concentration.

9. Although digested DNA is stable indefinitely when stored as described, low-mol-wt DNA will diffuse out of the agarose slice. This has not generally been found to be a problem in our experience, however, we have observed that DNA below approx 50 kb is lost when digested DNA is stored for several weeks.

10. Washing with 70% ethanol is a precaution against growth of algae or fungi that may produce nucleases resulting in DNA degradation. The ethanol is saved and reused. Alternatively, glass heat exchangers may periodically be autoclaved.

11. An alternative fragmentation process to acid depurination is nicking by UV radiation. This may be performed using a UV transilluminator or UV oven. As with acid depurination, the conditions of UV treatment must be optimized to give maximum hybridization signal and these conditions must then be faithfully maintained. The output from UV sources decreases with use, therefore recalibration will become necessary in time. If exhausted UV tubes are replaced in the transilluminator, then the newer tubes with higher output may cause an uneven exposure to DNA in the gel. Further information on optimization of DNA fragmentation may be found in Birren and Lai *(10)*.

Acknowledgments

We thank Ruth Charlton for critical reading of the manuscript.

References

1. Coffey, A. J., Roberts, R. G., Green, E. D., Cole, C. G., Butler, R., Anand, R., Giannelli, F., and Bentley, D. R. (1992) Construction of a 2.6-Mb contig in yeast artificial chromosomes spanning the human dystrophin gene using an STS-based approach. *Genomics* **12,** 474–484.

2. den Dunnen, J. T., Grootscholten, P. M., Bakker, E., Blonden, L. A. J., Ginjaar, H. B., Wapenaar, M. C., et al. (1989) Topography of the Duchenne muscular dystrophy (DMD) gene: FIGE and cDNA analysis of 194 cases reveals 115 deletions and 13 duplications. *Am. J. Hum. Genet.* **45,** 835–847.

3. Koenig, M., Beggs, A. H., Moyer, M., Scherpf, S., Heindrich, K., Bettecken, T., et al. (1989) The molecular basis for Duchenne versus Becker muscular dystrophy: correlation of severity with type of deletion. *Am. J. Hum. Genet.* **45,** 498–506.

4. Hu, X., Ray, P. N., Murphy, E. G., Thompson, M. W., and Worton, R. G. (1990) Duplicational mutation at the Duchenne muscular dystrophy locus: its frequency, distribution, origin, and phenotype-genotype correlation. *Am. J. Hum. Genet.* **46,** 682–695.

5. Boyce, F. M., Beggs, A. H., Feener, C., and Kunkel, L. M. (1991) Dystrophin is transcribed in brain from a distant upstream promoter. *Proc. Natl. Acad. Sci. USA* **88,** 1276–1280.

6. Hiraishi, Y., Kato, S., Ishihara, T., and Takano, T. (1992) Quantitative Southern blot analysis in the dystrophin gene of Japanese patients with Duchenne or Becker muscular dystrophy: a high frequency of duplications. *J. Med. Genet.* **29,** 897–901.

7. Galvagni, F., Saad, F. A., Danieli, G. A., Miorin, M., Vitiello, L., Mostacciuolo, M. L., and Angelini, C. (1994) A study on duplications of the dystrophin gene:

evidence of a geographical difference in the distribution of breakpoints by intron. *Hum. Genet.* **94,** 83–87.

8. Southern, E. M., Anand, R., Brown, W. R. A., and Fletcher, D. S. (1987) A model for the separation of large DNA molecules by crossed field gel electrophoresis. *Nucleic Acids Res.* **15,** 5925–5943.

9. Koenig, M., Hoffman, E. P., Bertelson, C. J., Monaco, A. P., Feener, C., and Kunkel, L. M. (1987) Complete cloning of the Duchenne muscular dystrophy (DMD) cDNA and preliminary genomic organization of the DNA gene in normal and affected individuals. *Cell* **50,** 509–517.

10. Birren, B. and Lai, E. (1993) *Pulsed Field Gel Electrophoresis: A Practical Guide.* Academic, San Diego, CA.

11. Abbs, S., Yau, S. C., Clark, S., Mathew, C. G., and Bobrow, M. (1991) A convenient multiplex PCR system for the detection of dystrophin gene deletions: a comparative analysis with cDNA analysis shows mistypings by both methods. *J. Med. Genet.* **28,** 304–311.

12. Nguyen, C., Djabali, M., Roux, D., and Jordan, B. R. (1991) Very high molecular weight DNA for pulsed field gel studies can be obtained routinely from conventional frozen blood aliquots. *Nucleic Acids Res.* **19,** 407.

18

Fluorescent Sequencing Protocols in Diagnosis

Colin A. Graham and Alison J. M. Hill

1. Introduction

1.1. Direct Fluorescent Sequencing

Direct sequencing of PCR products using the dideoxy chain termination procedure developed by Sanger et al. *(1)* is now the most commonly used method for defining specific mutations. The main benefits of this method lie in its ease of use, and this has been enhanced in recent years by the introduction of fluorescent labels and automated detection systems that obviate the need for radioactivity. Although the initial purchase price for automated sequencers is high, this is compensated for by single tube reaction chemistry and rapid analysis and base calling.

1.2. Instrumentation

At the present time only two commercial fluorescent sequencers are in common usage throughout the world; the 373A/377 fluorescent fragment analyzers (Perkin Elmer, Norwalk, CT/Applied Biosystems Division, Foster City, CA) and the ALF DNA sequencer (Pharmacia, Uppsala, Sweden). The 373A is the most widely used instrument and benefits from the use of multicolor fluorescence detection that enables single lane sequencing, and the company has developed very simple fluorescence dye-terminator sequencing kits. The methods described in this chapter are confined to the use of the 373A sequencer. The ALF instrument has the advantage of faster run times and the raw data does not require the mobility shift corrections used to compensate for differential dye mobilities in the 373A. However, it is restricted to running standard four lane sequencing and thus is more prone to electrophoretic irregularities.

From: *Methods in Molecular Medicine: Molecular Diagnosis of Genetic Diseases*
Edited by: R. Elles Humana Press Inc., Totowa, NJ

The 373A instrument contains a chamber for vertical polyacrylamide gel electrophoresis. This enables single base resolution of sequencing products. Fluorescently labeled fragments pass through a "read" window, 24 cm from the loading wells, which is scanned by an argon laser. The fluorochromes are excited by the laser emission and are detected with filter wheels and a photomultiplier. The fluorescent signals are passed to an Apple Macintosh computer that analyzes their position and strength and produces a chromatogram consisting of colored peaks. The area under the peak represents the strength of the signal and the peak color is specific for the base at that position. The software gives a base call A, T, C, or G at each position or assigns N if the position is unclear.

1.3. Comparison of Sequencing Protocols

The methods and examples given in this chapter concentrate on the *Taq (Thermus aquaticus)* polymerase dye terminator cycle sequencing system Fig. 1, as this is now becoming the most widely reported fluorescence sequencing method for the definition of mutations in human genes. An alternative method is *Taq* dye primer sequencing, the principles of which are outlined in Fig. 2. Some of the methodological details to be considered before setting up a sequencing procedure for diagnostic use are now considered bearing in mind that the method should be reliable, consistent, give good quality results, and be easy to use for a wide range of different sequences.

1.3.1. Sequencing Methods and Enzymes

Cycle sequencing using a thermostable DNA polymerase such as *Taq* is the method of choice. The benefits of this method are: a large number of reactions can be performed simultaneously using a thermal cycler, only a small amount (<1 µg) of template DNA is required to give good quality sequence, and the cycling nature of the reaction gives strong signal profiles and greatly reduces strand annealing and random priming events that produce background noise.

The use of *Taq* polymerase enables sequencing to be carried out at 60°C and this reduces secondary structure in the template and gives more efficient read through GC-rich regions. One of the disadvantages of *Taq* is that incorporation efficiencies for the fluorescent terminators are very sequence dependent and this leads to uneven signal profiles. This is illustrated in Fig. 3 (shown on page 317); chromatograms A and B as the profile of the arrowed base sequence CCACT varies dependent on the surrounding sequence. These panels also demonstrate how reproducible signal profiles are for a given sequence. If this is a problem then the Sequenase (USB) enzyme should be considered. A separate set of dye terminators has been produced by Perkin Elmer, Applied Biosystems division, for use with this enzyme. This enzyme gives more even dye terminator incorporation and thus more uniform signal profiles, but it cannot be used at 60°C and thus secondary structure problems lead to a portion of most sequences being unreadable.

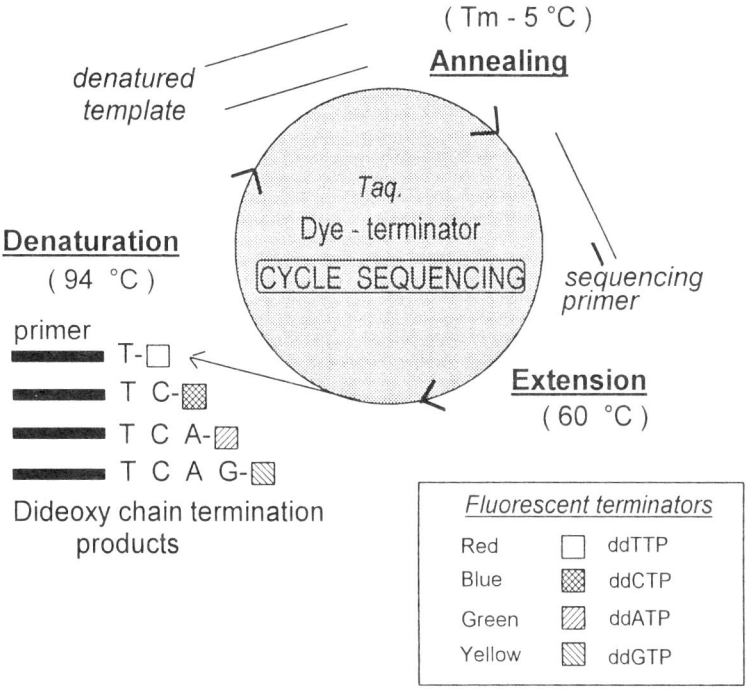

Fig. 1. *Taq* dye terminator cycle sequencing. Cycle sequencing is like a linear PCR reaction using single- or double-stranded DNA template and priming from a single sequencing primer. The dideoxy chain terminators carry four distinct fluorescent dyes, thus all the termination products can be loaded in a single lane and size separated on a polyacrylamide gel. The sequence is read as a color code using a laser and fluorescence detection system.

1.3.2. Dye Primer vs Dye Terminator

In dye primer sequencing the fluorescent labels have to be attached to the sequencing primer and four separate reactions are required matching a specific dye labeled primer with a specific dideoxy terminator. The products are then pooled and cleaned to remove dye primers prior to electrophoresis. With dye-terminator sequencing the dye labels are attached to the dideoxy terminator molecules and thus sequencing can be accomplished in a single tube reaction. Technicalities of the different sequencing chemistries are discussed by Hawkins *(2)*.

A comparison of these two sequencing chemistries is shown in Fig. 3C,D. This illustrates the main benefit of dye primer sequencing in that signal strengths are more uniform and A and T tract anomalies (Fig. 4A) and noise problems associated with dye terminator sequencing are greatly reduced. How-

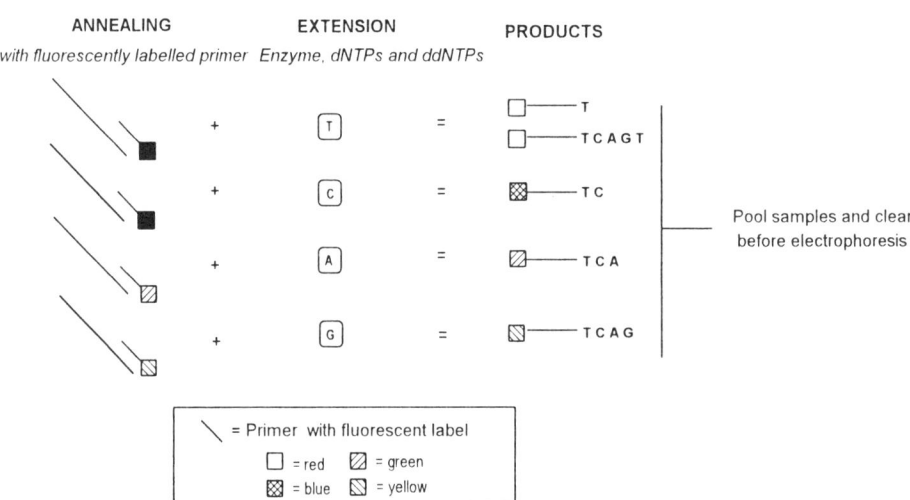

Fig. 2. Dye primer sequencing requires the sequencing primer to be fluorescently labeled with four distinct fluors. Each fluorescent primer is then matched with a specific dideoxy terminator and four separate sequencing reactions are required. The extension products can then be pooled, cleaned, and run in a single lane as with the dye terminator system.

ever, the cost and ease of use benefits of the dye terminator system make it the method of choice for the majority of PCR product sequencing requirements. If sequencing of an unknown fragment or repeated sequencing of the same region is required, then the dye primer method should be considered.

1.4. Primer Design and Synthesis

Primer base composition, secondary structure, stability, and specificity are all important in producing clear sequence data. The primer sequence should be specific to reduce binding to secondary sites and a minimum length of 20 bp is recommended. Primers with a high G/C content have higher annealing temperatures and will be more stable and effective in cycle sequencing. The

---

Fig. 4. *(opposite page)* Sequencing anomalies. (A) Some of the artifacts typically seen with *Taq* dye terminator sequencing. The arrows indicate the reduction in peak height observed after the first base in A and T tracts. The stars show the reduction in intensity observed following a G base, this is especially pronounced for C. (B) A simple polymorphism found in exon 10 of the CFTR gene. The star indicates the polymorphic base. (C) Forward (F) and reverse (R) sequence for the detection of the PKU mutation

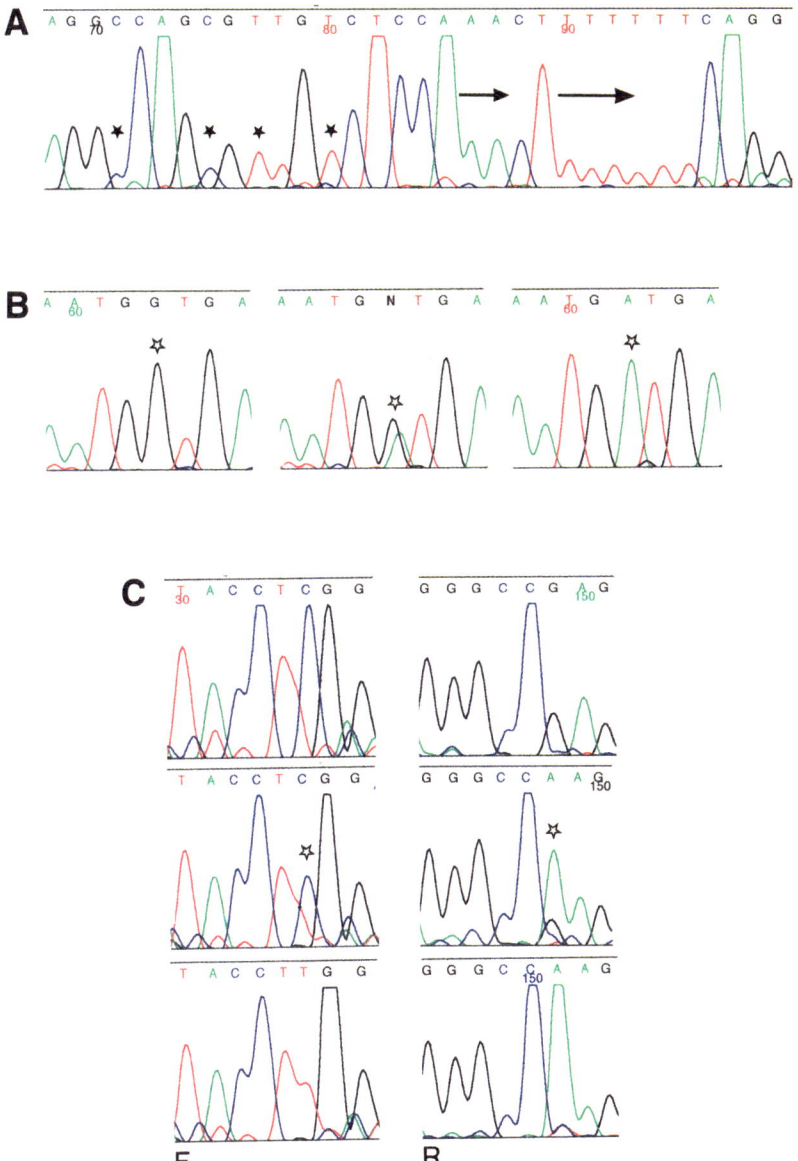

Fig. 4. *(continued)* R408W, a C > T base change in exon 12 of the PAH gene. The top panels show the normal profile and the bottom panels show a patient homozygous for the mutation. A patient heterozygous for the mutation is shown in the center panel and the mutant base is indicated with a star. In the forward sequence there is no sign of the mutant T base, although the intensity of the C peak is reduced. However, the mutant A base is seen readily in the reverse direction together with a reduced intensity G signal.

presence of a CG basepair at the 3' end of a primer can help to stabilize it during the cycling reaction. Computer packages, such as Primer Detective (Clonetech, Palo Alto, CA), can be used to identify suitable primers and will show any self- or cross-complementarity in the selected primers. Primer length, CG content, and product melt temperature are also considered. It can still be difficult to design reliable primers for some regions, mainly because the DNA sequence surrounding the area of interest contains repeat sequences or is AT rich. Poor quality primers can result in relatively good peak signal strengths but high background noise or noisy signal with no well-defined peaks, this can be due to random priming reactions if the primer is not specific or to impure primer. Primer synthesis for sequencing should be carefully monitored as short-mers and impurities may interfere with the sequencing reaction. For optimal results sequencing primers should be HPLC purified. If the primer, or template, concentration is too high, then reaction components can become exhausted during the cycle sequencing reaction with considerable reduction in signal intensity toward the end of longer fragments.

2. Materials

1. Centricon-100 concentrators (Amicon Inc., Danvers, MA).
2. Sterile, deionized water (water for injection, Antigen Pharmaceuticals, Roscrea, Ireland).
3. Ultrapure agarose (electrophoresis grade) (Gibco-BRL, Gaithersburg, MI).
4. Nusieve agarose (genetic technology grade) (FMC Bioproducts, Rockland, ME).
5. *Taq* DyeDeoxy Terminator Cycle sequencing Kit (Perkin Elmer).
6. PRISM (Ready Reaction) DyeDeoxy Terminator Cycle Sequencing Kit (Perkin Elmer).
7. Mineral oil (Sigma, St. Louis, MO).
8. Phenol:H_2O: chloroform (68:18:14 [v/v/v]) (Perkin Elmer).
9. 2.5M Sodium acetate (Perkin Elmer).
10. Absolute alcohol (AR) (Hayman Ltd., Witham, UK).
11. Alcinox detergent (Aldrich Chemical, Milwaukee, WI).
12. Sequagel-6 (premixed 6% sequencing gel, 19:1 acrylamide:bisacrylamide with urea and TBE buffer).
13. Ammonium persulfate: 10% stock solution (BioRad Laboratories, Hercules, CA).
14. Tris Borate EDTA (TBE buffer 10X) (Biowhittaker, Walkersville, MD).
15. Formamide (deionized) (Sigma).
16. EDTA: 50 mM stock solution pH 8.0 (Normapur, Prolabo, Paris, France).

3. Methods

The methods described are specifically designed for performing fluorescent sequence analysis on the Perkin Elmer, Applied Biosystems Model 373A. Use of the 373A sequencer and the relevant software is described in detail in the manufacturer's manual.

3.1. Template Preparation

The methods described in this chapter deal exclusively with template DNA produced using the polymerase chain reaction (PCR). The yield and purity of the amplified product are of critical importance for good quality sequence. Thus 5 μL of the amplified DNA is run out in 2% agarose gels to estimate concentration and purity. If nonspecific product is seen, the amplification reaction should be repeated under more stringent conditions, in the presence of dimethylsulphoxide (DMSO), or after band-stab gel purification as described in the following *(3)*.

3.1.1. Purification of PCR Amplified DNA by "Band-Stab"

This method of template purification allows amplification of specific regions of DNA without any nonspecific contaminating products, occasionally produced during the PCR reaction.

1. Amplify the section of DNA of interest by PCR and run out on a 2% agarose gel containing ethidium bromide (0.5 μg/mL).
2. Visualize the gel over a UV transilluminator and insert a sterile needle into the correct DNA band in the gel.
3. Redissolve DNA picked up by the needle in 50 μL of sterile deionized water in a clean microcentrifuge tube.
4. Use 5 μL of the resulting solution as template in a second PCR reaction with the same primers.
5. Check an aliquot of the second PCR product again for concentration and purity on an agarose gel.

3.1.2. Purification of Template DNA

The PCR product that is to be used as template for the sequencing reactions has to be purified in order to remove any residual primers or excess PCR reaction components that could interfere with the sequencing reactions. The use of ultrafiltration spin columns Centricon or Microcon (Amicon) has proved to be very effective (*see* Note 1).

3.1.2.1. CENTRICON-100 PURIFICATION COLUMNS

1. Assemble Centricon-100 columns as described in the manufacturer's manual.
2. Add 2 mL sterile, deionized water to the top of the column.
3. Gently layer the template DNA (30–40 μL of PCR product) on top of the water.
4. Attach the collection tube provided to the top of the assembled column.
5. Spin at 1000*g* for 30 min and remove lower collection chamber and discard fluid (a second spin with a further 2 mL of water is not required).
6. Invert the column and centrifuge for 2 min to collect the purified sample (~50 μL).
7. Transfer the sample to a clean, sterile microcentrifuge tube and store –20°C.

3.2. DyeTerminator Cycle Sequencing of Double-Stranded PCR Fragments

The method described here relates to the single tube sequencing of double-stranded DNA. Sequencing is carried out using the *Taq*DyeDeoxy Terminator Cycle Sequencing Kit or the reaction ready Prism *Taq*DyeDeoxy Terminator Cycle Sequencing Kit.

3.2.1. Cycle Sequencing Using the Taq*DyeDeoxy Terminator Cycle Sequencing Kit*

Each of the DyeTerminator sequencing kits contains reagents for 100 sequencing reactions. Unmixed reagents should be stored at –20°C. Reaction premixes can be made up according to the manufacturer's instructions and stored at 4°C for up to 1 mo. The amount of mix prepared should be scaled to average usage within this time. Preparing premixes should help to avoid variability between reactions. The primers used in the sequencing reactions may be the same used in the original PCR reactions or they may be specifically designed for sequencing and internal to the original primers. In either case they should be diluted to a working concentration of 3.2 pmol/μL.

1. Set up reaction mix in a clean, sterile microcentrifuge tube. Reaction mix: $N \times 9.5$ μL reaction premix, $N \times 1.0$ μL sequencing primer, $N \times 2.5$–4.5 μL sterile, deionized H_2O (where N = no. of samples + 1).
2. Aliquot 13 μL of the reaction mix into individual PCR tubes (0.6 mL).
3. Add 5–7 μL template DNA, depending on gel estimate of concentration.
4. Overlay reactions with one drop of mineral oil and place on the thermal cycler preset with the appropriate cycle sequencing reaction conditions (*see also* Note 2).

3.2.1.1. TYPICAL CYCLE SEQUENCING REACTION

1. Initial denaturation: 94°C for 2 min and 94°C for 30 s.
2. Twenty-five cycles: primer T_m –5°C for 15 s and 60°C for 4 min.
3. Final cooling: 4°C for 10 min.

3.3. Purification of Sequencing Reaction Products

After cycle sequencing the huge excess of fluorescent dye terminators used to drive the reaction must be efficiently removed for good quality electrophoretic separation of the termination products and effective analysis of the initial 50 bases after the primer. A variety of methods are available to achieve this, two of which are described in the following.

3.3.1. Phenol:Chloroform Extraction Method

1. Transfer the 20 μL of sequence reaction to a clean 0.6-mL microcentrifuge tube taking care not to transfer any of the mineral oil overlaying the reaction.
2. Add 80 μL sterile deionized water and vortex to mix.
3. Add 100 μL phenol:H_2O:chloroform (68:18:14) and vortex.

4. Centrifuge briefly. Remove and discard the lower organic phase.
5. Repeat the organic extraction process and centrifuge for 1 min.
6. Transfer the upper aqueous layer to a clean tube and place sample on ice.
7. Precipitate the extension products with 20 µL 2.5*M* sodium acetate, pH 4.5, and 300 µL of 100% ethanol stored at –20°C (*see* Note 3).
8. Place samples at –70°C for 10–15 min and collect the precipitate by centrifugation at room temperature for 15 min.
9. Wash the pellet gently with 70% ethanol. *Do not resuspend.* Centrifuge at room temperature for 15 min.
10. Remove ethanol and vacuum dry the pellet.

3.4. Polyacrylamide Gel Preparation and Electrophoresis

The glass plates used for fluorescent sequencing are made of glass that does not contain any fluorescent elements and are obtained from Perkin Elmer, Applied Biosystems division. They should be free of dust and grease and are cleaned using the detergent Alcinox. After washing, the plates are rinsed extensively in tap water and 100% ethanol and allowed to air dry. The plates are separated using 0.4-mm spacers and poured horizontally on a level surface. If vertical pouring is preferred then the plates are taped along the outer edges.

3.4.1. Gel Casting

1. Mix 50 mL of Sequagel-6 (premixed 6% sequencing gel, 19:1 acrylamide:bis-acrylamide with TBE buffer) (*see* Note 4) with 400 µL fresh ammonium persulfate (10% solution).
2. Set the plates on a level surface and add the gel mix from the top center using a 20-mL syringe, tapping the plates occasionally to ensure air bubbles are not trapped. Small air bubbles at the edges are not a problem.
3. Insert and clamp the well-former and clamp the top edges of the plates with "bulldog" clips.
4. Allow the gel to polymerize for 1–2 h. If storing overnight keep the gel at 4°C.
5. Check the plates for any dust or spilled acrylamide as described in the user's manual. If necessary clean the outside of the plates. Scratches on the plate or irregularities cast in the gel can be lifted above the scan window by placing cardboard under the buffer chamber.
6. Carefully remove the well-former and insert the shark's tooth comb with the teeth of the comb just touching the surface of the gel (24 and 36 well combs are available).
7. Set up the 373A DNA sequencer according to the manufacturer's instructions and prerun the gel at 30 W for up to 1 h.

3.4.2. Preparation of Samples for Gel Electrophoresis

Dried pellets may be resuspended in loading buffer and stored at 4°C for 1–2 h.

1. Prepare fresh loading buffer: 5 µL formamide and 1 µL 50 m*M* EDTA (pH 8.0) per sample.
2. Dissolve the pellet in 4-µL loading buffer and denature the samples at 90°C for 3 min and place on ice.

3. Wash out the wells with 1X TBE using a syringe with spade tip to remove urea, and load samples into the odd-numbered wells only. Run samples into the gel for 10 min. Interrupt the run and load the even numbered samples. Staggered loading allows the sequencer software to more easily identify individual sample lanes for tracking purposes.
4. The electrophoresis settings are 25–30 W and 1500 V with the power limiting.
5. Click on COLLECT on the computer screen to ensure data collection.

3.5. Analysis of Results

The sequencing software analyzes a run by looking for a first fluorescent band, which is followed within a given time period by a second band. On this basis, the software designates the first band as base "1." It can, however, be confused by salt fronts running ahead of the main data or by the presence of unincorporated terminators that give high signal dye "blobs" and result in inappropriate base calling and reduction of the observed signal strength in the true sequence data. In addition, the first 20 or 30 base calls can be difficult to read because of high signal levels and it is therefore important to be able to assign base "1" accurately and reanalyze that portion of the sequence giving the best data. This can be achieved by the postrun operator controlled removal of nonspecific data before and after the usable sequence.

It is also important for the software to recognize each individual lane and to stay tracked within the center of the lane. Tracking can be affected adversely by uneven polymerization of the gel or large residual amounts of salt in the samples. The dye blobs associated with unincorporated dye terminators can also spill fluorescence into adjacent lanes and confuse tracking. It is necessary therefore to check that the assigned tracks remain in the center of the lane for the length of the run and if not then they should be reassigned and the lanes reanalyzed. This type of operator controlled reanalysis can significantly improve the data quality.

3.5.1. Signal Strength

As mentioned previously the incorporation efficiency of fluorescent dye terminators by *Taq* polymerase is variable and the C terminator is the least efficient. Thus the C signal level is usually the lowest unless the sequence is very C rich. If C is <20 there will be a lot of C noise in the chromatogram profile as the C signal is amplified to give a reasonable profile. Such sequence profiles are best disregarded and the sequencing repeated with an increase in the amount of template or reduction in the annealing temperature.

3.5.2. Base Spacing and Base Calling

In order to accurately call the bases in a sequence, the sequencing software needs to determine average peak intensities and spacings over a minimum of approx 150 bp. Fragments shorter than that minimum result in the software not being able to accurately assign base spacing. When this happens the software is more susceptible to effects of gel compressions that are thought to be caused by the presence of hairpin loop structures at the ends of fragments. The mobility of shorter fragments is more affected by these secondary structures than longer fragments and thus they are more likely to show compression effects. These manifest themselves as uneven spacing in the chromatogram and, in the worst instance, the computer software will insert a base into the gap that it assumes should be filled. If the background noise is high in the gap then the the software might call a base. In many instances, however, it will make an equivocal call (N). The base spacing can only be called if the scans per base fall between 9 and 15; this is determined by the rate of electrophoresis that can be adjusted by altering the electrophoresis power or optimizing the polymerization of the acrylamide. Base calling also can be compromised by high noise levels because of low signals or false priming.

3.5.3. Sequence Alignment and Comparison Software

An analysis package called SeqED (Perkin Elmer, Applied Biosystems division) can be used to align similar sequence data from different tracks or runs and can display aligned data and chromatograms. However, it has very limited ability to perform multiple alignments and this together with an inefficient means of heterozygote detection make the program poor for heterozygote mutation detection. A follow-on program called Sequence Navigator (Perkin Elmer, Applied Biosystems division) was produced as a more comprehensive analysis package. This program can perform multiple alignments much more efficiently and considers peak size for heterozygote detection. A composite normal can be produced that can then be compared with abnormal samples for heterozygote detection and the level of recognition of the second base can be set by the user.

3.5.4. Data Storage

For each 373A instrument it is advisable to have a Macintosh computer dedicated to collection of data and initial automated analysis, this allows two to three runs per 24 h period with virtually continuous data collection. For data collection it is recommended that there is at least 40 Mb free hard disk space on the computer prior to collection and that the disk is regularly monitored with a repair program such as Norton Utilities. In order to process this amount of data from the instrument, it is necessary to have two additional computers for detailed sequence analysis, comparison, and printing of hard copies. Networking of the computers is preferred as transfer of large files (up to 20 Mb) is required. This can be otherwise achieved by the use of removable hard or optical drives. Once analysis of the large gel file is complete, this file can be discarded and only the results files require archiving. A result file for a single track in a gel occupies 96 kb of disk space, thus two floppy disks (1.4 Mb) are required to store result data from a 24-lane gel. It is recommended that bulk archiving is carried out using removable hard or optical disks with capacities from approx 40–200 Mb. Optical drives probably are more reliable and cheaper per megabyte storage, however the drive unit is considerably more expensive. We have found removable hard disks (Syquest 88 Mb with a Prodrive 80 drive unit, Formac) to be satisfactory. However, essential results should also be stored on floppy disk. Networking to a main frame computer for storage is another option that should be discussed with your local information technology department.

3.6. Examples and Interpretation of Fluorescent Sequencing Gels for Heterozygote Detection in Diagnosis

Visual pattern recognition is very efficient for identifying sequence profile irregularities providing that the *Taq* dye-terminator sequencing anomalies and the heterozygote detection criteria defined are considered (*see* Notes 5–8). A color inkjet printer such as the Hewlett Packard 500c series is more suitable for printing sequence chromatograms than the thermal wax printers supplied with the machine because of cost and the color definition is better.

3.6.1. Phenylalanine Hydroxylase (PAH) Gene Mutations

Phenylketonuria is an autosomal recessive disorder caused by mutations in the PAH gene. The gene is composed of 13 exons coding for a 2.2-kb mRNA. The mutational spectrum is diverse with point mutations occurring throughout the gene. We have used fluorescence dye terminator cycle sequencing to screen all exons of the gene and have identified 35 different missense and nonsense mutations accounting for 99% of gene defects *(5)* and several polymorphisms. Anomalies observed in the detection of the main mutation R408W are shown in Fig. 4C.

3.6.2. Cystic Fibrosis Transmembrane Conductance Regulator (CFTR) Gene Mutations

Cystic fibrosis is an autosomal recessive disorder caused by mutations in the CFTR gene. The gene is composed of 27 exons coding for a 6.5-kb mRNA *(6)*. The main mutation is a 3-bp in frame deletion in exon 10. The sequence pattern for a patient heterozygous for this mutation, ΔF508, is shown in Fig. 5C. The mutational spectrum is very heterogeneous and over 500 mutations have been reported to date, covering all exons of the gene, intron splice regions and the 5' promoter.

Fig. 5. *(opposite page)* Deletion mutations. All chromatograms are of *Taq* dye terminator cycle sequencing of PCR products. **(A)** A single base deletion in exon 4 of the CFTR gene (557 del T). **(B)** The reverse sequence for a 2-base deletion in exon 6 of the p53 gene (1214 del TT). **(C)** A 3-base deletion in exon 10 of the CFTR gene (ΔF508, 1652 del CTT). In each case the normal profile is shown in the

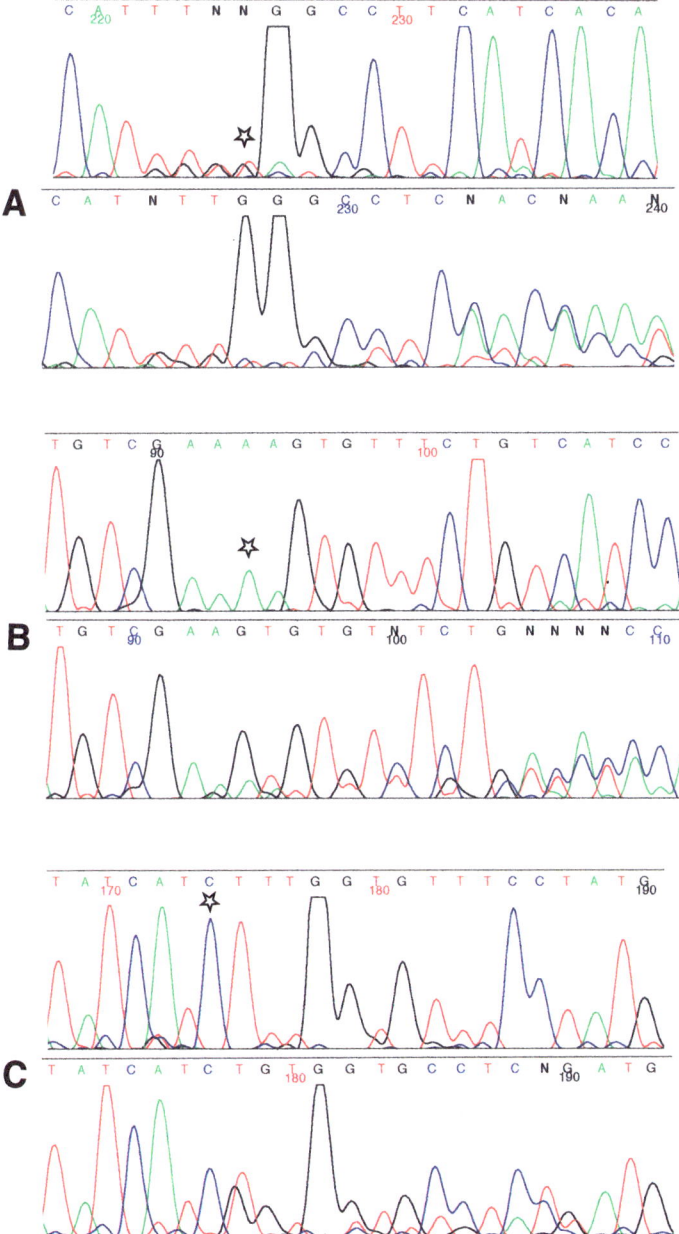

Fig. 5. *(continued)* top panel and the start of the deletion is indicated with a star. The deletions are only present in one allele (heterozygous). Thus the profiles are staggered by 1, 2, and 3 bases after the site of the deletion.

Thus comprehensive mutation detection for this disorder requires analysis of the common mutations followed by screening of all the exons and splice sites. We have used direct fluorescent dye terminator cycle sequencing to screen all exons of the gene. Over 40 different mutations and several polymorphisms have been detected using this method. A polymorphism in exon 10 is shown in Fig. 4B. A rare single base deletion in exon 4 *(7)* and a stop mutation in exon 3 are illustrated in Figs. 5A and 6A, respectively.

3.6.3. LDLR Gene Mutations

Familial hypercholesterolemia is a codominant disorder caused by mutations in the low density lipoprotein receptor gene (LDLR). The gene is composed of 18 exons coding for a 5 kb mRNA. Over 150 different mutations have been described to date *(8)*. In approx 5% of cases the condition is caused by gross deletion in the gene, however, the majority of cases are caused by small deletions and single base changes. Automated fluorescent sequencing has enabled us to identify over 70% of gene defects in patients heterozygous for this condition and two missense mutations in consecutive codons in exon 10 are shown in Fig. 6B *(9)*. *See* Notes 9–13 for general interpretative points in heterozygote detection.

3.6.4. p53 Gene Mutations

Mutations in the p53 gene represent the most common genetic abnormality described in human cancers to date. The prevalence of p53 mutations varies among tumor types, ranging from 0–60% in major cancers, and is over 80% in some histological subtypes. The p53 gene consists of 11 exons; exon 1 is noncoding, exons 2–11 code for the protein of 393 amino acids. There are a wide variety of p53 mutations, dispersed over several hundred basepairs of the gene *(10)*. The majority of p53 mutations (approx 90% of all mutations) occur in exons 5–8, corresponding to the regions of the gene that are highly conserved through evolution. Missense mutations are the most common type (79% of mutations) in this conserved midregion, but occur less frequently in the amino and carboxy termini where nonsense mutations predominate (77% of mutations) *(11)*.

Direct fluorescent sequencing of exons 5–8 has proved to be an effective method for the detection of mutations in the p53 gene, a 2-bp deletion in exon 6 is illustrated in Fig. 5B.

Fig. 6. *(opposite page)* Missense mutations. All chromatograms are of *Taq* dye terminator cycle sequencing of PCR products. **(A)** A G > T change in codon 60, exon 3 of the CFTR gene. **(B)** Codons 460–462, exon 10 of the LDLR gene. The top panel shows a G > A change and the bottom panel a T > C change. In the given examples the heterozygote shows roughly equal intensities for the mutant and normal bases and the normal base is reduced relative to the control. **(C)** Codons 57–59, exon 2 of the HLA DRB1 gene. The top panel shows the normal profile of the 0401 type. The bottom panel shows a G > C change in the 0416 type. A DR4 specific primer was used in the PCR reaction thus only that allele was amplified and the sequence change shows as a homozygote.

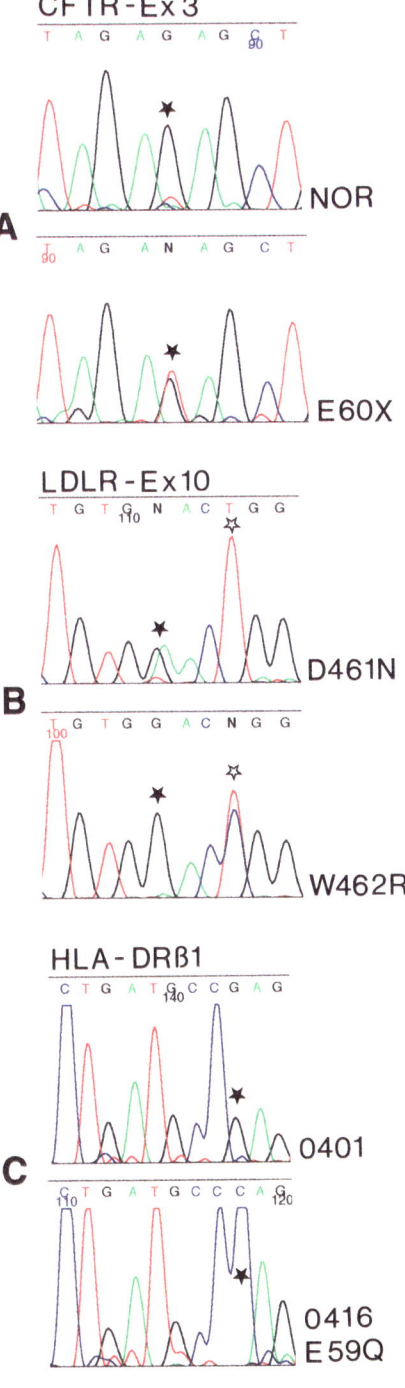

Fig. 6.

3.6.5. HLA DR and DP Typing

Automated fluorescence sequencing is now being considered as a possible alternative to oligotyping for the DR and DP loci. These regions are highly polymorphic and a sequencing method would require a very efficient means of semiautomated heterozygote detection. The use of Sequence Navigator may accomplish this. We have used allele-specific PCR and dye-terminator sequencing to define a rare subtype detected by oligotyping (Fig. 6C).

3.6.6. Discussion

Automated fluorescent sequencing using the dye-terminator chemistry is increasingly being used in diagnostic laboratories to define rare mutations detected by rapid screening procedures such as DGGE *(12)* or SSCP *(13–15)*. The main benefits of this system are single tube and single lane reaction chemistry, cycle sequencing for easy sequencing of PCR products, fluorescent detection that eliminates the need for radioactivity, automated base calling and semi-automated analysis, hard copy printouts of the signal profiles, and mass data storage.

4. Notes

1. The purified samples should be checked on 2% agarose gels to ensure efficient sample recovery from the column. Alternative methods can be used for template purification *(4)* including ion-exchange columns such as QIAquick-spin columns (Quiagen); "gene cleaning" methods using glass powder suspensions such as Geneclean (Stratech Scientific, Teddington, UK) or similar DNA binding agents as used in Magic PCR preps (Promega, Madison, WI). These methods may be less expensive than the ultrafiltration method described earlier, however, they are more labor intensive and we have not found them to give good results as consistently. Overall the Centricon-100 procedure gives the most consistent results in our hands and is recommended for diagnostic sequencing. This method efficiently purifies PCR products of >100 bp.

2. The PRISM kits marketed by Perkin Elmer, Applied Biosystems division, are ready mixed versions of the *Taq*DyeDeoxy Terminator Kits and are used in exactly the same manner but without the preparation of the premix. The cycling reaction should take approx 2 h 45 min. If the thermal ramping time is too fast or too slow, the resulting data may be poor, with high levels of background noise. The annealing temperature should be adjusted according to the primer sequence and is usually optimal 5–7°C below the estimated melt temperature of the primer $[T_m = 2(A + T) + 4(G + C)]$. The following thermal cyclers have been found to give good quality cycle sequencing Perkin Elmer 480 and Aztec PC-700 (Hoefer, San Francisco, CA).

3. The precipitation step is vital for efficient recovery of termination products after phenol:chloroform extraction and it is necessary to use fresh sodium acetate (<1 mo at 4°C after opening) to obtain good product yield. It is also *not* recommended to resuspend the pellet during the 70% ethanol rinse to remove the sodium acetate prior to electrophoresis, as this can result in a low yield and poor

signal. When used efficiently spin columns can prove an effective and quick method for terminator removal. Select-D, G50 columns have been used and proved to be satisfactory with careful use. With the spin column procedure avoid touching the side of the column when loading the samples, as this material can shunt through and contaminate the eluate. Inconsistency in column preparation can also affect the efficiency of terminator removal. In general the phenol:chloroform extraction method is preferred.

4. The use of a low fluorescence commercial sequencing gel mix is highly recommended, as these are batch tested and thus gel consistency can be assured within a batch. This also eliminates gel variation problems if the machine is being operated by multiple users. The Sequagel-6 gel mix does not require degassing for optimal polymerization.

Notes 5–8 refer to *Taq* dye terminator sequencing anomalies.

5. Peak profiles are irregular but highly consistent for given sequence (*see* Fig. 3A,B).

6. Reduction in signal strength occurs after the first base in A and T tracts (*see* Fig. 4A).

7. Bases following a G base often have a reduced signal, especially C (*see* Fig. 4A★).

8. Multiple Gs often show a signal reduction at the second or third base (*see* Fig. 3A,B).

Notes 9–11 refer to interpretive points in heterozygote detection.

9. Print sequence profiles in color at four to five panels per page and 500–800 points per panel.

10. Signal strength reduction of the normal base is the most consistent feature denoting a heterozygous base position (*see* Figs. 4B,C and 6A,B).

11. The appearance of the second base in a heterozygote is often not detected by the base calling software. Compare the center panel of the sequence in Fig. 4B with the center panel of the R sequence in Fig. 4C.

12. The base after the heterozygote position will often show an altered signal strength (*see* Fig. 4B T after the G > A polymorphism).

13. Heterozygotes that show only peak reduction in one direction generally show the mutant base clearly in the other direction (*see* Fig. 4C).

14. In August 1995 Perkin Elmer, Applied Biosystems division, released a new generation of PRISM kits, including the ABI PRISM Dye Terminator Cycle Sequencing Ready Reaction Kit (with Ampli*Taq* DNA Polymerase, FS Product No. 402079) all of which utilize a thermal stable enzyme specially modified for fluorescent sequencing. All the necessary reagents are premixed and ready for use in the sequencing of single- and double-stranded DNA and PCR fragments. There are however some differences in the techniques used and the results obtained with these kits. This section again concentrates on *Taq*-FS dye terminator cycle sequencing of double-stranded PCR products.

a. Template: Double-stranded PCR template is produced and purified as described (*see* Section 3.1.). Use of the new Ampli*Taq*FS enzyme has resulted in an increase in the efficiency of the fluorescent cycle sequencing reaction. It is therefore only necessary to use approximately half of the original amount of template, i.e., 2–4 µL or 250–500 ng.

b. Terminator incorporation: Ampli*Taq* DNA Polymerase (FS) is a mutant form of the original *Taq* DNA polymerase. It has very little 5'–3' exonuclease activity and incorporates all four dideoxynucleotides with equal ease thus removing the need for very high concentrations of dye-labeled terminators. The concentrations of dideoxynucleotides and dye terminators have therefore been set such that the A, T. C, and G signals should be relatively uniform between bases 10 and 700. In addition dGTP has been replaced with dITP in an effort to reduce band compression effects.

c. Purifying cycle sequencing products: The reduction in the amount of dye-labeled terminators in the sequencing reaction has resulted in the removal of the phenol:chloroform extraction step and its replacement by a simple ethanol precipitation or spin column purification, both of which have been recommended by the manufacturer. The ethanol precipitation is inexpensive and effective and gives clean, reproducible sequence.

   i. Add 2 µL 3*M* sodium acetate, pH 6.0 and 50 µL of 95% ethanol to a microcentrifuge tube.

   ii. Transfer the 20 µL sequencing reaction product to this tube and mix thoroughly. Place at 4°C for 10–15 min.

   iii. Microcentrifuge at high speed for 20–25 min.

   iv. Gently remove the supernatant using a plastic Pasteur pipet attached to a fine pipet tip, taking care not to disturb the pellet, which is not usually visible.

   v. Rinse the pellet with 250 µL of cold 70% ethanol.

   vi. Remove the 70% ethanol as previously described and carefully dry the inside of the tube using a tissue.

   vii. Dry the pellet in a vacuum centrifuge and store at –20 or +4°C, until ready for electrophoresis.

d. The changes described in the concentrations and effectiveness of incorporation of the dideoxynucleotides and dye terminators has resulted in more even dye terminator incorporation and thus more even signal profiles. However the signal profile for a given sequence differs markedly between the old and new kits as illustrated in Fig. 7. Thus it is not possible to directly compare old and new version sequences especially for heterozygote detection. Specific improvements with the new kit include better read through A and T tracts and no signal drop off after G bases. However there is now a drop in signal strength after A bases particularly for G bases.

Fig. 3. *(opposite page)* Signal profiles in fluorescent sequencing. **(A,B)** *Taq* dye terminator cycle sequencing of PCR product for exon 4 of the LDLR gene in two patients. The peak profiles produced for a given sequence are virtually identical from one individual to another. The arrow indicates how the position of specific bases, e.g., CCACT within a sequence can determine their exact profile. **(C,D)** *Taq* dye terminator vs *Taq* dye primer cycle sequencing of PCR product for exon 13a of the CFTR gene. The dye primer sequencing gives more even peak heights and does not suffer from the A and T tract peak reductions seen with dye terminators.

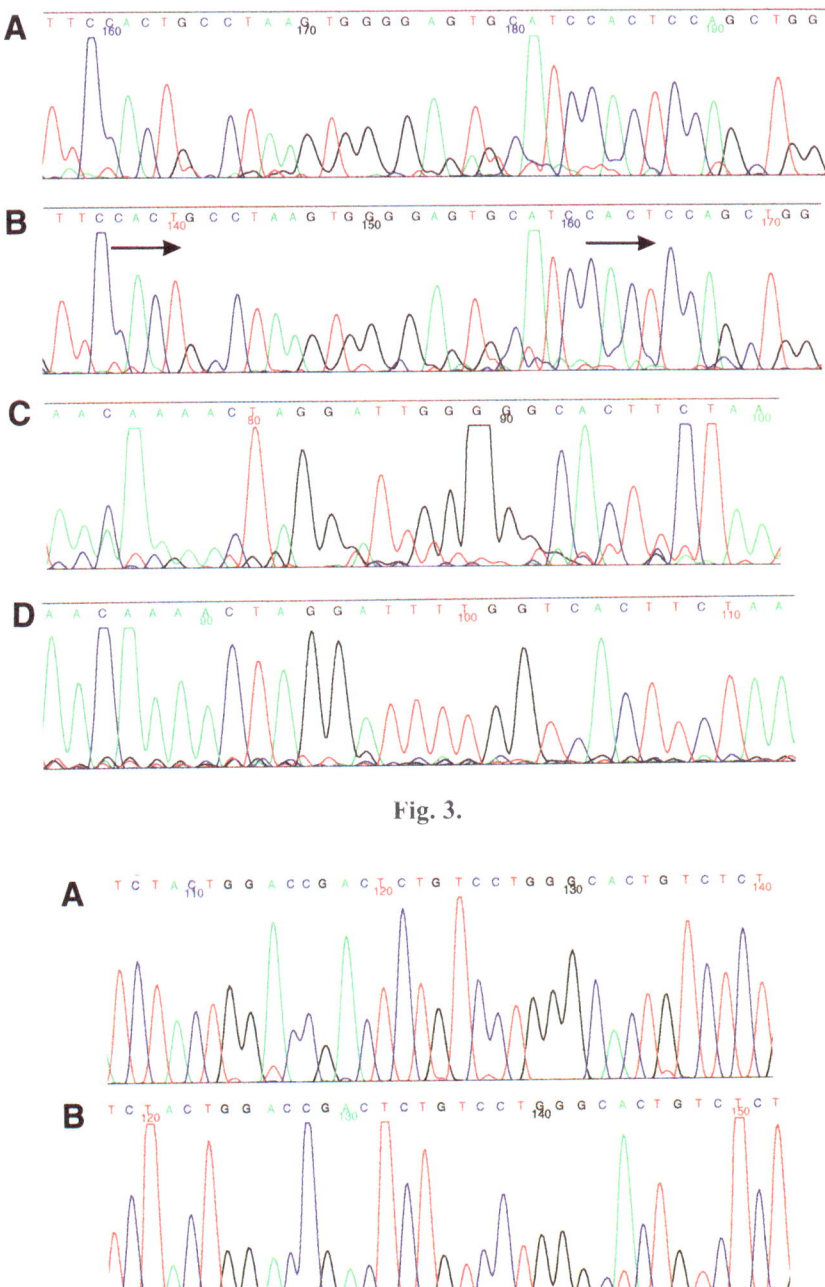

Fig. 3.

Fig. 7. Comparison of the *Taq*-FS **(A)** and *Taq* **(B)** version dye terminator sequencing kits for PCR product sequencing. Note the more consistent signal profile with the newer version *Taq*-FS kit. Over a 70-base region of this exon (LDLR exon 10), 94% of peaks were >25% of the panel height with *Taq*-FS compared to 73% with *Taq*.

Acknowledgments

We thank our colleagues Johannes Zschocke, Alana Ward, Kate Gleeson, and David Hughes for providing data and for helpful discussions during the preparation of this chapter. The following have provided financial support for our sequencing projects: The Cystic Fibrosis Research Trust; The Northern Ireland Chest, Heart and Stroke Association; and the Medical Research Council.

References

1. Sanger, F., Nicklen, S., and Coulson, A. R. (1977) DNA sequencing with chain terminating inhibitors. *Proc. Natl. Acad. Sci. USA* **74,** 5463–5467.
2. Hawkins, T. L., Du, Z., Halloran, N. D., and Wilson, R. K. (1992) Fluorescence chemistries for automated primer-directed DNA sequencing. *Electrophoresis* **13,** 552–559.
3. Bjourson, A. J. and Cooper, J. E. (1992) Band-stab: a simple technique for the purification of individual PCR products. *Nucleic Acids Res.* **20,** 4675.
4. Rao, V. B. (1994) Direct sequencing of polymerase chain reaction-amplified DNA. *Anal. Biochem.* **216,** 1–14.
5. Hobbs, H. H., Brown, M. S., and Goldstein, J. L. (1992) Molecular genetics of the LDL receptor gene in familial hypercholesterolaemia. *Hum. Mutat.* **1,** 445–466.
6. Graham, C. A., Ward, A. J., Nevin, N. C., Young, I., O'Kane, M., and Nicholls, D. P. (1994) Automated sequencing has identified 70% of mutations in 30 patients with familial hypercholesterolaemia in Northern Ireland. *Atherosclerosis* **112,** 262.
7. Zschocke, J., Graham, C. A., Stewart, F. J., Carson, D. J., and Nevin. N. C. (1994) Automated sequencing detects all mutations in Northern Irish patients with phenylketonuria and mild hyperphenylalaninaemia. *Acta Paediatr.* **407(Suppl.),** 37,38.
8. Kerem, B., Rommens, J. M., Buchanan, J. A., Markiewicz, D., Cox, T. R., Chakravati, A., et al. (1989) Identification of the cystic fibrosis gene: genetic analysis. *Science* **245,** 1073–1080.
9. Graham, C. A., Goon, P. K. C., Hill, A. J. M., and Nevin, N. C. (1992) Identification of a frameshift mutation (557delT) in exon 4 of the CFTR gene. *Genomics* **12,** 854,855.
10. de Fromentel, C. C. and Soussi, T. (1992) TP53 tumor suppressor gene: a model for investigating human mutagenesis. *Genes, Chromosom. Cancer* **4,** 1–15.
11. Hollstein, M., Rice, K., Greenblatt, M. S., Soussi, T., Fuchs, R., Sorlie, T., et al. (1994) Database of p53 somatic mutations in human tumors and cell lines. *Nucleic Acids Res.* **22,** 3551–3555.
12. Guldberg, P., Henriksen, K. F., and Guttler, F. (1993) Molecular analysis of phenylketonuria in Denmark: 99% of the mutations detected by denaturing gradient gel electrophoresis. *Genomics* **17,** 141–146.
13. Chillon, M., Casals, T., Gimenez, J., Nunes, V., and Estivill, X. (1994) Analysis of the CFTR gene in the Spanish population: SSCP-screening for 60 known mutations and identification of four new mutations (Q30X, A120T, 1812-1 G > A and 3667del4). *Hum. Mutat.* **3,** 223–230.

14. Nunes, V., Chillon, M., Dork, T., Tummler, B., Casals, T., and Estivill, X. (1993) A new missense mutation (E92K) in the first transmembrane domain of the CFTR gene causes a benign cystic fibrosis phenotype. *Hum. Mol. Genet.* **2,** 79,80.

15. Hagemann, T. L., Chen, Y., Rosen, F. S. and Kwan, S.-P. (1994) Genomic organization of the *Btk* gene and exon scanning for mutations in patients with X-linked agammaglobulinaemia. *Hum. Mol. Genet.* **3,** 1743–1749.

19

High Throughput Modifications of Single-Strand Conformation Polymorphism Analysis

Mutation Detection in Familial Hypercholesterolemia

Steve E. Humphries, Vilmundur Gudnason, Ros E. Whittall, and Ian N. M. Day

1. Introduction

In most patients with familial hypercholesterolemia (FH) the disorder is caused by a mutation in the gene coding for the low density lipoprotein receptor (LDL-R) *(1)*. The variety of different defects observed in receptor function at the cellular level reflects mutations in different domains of the gene, and there is an increasing number of pointers to suggest that genetic factors influence clinical severity. The diagnosis of FH on clinical grounds is not 100% accurate, and some hypercholesterolemic individuals may not have a mutation in the LDL-R gene, whereas some individuals who would not be included in the clinical criteria do have such a mutation. The purpose of this chapter is to illustrate the use of the single-strand conformational polymorphism (SSCP) technique for mutation screening in the LDL-R gene and to discuss several adaptations of published methods that improve throughput, and that we believe are appropriate for a disorder such as FH. In the next few years such techniques will help to tackle molecular diagnosis and family tracing in the large number of FH patients present in Europe and North America.

1.1. General Principles of the (SSCP) Technique

Several methods have been published that allow rapid comparison of the sequence of specific fragments of DNA amplified by polymerase chain reaction (PCR) from different individuals *(2,3)* and we have found the SSCP analysis to be the most useful.

From: *Methods in Molecular Medicine: Molecular Diagnosis of Genetic Diseases*
Edited by: R. Elles Humana Press Inc., Totowa, NJ

The SSCP technique *(4)* is a method capable of identifying most sequence variations in a single strand of DNA, typically between 150 and 250 nucleotides in length. Under nondenaturing conditions a single strand of DNA will adopt a conformation (presumably dependent on internal basepairing between short segments by foldback) that is uniquely dependent on its sequence composition. This conformation usually will be different, if even a single base is changed. Most conformations seem to alter the physical configuration or size sufficiently that, even though the variant sequence has the same charge, the configuration-to-charge (size-to-charge) ratio is different enough to be detectable as a mobility difference on electrophoresis through a retarding matrix such as polyacrylamide gel. Although the samples have been denatured, the buffer in the wells and nondenaturing environment into which the sample concentrates immediately on entry into the gel will allow some double-strand reannealing to take place, as well as adoption and resolution of the various single-strand conformations. The considerations implicit in classical "Cot" studies of reannealing (concentration of each single strand, DNA complexity, and time) apply *(5)*.

The "classical" SSCP protocol is a denatured sample, [^{32}P]-labeling for maximal detection sensitivity in the diluted sample and long track length for maximal resolution of small mobility differences *(see* Fig. 1). However, in the interests of higher efficiency of detection, greater convenience, or safety, a number of studies have been made using other protocols. Restriction digestion of a large PCR fragment prior to SSCP has been described *(6)*. Multiplex PCR is also possible and SSCP can be combined with allele-specific PCR *(7,8)* to select alleles in complex sets (e.g., HLA genes), and can also be combined with dideoxy chain termination to localize the approximate position of an SSCP variation in a sequence *(9)*.

In SSCP analysis, heteroduplex bands are often seen on the gel as a useful byproduct of the procedure *(10)*. Reannealing of double-strand DNA has been discussed herein, and when higher concentrations of single-stranded DNA are loaded, for example, for nonisotopic detection methods, the double-strand band is the predominant band. For human DNA (except for the sex chromosomes in males), a PCR product usually represents amplification from two alleles, derived from each autosome of a pair. When a sequence variation is present in the heterozygous state, the classical SSCP picture would be of four single-stranded bands, the sense and antisense strands of the "normal" allele, and the altered mobility sense and antisense strands of the "variant" allele. In addition, reannealing to double strands permits four possible products, "normal" double strand, "variant" double strand, and two heteroduplexes ("normal" sense/"variant" antisense; and "normal" antisense/"variant" sense). The heteroduplexes have a mismatch "bubble" that often alters their mobilities relative to

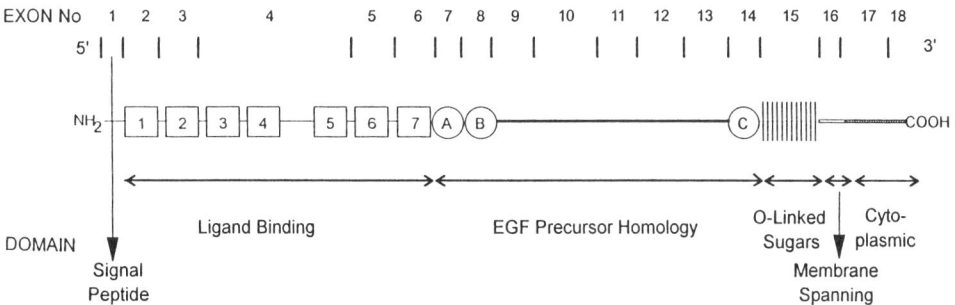

Fig. 1. A map of the LDL-R protein, its mRNA and gene. Vertical bars denote the exon–exon junctions. Numbered boxes and circles denotes the cysteine-rich repeats. The primary coding sequence is 2580 nucleotides long. The 3' untranslated region is not shown on the scale of the figure *(1)*.

homoduplex, resulting in further additional bands (*see* Fig. 2). The combined efficiency of SSCP plus heteroduplex analysis for detection of sequence variations should be well in excess of the 80% estimated for each technique considered individually *(2)*.

Since RNA basepairing is more stable than RNA-DNA basepairing, RNA might be expected to adopt more conformational structure and hence be more sensitive to sequence changes. Published evidence suggests that this is the case *(11)*, with detection of up to 95% of variations, but the inconvenience of making RNA strands (which involves the complexity and expense of introducing RNA polymerase promoters and extra reaction steps) for SSCP has precluded widespread use. For analysis of FH, used as a model system in this chapter, a suitable source of RNA would be from lymphocytes, but success is dependent on equal representation of mRNA levels from the normal and mutant allele, and in the presence of premature stop codons or splice-site mutations this may not be the case (V. Gudnasson, unpublished).

1.2. FH

FH is characterized clinically by elevation in the concentration of LDL cholesterol in blood, tendon xanthomata, and an increased risk of myocardial infarction. It is present in 5–10% of individuals who develop coronary artery disease (CAD) under the age of 55 yr in the United Kingdom and the United States *(1,12)*. Based on the estimated population frequency of carriers of 1/500, there are more than 100,000 FH heterozygous individuals in the United Kingdom, of which probably less than 3000 have been identified to date. Once identified, the hyperlipidemia of these patients is responsive to treatment by

Humphries et al.

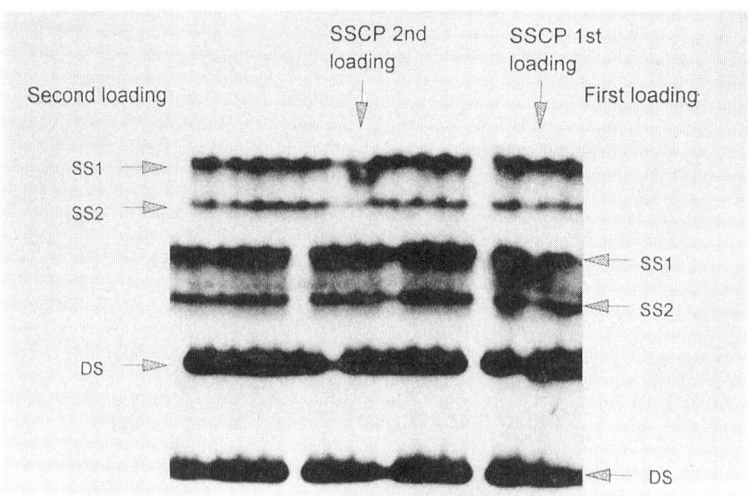

Fig. 2. Autoradiograph of a double-loaded SSCP gel of exon 3 of the LDL-R gene. Exon 3 was amplified by PCR using primers flanking exon 3. The sequence of the 5' primer is 5'-TGACACTTCAATCCTGTCTCTTCTG and for the 3' oligonucleotide 5'-ATAGCAAAGGCAGGGCCACACTTAC, to give a product of 172 bp *(4)*. Oligonucleotides were obtained from Genosys. The amplifications were performed in an automated thermal cycler (Hybaid Omnigene) using *Taq* DNA polymerase (Gibco BRL) in a total volume of 20 µL and overlaid with 20 µL paraffin oil, using previously described cycling conditions *(11)*. The fragment was labeled by PCR amplification, with the addition of [α-^{32}P] deoxycytosine triphosphate (800 Ci/mmol, 10 µCi/µL; Amersham). A quantity of 5 µL of the PCR mixture was diluted with 25 µL of 0.1% SDS and 10 mM EDTA. Five microliters of this dilution was mixed with 5 µL formamide dye (95% formamide, 20 mM EDTA, 0.05% bromophenol blue, 0.05% xylene cyanole; FF). The PCR DNA was denatured by boiling at 100°C for 3 min and then chilled immediately on ice. Samples (4 µL) were loaded onto a 4.5% polyacrylamide nondenaturing gel (ratio of acrylamide to bisacrylamide 49:1) in 1X TBE buffer, with 10% glycerol. Gels were 40 cm × 30 cm × 0.4 mm. Electrophoresis was at 20 mA for 16 h at room temperature on 4.5% polyacrylamide gels with 10% glycerol. The gel was then transferred onto Whatman 3MM chromatographic paper, dried, and exposed to hyperfilm β max (Amersham) for 12–24 h at –70°C before developing. The samples are run toward the anode (+). The single and double strands of the first and second loadings are designated, respectively, on right and left, SS1, SS2, and DS, the double strands having migrated approx 30 cm and the single strands approx 20 cm in the gel. SSCP variants are apparent in one sample from the first loading and in one from the second loading, as indicated.

diet and drugs *(13)*, and such treatment reduces subsequent morbidity and mortality *(14)*. FH results from different genetic defects in a cell surface receptor that normally controls the uptake of plasma LDL *(1)*, or in a small proportion of patients one particular defect in apolipoprotein B, the ligand for the receptor *(15)*. This disorder, which is called Familial Defective apoB, has been reported to occur in about 3% of FH patients in the United Kingdom, and the mutation in the apoB gene causing it can be detected easily by PCR and ASOs (allele-specific oligonucleotides). Children who have inherited two defective alleles of the LDL-R (homozygous FH phenotype, but usually compound heterozygous for two different defects) represent 1/million of the population. In these children there is usually little useful lowering of plasma LDL-cholesterol levels in response to diet or drugs, and many suffer a major coronary event in the first or second decade of life, but life expectancy can be extended by appropriate treatment. Current treatment is usually by plasma exchange or LDL apheresis, but patients alternatively may be treated by transplantation of a donor liver, possibly in conjunction with a heart transplant *(16)*. In the future it may be possible to treat such children using "gene therapy" methods *(17)*.

For many heterozygous FH individuals a clear diagnosis can be made on the basis of elevated plasma cholesterol. However, several studies *(18)* have shown that measures of total cholesterol or LDL cholesterol alone do not allow unequivocal diagnosis of FH in 10–15% of cases, even in the children of a parent with FH. It has been suggested that a monocyte or lymphocyte assay may be a useful tool for identifying individuals with defective LDL-R function, and there are several reports of such methods *(19)*. However, there are considerable technical difficulties with these approaches that prevent their application for routine screening at the present time. In particular, as with all other tests used for diagnosis of FH, there is still overlap between the values obtained for some "normal" individuals and patients with a defect in the receptor, whereas a genetic approach to identify LDL-R defects gives an unequivocal result. An additional concern about such nongenetic tests is the frequency of false-negative results, and some children whose lipid levels initially are within the normal range for their age and gender, show a greater than average rise in lipid levels over time, to a point where it is evident that they have inherited the LDL-R gene mutation *(20)*. Although the frequency of this problem is unknown, there is no doubt that the equivocal nature of the tests currently available to identify children with FH is one of the factors that deter some clinicians from actively pursuing such diagnosis in the relatives of a patient with FH. The advantage of an unequivocal DNA test would be both to allay fears for half the relatives, and to identify children where monitoring dietary advice and appropriate therapy should be started.

1.3. The LDL-R
and LDL-R Gene Mutations

The LDL-R is a membrane protein of 839 amino acids that is responsible for cholesterol uptake into cells via receptor-mediated endocytosis of cholesterol-rich lipoproteins secreted by the liver *(1)*. The LDL-R binds two different ligands, apoB, which is the sole apoprotein of LDL, and apoE, which is found on the triglyceride-rich lipoproteins and their remnants. Once the LDL-R has bound a ligand, it clusters in coated pits, where it is taken up by the cell, via endocytosis. The ligand is released from the receptor in the lysosome and the receptor is then recycled to the cell surface where it can bind a ligand again.

The human LDL-R gene was cloned and characterized more than 10 yr ago *(1)*. It is located on the short arm of chromosome 19 (p13.1–p13.3), and as shown in Fig. 1, it spans 45 kb and comprises 18 exons and 17 introns. Five classes of mutations at the LDL-R locus have been identified on the basis of the phenotypic behavior of the mutant protein, and to date there have been over 200 different mutations of the LDL-R gene characterized at the DNA level *(21)* and they have given valuable insights into the function of the different domains in the LDL-R. Within a geographically or culturally isolated population, or where a large proportion of people are related by descent because of migration, there may be a single mutation causing FH in many of the patients. For example, in the Christian Lebanese one mutation is responsible for the disorder in 98% of all FH patients, whereas in Afrikaaners in South Africa three mutations are responsible for over 95% of FH patients, with the most common mutation being found in two-thirds of all patients. In French-Canadians a common founder deletion occurs in 60% of FH patients, and in Finland two mutations account for most FH *(1,21)*. In the United Kingdom, where there is a very heterogeneous population, *a priori* it is unlikely that any mutations will be present at a high frequency, and so far no mutation detected has been present at a frequency greater than 2–3% *(22–29)*. However, it is of interest that a point mutation in exon 3 of the gene was present in 2% of the London sample, but 15% of a sample of patients from Manchester *(25)*, and therefore some mutations may be relatively high in certain local areas. We predict that there may be more than 100 different mutations in the United Kingdom, of which so far more than 20 have been detected *(22–29;* unpublished), and although it would be feasible to develop methods to screen for reported mutations, our calculations demonstrate that it is more cost and time effective to use an approach that will enable any mutation in the LDL-R gene to be detected, rather than to screen specifically for all mutations.

1.4. Mutations in Repeat Five
of the Ligand Binding Domain of the LDL-R

The first 292 residues of the receptor contain seven imperfect repeats of 40 amino acids that make up the binding domain *(1)*. Mutational analysis of the binding domain *(30)* has shown that repeat one is not required for binding of either apoB or apoE. Repeats two and three as well as six and seven are required for maximal binding of an apoB-containing lipoprotein such as LDL, but not for apoE lipoproteins, and a naturally occurring mutation in repeat four (S156L), abolishes the binding of LDL but not that of VLDL *(31)*. On the other hand, repeat five is required for both ligands, and this is encoded by the 3' end of exon 4. We have applied SSCP to detect mutations in this region *(17)*, and in 311 FH patients investigated, seven different mutations were detected in a total of 29 patients (9.3%). Three of the mutations show very similar changes in mobility and cannot be distinguished easily from each other by the SSCP pattern alone and need separate tests for confirmation (e.g., restriction digestion, ASOs, or sequencing).

1.5. Current Progress of SSCP Analysis on FH Research

With the modifications in sample handling described in this chapter, it has been possible to screen DNA from 800 FH patients for mutations in the LDL-R at the rate of one exon per week, which occupies 3.5 research assistant days/ week. The LDL-R gene has 18 exons, and pairs of oligonucleotides and amplification conditions have been reported *(11)*, which allow the amplification of the promoter plus coding portions of the entire gene in 20 fragments (exon 4 has to be amplified in two parts owing to its size). In all cases the amplifying oligonucleotides are complementary to intron sequences, which therefore also allow comparison of the intron–exon boundary junction in patients, where mutations may cause defects in correct splicing of nuclear RNA. This has resulted in more than 170 SSCP variants identified at a rate of 10–12/wk. The frequency of detected SSCPs in the different exons of the gene is shown in Fig. 3.

1.6. Future Developments
in SSCP Mutation Screening for FH

Some patients will have no defect identified by the SSCP technique, although published data *(20)* suggests the sensitivity of the method is extremely high (80–90%). Some patients may have a major deletion or rearrangement of the gene, and in the English population the frequency of gross alterations (insertions and deletions) is approx 5% *(13)*. Many of these gross alterations have occurred because of recombination between repetitive *Alu* type elements, and detailed analysis indicates nonhomologous recombination involving *Alu* sequences as the mechanism of the rearrangements. In the LDL-R gene the deletions and insertions described are distributed over the whole of the gene, so

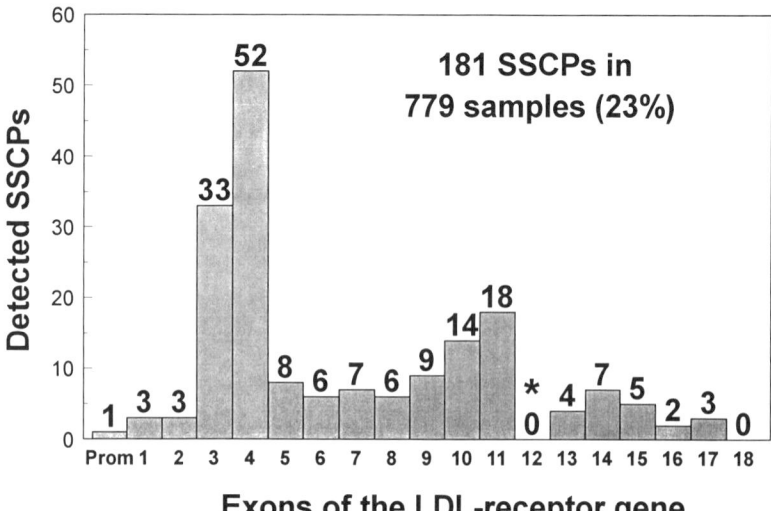

Exons of the LDL-receptor gene

Fig. 3. Frequency of detected SSCPs in the LDL-R gene in 779 UK patients with FH. *, SSCP interpretation difficult because of two common polymorphisms. From Day et al., in preparation.

there are no isolated hotspots that could be used to develop a simple rapid strategy for gross rearrangement detection. When screening large numbers of patients for mutations in the LDL-R gene, Southern blotting will become the last line of investigation after identification of point mutations by faster and easier means, such as SSCP. In the case of already known rearrangement, PCR-based tests can be constructed to identify patients with that particular mutation. These PCR-based tests may also eventually replace Southern blotting for assays for gene rearrangement, analogous with methods established for the dystrophin (Duchenne) gene *(32)* (*see* Chapter 2).

At the present time the majority of detected mutations are novel, indicating that general screening methods such as SSCP will continue to be useful for FH for some time. However, it can be seen from Fig. 3 that in patients in the United Kingdom, roughly 30% of all detected SSCPs occur in exon 4 and 18% in exon 3. This suggests that a useful strategy will be to focus on exons 3 and 4. This would lead to the rapid detection of the specific mutation in 10% of patients. In other parts of the world where founder mutations have been identified, or in the United Kingdom if common mutations or "region-specific" mutations are detected, it is possible that, as with mutations causing thalassemia, a targeted, or sequential approach to specific mutation testing will be useful in the future (*see* Chapter 9).

2. Materials
2.1. PCR

1. *Taq* DNA polymerase (Gibco, Paisley, UK). Stored at –20°C.
2. 1X *Taq* DNA polymerase reaction buffer: 10 mM Tris-HCl, pH 8.3, 50 mM KCl, 0.001% gelatin, 0.2 mM dATP, 0.2 mM dGTP, 0.2 mM dTTP, and 0.02 mM dCTP. 10X stock is prepared and stored in aliquots at –20°C.
3. MgCl$_2$ is kept as stock of 50 mM in aliquots at –20°C.
4. W-1 ("detergent" from Gibco) stored at –20°C.
5. Redivue [^{32}P]-αdCTP (Amersham, Amersham, UK) stored at 4°C.
6. Oligonucleotide primers (Genosys). Store in aliquots at –20°C.
7. Paraffin oil (light liquid, BDH, London, UK).

2.2. Gel Running

1. 30% Polyacrylamide gel solution with bis acrylamide to acrylamide ratio of 1:49. (Severn Biotech Ltd, UK). Store at 4°C.
2. TEMED (N,N,N',N'-tetramethylethylenediamine) (BDH). Store at 4°C in the dark.
3. 25% Ammonium persulfate (BDH).
4. Glycerol.
5. Formamide dye mix: 95% formamide, 10 mM EDTA, 0.025% bromophenol blue, 0.025% xylene cyanol FF.
6. 0.1% (w/v) Sodium dodecylsulfate (SDS) containing 10 mM EDTA.
7. 10X TBE: 0.89M Tris-base, 0.89M boric acid, 20 mM EDTA, pH 8.0.
8. Repelcote (BDH).

3. Methods
3.1. Rapid Throughput Modifications for Sample Handling

We have made several major improvements in the techniques used for sample handling that allow SSCP or other such mutation analyses to be carried out in an extremely rapid manner *(33,34)*. Tube handling and labeling time has been reduced by storing DNA from individual patients in a 96-well format. These arrays can easily be "replicated" 20–30 times in 96-well microtiter plates, for subsequent PCR amplification and mutation screening or other genotyping. The use of 96-well microtiter arrays and compatible multichannel devices are well established for cell culture and for analytical reactions. There is no labeling of tubes and the plate is also the storage rack (with identity of sample being related to its position in the array). The storage of many such plates, each containing a small volume of pre-PCR template in refrigerators or freezers is inconvenient and expensive. To overcome this problem, we allow the DNA templates to dry overnight at room temperature and store all such plates at room temperature. There are the additional advantages that because the template DNA is dry, it has no volume to be taken into account when setting up the PCR reaction and it also reduces the probability of cross-contamination when using an automatic multipipet to aliquot the PCR mix. Several wells are left empty of DNA in each array, so that cross-contamination can be monitored and control samples can be added when necessary. In several months using this procedure we have not found any cross-contamination. For samples from which repeated and different PCRs will be undertaken, this enormously reduces staff time and reduces the requirement for laboratory equipment for storage. We routinely adjust the DNA concentration in the master array to an average of 16 ng/µL water, so that to obtain 40 ng dried DNA requires repeated pipeting of 2.5-µL aliquots using multichannel pipets: It is much easier to pipet repeatedly 2.5 µL rather than 1 µL of a more concentrated stock using standard tips and 2.5 µL is a small enough volume to dry in a few hours on standing at room temperature. Twenty replicas from one master array, consuming 96 tips in total rather than 20 × 96 tips, can be prepared with an eight-channel pipet by one worker in 2 h. Storage of pre-PCR dried plates at room temperature makes it possible to prepare many identical replicas in advance, where many different PCRs are planned from a given master array, whereas advance preparation of replicas would not be possible if there were a requirement for refrigeration or freezing.

The setup of these PCRs is extremely simple, in that the sample has zero volume, so that unless the exact quantity of template DNA is critical, any volume of a PCR master mix containing all components except template DNA can be added to the well. The coefficient of variation introduced by pipeting is also minimized. Thus, as well as ease of setup, robustness to drop-out of PCRs is improved. The making and distributing of a PCR mix and oil to all wells of a dried plate using a repeating dispenser takes one worker approx 10 min. We have also recently described, for PCR checking and other analyses, a system for preparing, and stacking open-faced horizontal polyacrylamide gels, in which the wells retain the 96-well array (microtiter array diagonal gel electrophoresis, MADGE) (*35;* Chapter 16).

3.2. All Exon SSCP Screen

In some situations, we wish to undertake a large number of different PCRs simultaneously on the same DNA sample or on a small set, e.g., samples from four newly diagnosed FH patients. Instead of drying a different template in each well, drying a different premixed pair of PCR primers in each well is

Prom Ex 1 Ex 2 Ex 3   4-5' 4-M   4-3' Ex 5   Ex 6 Ex 7 Ex 8 Ex 9

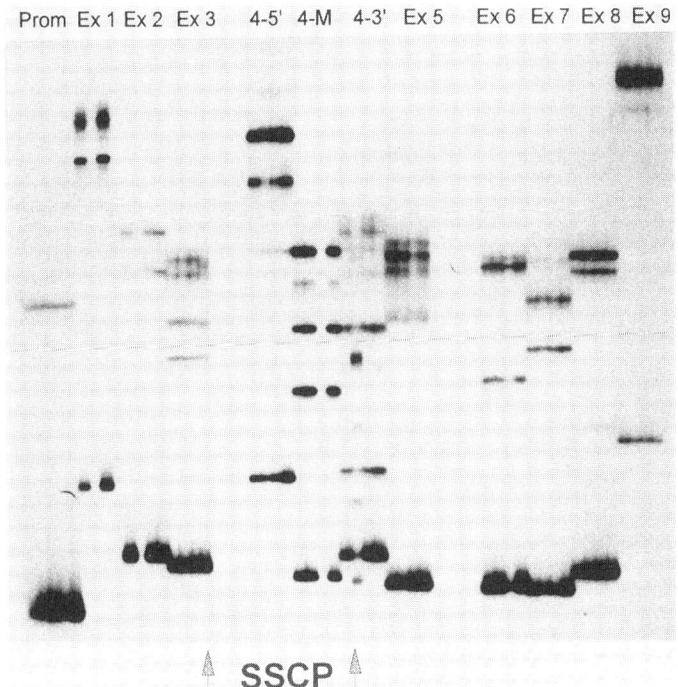

SSCP

Fig. 4. Electrophoresis of PCR products from four independent human DNAs, using dried arrays of PCR primer pairs. The PCR products are electrophoresed under standard SSCP technique conditions and are grouped by PCR. It can be noted that almost all PCR reactions yielded PCR product. The lowermost band represents double-stranded DNA, the upper bands represent single strands: There are polymorphisms or mutations in the third, fourth, and seventh sets of PCR reactions counting from the left. Note SSCP arrow indicating Ex2 SSCP.

equally efficient in PCR yield. This suggests that little of the oligonucleotide is irreversibly bound to the plastic. The PCR premix is arranged to contain a template DNA instead of a primer pair, and an example of an SSCP autoradiograph from the simplified setup of 21 PCRs from the LDL-R gene in four patients with familial hypercholesterolemia is shown in Fig. 4. Typical PCRs in this laboratory are set up in a volume of 20 µL, using 40 ng template DNA and 8 picomoles of each PCR primer. Eight pmol of a 20-mer primer represents approx 48 ng, so that a dried DNA template plate contains 40 ng DNA per well, a dried primer-pair plate contains 96 ng oligonucleotide per well. Thus, on a weight basis, the layer of DNA dried onto the plastic is of the same order for the two strategies.

3.3. PCR Setup
Using Microtiter Arrays of Dried Template DNA

1. Dilute DNA samples to a concentration of approx 10 ng/μL in 0.5 μL in 96-well arrays. This forms the master plate.
2. Transfer 2.5 μL of this to 96-well microtiter plates (Hybaid Omnigene, UK, microtiter plates for PCR) using an eight-channel multipipet. Many copies from the master plate can be made, left to dry overnight, and stored at room temperature for future use.

3.4. Minimization of ^{32}P Usage

1. Make up a modified PCR polymerase mix containing one-tenth the usual concentration of dCTP (0.2 mM dATP and so forth, 0.02 mM dCTP). This may be used in conjunction with a 10-fold reduction in the concentration of [α-^{32}P]dCTP compared with earlier protocols *(14,19)*.
2. Prepare the complete polymerase mix including oligonucleotides, *Taq* polymerase, deoxynucleotides, buffer, W1, and radioisotope for distribution into the wells of plates containing dried DNA templates.
3. Perform the amplifications in an automated thermal cycler (Hybaid Omnigene) using Thermus Aquaticus (*Taq*) DNA polymerase (Gibco BRL) in a total volume of 20 μL and overlay with 20 μL paraffin oil, using previously described cycling conditions *(11)* (*see* Note 1).

3.5. SSCP Double Gel Setup

1. Pour two gels between one large glass sequencing plate (33 × 42 cm) and two outer smaller plates (33 × 39 cm), so that the two gels can be subjected to electrophoresis simultaneously on one apparatus (*see* Note 2). The three plates are defined: "lowest," which is the large plate and the outermost one when the arrangement is clamped to the vertical electrophoresis apparatus; "middle;" and "uppermost." The terms refer to the plates as arranged horizontally on a leveling table for gel pouring.
2. Prior to gel pouring, silanize the four glass faces which will contact the gel with Repelcote.
3. Spread 2 mL evenly over the surface with the edge of another glass plate. Arrange the plates with their sides aligned, with a pair of 0.4 × 10 × 400 mm spacers supporting the sides of both the middle and uppermost glass plates. The edge of the middle plate that will contact the bottom gel tank is arranged to be recessed 5 mm relative to the other plates. This leaves a 5-mm "platform" at the top, which better facilitates the insertion of the comb for the upper gel.
4. Clamp the three plates at the sides with bulldog clips.
5. Pour the bottom gel (on the large plate) first (by injection between the plates using a large syringe, with firm tapping to avoid the formation of bubbles during pouring).
6. Insert the comb and leave the gel to set for 30–60 min.

7. Prepare the second gel in an identical manner. The gels can be stored for several days with TBE-saturated tissues and cling film covering the ends. Care must be taken when clamping the gels to the apparatus to ensure that no air bubbles are trapped in the recess between outermost and innermost plates in the bottom tank.

3.6. SSCP Analysis on Nondenaturing Gels

1. Add 2 μL of the PCR product to 12 μL of a 7:5 ratio mix of formamide dye mix and a solution of 0.1% (w/v) SDS containing 10 mM EDTA.
2. Denature the amplified DNA sample at 95°C for 5 min and chill immediately on wet ice (*see* Note 3). Load 7.5 μL samples on to a 7.5% polyacrylamide nondenaturing gel (ratio of acrylamide to bisacrylamide of 49:1) in 1X TBE buffer with 5% glycerol, 10 mM EDTA. Gels were 40 cm × 30 cm × 0.4 mm.
3. Conduct electrophoresis at a constant voltage of 200 V overnight at room temperature (usually 21–25°C) (but *see* Note 4) until the xylene cyanol migrates 20 cm.
4. Transfer the gels onto Whatman 3MM chromatographic paper, dry, and expose to Hyperfilm β max (Amersham, Maidstone, UK) for 1–4 d at –70°C with one intensifying screen before developing the film (*see* Note 5).

3.7. Double Loading Gels

1. After first loading the gel, the samples are electrophoresed at 400 V until the bromophenol blue runs 2.5–3 cm, at which point the electrophoresis may be stopped and a second set of SSCP samples loaded in the same way as the first samples.
2. Before loading the second time, the sharktooth comb must be removed and repositioned half a well across from its original position. This enables the first and second loading bands to be distinguished more easily (*see* Note 6).

3.8. Sharktooth Comb

1. Sharktooth combs are custom cut with 4.5-mm spacing tooth-to-tooth to enable the use of a multichannel pipet compatible with microtiter plates (9-mm well-to-well spacing) for loading the SSCP gels. This results in every second well being loaded with a multichannel pipet so that two adjacent columns or rows of a microtiter plate are interleaved when loading (*see* Note 6).

4. Notes

1. Single-strand length: The optimal length of single strand seems to be approx 150–200 nt *(36)*. In this size range 70–90% of single base substitutions are apparent on SSCPs. Presumably, longer strands exhibit relatively less conformational change by a single base substitution, and shorter strands adopt less complex conformations. On average, the reverse complement of a particular four-base sequence will occur once every $4 \times 4 \times 4 \times 4 = 256$ nucleotides: Thus, it would be expected that a PCR single strand would contain quite a few possible sequences to form four-base double-stranded stems, but few stems of significantly longer perfect-match duplexes. Such segments would be expected to melt and hence

lose any sequence-specific conformation below the melting temperatures (25–35°C) at which 10–15-mer oligonucleotides dissociate from their target *(37)*. The behavior of stem-loop folds would also be expected to depend on guanosine plus cytosine content, since the three hydrogen bond basepair, GC, is more stable to temperature than the two hydrogen bond basepair, AT. We have observed that for exon 4 mutations in the LDL-R gene, mobility shifts are more frequently apparent in the upper strand. One explanation for this might be that the faster migrating single strand, which is assumed to be more compact, has sufficient stability not to be so markedly affected by a base change at the temperatures used. A better understanding of these factors would be of value in order to make predictive analyses of specific sequences and maximize the mutation detection efficiency of SSCP in a fashion similar to the preplanning of DGGE experiments *(38)*.

2. Effect of temperature: Several studies have reported the use of different temperature running conditions for SSCP, and typical conditions are either at room temperature, or 4°C with 5 or 10% glycerol. As discussed earlier, the small regions of basepairing that are responsible for the conformation of the single strands and thus the potential polymorphisms are likely to have a melting temperature at or below the UK average room temperature, and our experience is that during hot weather the migration of bands changes considerably such that certain SSCPs are no longer detected. The use of 4°C standardizes these conditions, but although we have not systematically investigated the effect of temperature control on band sharpness or detection rate of SSCPs, we and others have not found many additional SSCPs in samples run at other than our standard conditions *(39,40)*. Gels are routinely run at 5 V/cm overnight at "room" temperature in an air conditioned room, which is typically approx 22°C, with temperature fluctuations between 20 and 25°C. At this voltage, power per gel is about 4 W, and gel warming is insignificant. A more expensive option would be the use of a water-jacketed gel plate with a circulating water bath.

3. PCR product denaturation: For convenience, PCR products are used without purification, but spurious bands may result if the number of cycles is excessive or if there is excessive residual primer which may anneal to single strands *(41)*. Using high detection sensitivity for DNA (i.e., ^{32}P) the number of PCR reaction cycles can be reduced (e.g., to 20) and the sample can be diluted 10–30-fold, which will minimize annealing between single strands or between single strands and PCR oligonucleotides. However, if less sensitive detection methods are to be used *(see the following)* less dilution is possible and stronger denaturants added to the sample may help. Formamide, sodium hydroxide, urea, and methylmercuric hydroxide have been used *(42)*. Although toxic and requiring a fume hood, methylmercuric hydroxide appears to be the most effective. Most protocols involve heating the sample, immediate chilling on ice, then loading onto an apparatus of temperature between 4 and 25°C. A top layer of gel with formamide incorporated has also been proposed to aid sample denaturation *(43)*, but this does not avoid the strand reannealing that will take place when the single strands first enter the nondenaturing gel.

4. Characteristics of the gel: Polyacrylamide is the commonly used matrix for DNA fragments in the SSCP size range. The ratio of acrylamide to *bis*-acrylamide crosslinker, and the total acrylamide concentration, determines the sieving properties of the gel. The buffer conductivity and concentration also influence SSCP mobility, as do gel temperature and other additives such as glycerol. Several publications have detailed the different effects that these conditions can have on resolving a particular sequence variation. Reduced crosslinker ratio (*bis*: acrylamide 1:49) and 5–10% (v/v) glycerol are popular *(44)*, although other protocols such as high percentage gels can be useful *(45)*. We have found (Gudnason, unpublished) that the latter is true for a 340 bp PCR fragment representing the 5' end of exon 4 of the LDL-R gene. However, there is no adequate theoretical basis to explain the substantial influence of particular conditions in resolving certain SSCPs although some studies of folding and single-strand mobility have been performed under nondenaturing and denaturing conditions *(46,47)*. Hydrolink is an acrylamide-like matrix polymerized by TEMED and ammonium persulfate, which is reported to have a more uniform pore size and is claimed to give narrower bands and hence better resolution than acrylamide *(27)*.

Reported gel lengths range between 5 and 50 cm. At present, most results are read by eye and therefore visible resolution is necessary. Although clearcut mobility shifts (e.g., 10%) are demonstrable on short gels, a long electrophoresis may be necessary to resolve a 0.5% mobility difference. Long electrophoresis has the disadvantages that it needs a large apparatus, a higher voltage power pack, and more complex arrangements to set up and control temperature. A longer run broadens a band in accord with basic theory (effects of an imperfect matrix and diffusion) and this may be compounded for SSCP without proper temperature control (i.e., nonuniform conformation and hence nonuniform mobility). Nevertheless, where it is important to avoid false-negative results, long track length is advisable.

5. Detection methods for SSCP single strands: Autoradiography of dried gels for ^{32}P incorporated during PCR as [α-^{32}P]dNTP (or by [γ-^{32}P]ATP end-labeling primers (or PCR product) involves the hazards and inconvenience of radioisotope usage. The main options that have been explored are silver staining *(48,49)* and ethidium bromide fluorescence *(43)*. Ethidium bromide intercalates with 5–10-fold higher affinity in double-stranded DNA, and is therefore not well suited to single-strand detection. Nevertheless, ethidium bromide staining is a one-step process and conditions to load sufficient single-strand DNA have been achieved *(42,43)*. Sensitive silver staining protocols are available for DNA, with detection down to 1–10 pg/mm^2 *(50)*. The catalytic process of silver reduction is initiated on DNA bases. A typical protocol involves deposition of silver nitrate on bands, then reduction of silver by formaldehyde and sodium carbonate to give a brown color (*see* Chapter 3 for protocol). The reaction is stopped by acetic acid.

Large gels (e.g., 30 × 40 × 0.04 cm are difficult to handle for postelectrophoretic staining. Binding the gel to one glass plate with γ-methacryloxypropyltrimethoxysilane is used for silver staining, but this renders gel recovery (as a dried image on Whatman 3 MM paper) very difficult. A photographic film based process can take a direct imprint from the gel while amplifying the signal (Promega Corp., Southampton, UK). We find that our staining protocol can be used, with complete adherence of the gel to a glass plate, using 4 μL/cm^2 of 0.5% γ-methacryloxypropyltrimethoxysilane/0.5% glacial acetic acid/ethanol, and that the gel can then be reliably recovered onto Whatman 3 MM paper. The single-strand band intensity depends on PCR fragment sequence and size (some reanneal more readily than others) and tends to be faint.

A further possibility, not yet fully explored is to blot the gel, most conveniently by "direct blotting." DNA is electrophoresed off the end of the gel onto a revolving blot (51) and then one of the several methods of detection by hybridization is used.

Automated DNA sequencers perform electrophoresis and detection on gels similar to manual sequencing gels. However, the detection system is usually fluorescence either using oligonucleotides with fluorescent labels attached, or incorporating fluorescent nucleotide analysis during polymerase reactions. It has been shown that such apparatus also can be applied to SSCP using fluorescent labels (52). The arguments pertinent to throughput, sensitivity of detection, and resolution are similar to those for automated sequencing (53). The main shortfalls are that one sequencer can only run one gel at a time; that there is high capital expenditure; that access to "primary data" is impossible if computer corrections for the differential effect of different dyes on mobility are involved; and that there is the need for additional sophisticated workstations for secondary editing and interpretation of the data.

6. The first and second loading single and double strands need to be nonoverlapping if the gel is to be informative. The calculation of the timing of the second loading is possible if the relative mobilities of the two single strands, one double strand, and marker dyes are already known for the set of conditions to be used. These mobilities may be determined in a prior experiment with single loading. In order that repetitive loading can be applied both to the same and different exons, we have prepared a computer simulation that solves the equations relating relative mobilities, boundary conditions including timing of loading, range of migration distance desired and time delays between loadings (available from G. P. Weavind, 73064,3063@compuserve.com by e-mail request). Double loading the gel means that a whole 96-well microtiter array of samples may be analyzed on one gel.

Acknowledgments

I. N. M. Day is the recipient of a British Heart Foundation Intermediate Fellowship. S. E. Humphries is supported by a Chair award and Program grant RG16 from the British Heart Foundation, and V. Gudnason by the Icelandic Council of Science. The work was also supported by the Sir Halley Stewart Trust, Helen Eppel Fund, and John Pinto Foundation.

References

1. Goldstein, J. L. and Brown, M. S. (1989) Familial hypercholesterolemia, in *The Metabolic Basis of Inherited Disease*, 6th ed. (Scriver, C. R., Beaudet, A. L., Sly, W. W., and Valle, D., eds.), McGraw-Hill, New York, pp. 1215–1250.
2. Cotton, R. G. H. (1993) Current methods of mutation detection. *Mutat. Res.* **285**, 125–144.
3. Condie, A., Eeles, R., Borreson, A.-L., Coles, C., Cooper, C., and Prosser, J. (1993) Detection of point mutations in the P53 gene: comparison of single-stand conformation polymorphism, constant denaturant gel electrophoresis, and hydroxylamine and osmium tetroxide techniques. *Hum. Mutat.* **2**, 58–66.
4. Orita, M., Suzuki, Y., Sekiya, T., and Hayashi, K. (1989) Rapid and sensitive detection of point mutations and DNA polymorphisms using the polymerase chain reaction. *Genomics* **5**, 874–879.
5. Britten, R. J. and Davidson, E. H. (1985) Hybridisation strategy, in *Nucleic Acid Hybridisation: A Practical Approach* (Hames, B. D. and Higgins, S. J., eds.), IRL Press, Oxford, UK, pp. 3–15.
6. Lee, H.-H., Lo, W.-J., and Choo, K.-B. (1992) Mutational analysis by a combined application of the multiple restriction fragment-single strand conformation polymorphism and the direct linear amplification DNA sequencing protocols. *Anal. Biochem.* **205**, 289–293.
7. Suzuki, Y., Sekiya, T., and Hayashi, K. (1991) Allele-specific polymerase chain reaction: a method for amplification and sequence determination of a single component among a mixture of sequence variants. *Anal. Biochem.* **192**, 82–84.
8. Lo, Y.-M. D., Patel, P., Mehal, W. Z., Fleming, K. A., Bell, J. I., and Wainscoat, J. S. (1992) Analysis of complex genetic systems by ARMS-SSCP: application to HLA genotyping. *Nucleic Acids Res.* **20**, 1005–1009.
9. Sarkar, G., Yoon, H.-S., and Sommer, S. S. (1992) Dideoxy fingerprinting (ddF): a rapid and efficient screen for the presence of mutations. *Genomics* **13**, 441–443.
10. Keen, J., Lester, D., Inglebearn, C., Curtis, A., and Bhattacharya, S. (1991) Rapid detection of single base mismatches as heteroduplexes on Hydrolink gels. *Trends Genet.* **7**, 5.
11. Sarkar, G., Yoon, H.-S., and Sommer, S. S. (1992) Screening for mutations by RNA single-strand conformation polymorphism (rSSCP): comparison with DNA-SSCP. *Nucleic Acids Res.* **20**, 871–878.
12. Patterson, D. and Slack, J. (1972) Lipid abnormalities in male and female survivors of myocardial infarction and their first degree relatives. *Lancet* **i**, 1393–1399.
13. Betteridge, D. J., Dodson, P. M., Durrington, P. N., Hughes, E. A., Laker, M. F., Nicholls, D. P., et al. (1993) Management of hyperlipidaemia: guidelines of the British Hyperlipidaemia Association. *Postgrad. Med. J.* **69**, 359–369.
14. Kane, J. P., Malloy, M. J., Ports, T. A., Phillips, N. R., Diehl, J. C., and Havel, R. J. (1990) Regression of coronary atherosclerosis during treatment of familial hypercholesterolemia with combined drug regimens. *JAMA* **264**, 3007–3012.
15. Tybjaerg-Hansen, A. and Humphries, S. (1992) Familial defective apolipoprotein B-100: a single mutation that causes hypercholesterolaemia and premature coronary artery disease. *Atherosclerosis* **96**, 91–107.

16. Starzl, T. E., Bilheimer, D. W., Bahnson, H. T., Hardesty, R. L., Griffith, B. T., Iwatsuki, S., et al. (1984) Heart–liver transplantation in a patient with familial hypercholesterolaemia. *Lancet*, **23**, 1382,1383.

17. Grossman, M., Raper, S. E., Kozarsky, K., Stein, E. A., Engelhardt, J. F., Muller, D., et al. (1994) Successful *ex vivo* gene therapy directed to liver in a patient with familial hypercholesterolaemia. *Nat. Genet.* **6**, 335–341.

18. Leonard, J. V., Whitelaw, A. G. L., Wolff, O. H., Lloyd, J. K., and Slack, J. (1977) Diagnosing FH in children by measuring serum cholesterol. *Br. Med. J.* **i,** 1566–1568.

19. Schmitz, G., Bruning, T., Kovacs, E., and Barlage, S. (1993) Fluorescence flow cytometry of human leukocytes in the detection of LDL receptor defects in the differential diagnosis of hypercholesterolemia. *Arterioscl. Thromb.* **13**, 1053–1065.

20. Kessling, A. M., Seed, M., Taylor, R., Wynn, V., and Humphries, S. E. (1990) Rising cholesterol levels in children with familial hypercholesterolaemia. *Biomed. Pharmacother.* **44**, 373–379.

21. Hobbs, H. H., Brown, M. S., and Goldstein, J. L. (1992) Molecular genetics of the LDL receptor gene in familial hypercholesterolaemia. *Hum. Mutat.* **1**, 445–466.

22. King-Underwood, L., Gudnason, V., Humphries, S., Seed, M., Patel, D., Knight, B., et al. (1991) Identification of the 664 proline to leucine mutation in the low density lipoprotein receptor in four unrelated patients with familial hypercholesterolaemia in the UK. *Clin. Genet.* **40**, 17–28.

23. Sun, X.-M., Webb, J. C., Gudnason, V., Humphries, S., Seed, M., Thompson, G. R., Knight, B. L., and Soutar, A. K. (1992) Characterization of deletions in the LDL receptor gene in patients with FH in the UK. *Arterioscl. Thromb.* **12**, 762–770.

24. Gudnason, V., King-Underwood, L., Seed, M., Sun, X-M., Soutar, A. K., and Humphries, S. E. (1993) Identification of recurrent and novel mutations in exon 4 of LDL receptor gene in patients with familial hypercholesterolaemia in the United Kingdom. *Arterioscl. Thromb.* **13**, 6–63.

25 Webb, J. C., Sun, X.-M., Patel, D. D., McCarthy, S. N., Knight, B. L., and Soutar, A. K. (1992) Characterisation of two new point mutations in the low density lipoprotein (LDL) receptor genes of an English patient with homozygous familial hypercholesterolemia. *J. Lipid Res.* **33**, 689–698.

26. Gudnason, V., Mak, Y.-T., Betteridge, J., McCarthy, S. N., and Humphries, S. (1993) Use of the single strand conformational polymorphism method to detect recurrent and novel mutations in the low density lipoprotein receptor gene in patients with familial hypercholesterolaemia: detection of a novel mutation Asp^{200} → Gly. *Clin. Invest.* **71**, 331–337.

27. Gudnason, V., Day, I., and Humphries, S. E. (1994) Effect on plasma lipid levels of mutations in exon 4 of the low-density lipoprotein receptor gene in patients with familial hypercholesterolaemia. *Arterioscl. Thromb.* **14**, 1717–1721.

28. Sun, X.-M., Patel, D. D., Bhatnagar, D., Knight, B. L., and Soutar, A.K. (1995) Characterization of a splice-site mutation in the gene for the LDL receptor associated with an unpredictably severe clinical phenotype in English patients with heterozygous FH. *Arterioscl. Thromb.* **15**, 219–227.

29. Graham, C. A., Ward, A. J., Nevin, N. C., Trinick, T.,Young, I., O'Kane, M., and Nicholls, D. P. (1995) Automated sequencing has identified 70% of mutations in 30 patients with familial hypercholesterolaemia in Northern Ireland. *Atherosclerosis* **112,** 261–267.

30. Esser, V., Limbird, L. E., Brown, M. S., Goldstein, J. L., and Russell, D. W. (1988) Mutational analysis of the ligand binding domain of the low density lipoprotein receptor. *J. Biol. Chem.* **263,** 13,282–13,290.

31. Hobbs, H. H., Leitersdorf, E., Leffert, C. C., Cryer, D. R., Brown, M. S., and Goldstein, J. L. (1989) Evidence for a dominant gene that suppresses hypercholesterolemia in a family with defective low density lipoprotein receptors. *J. Clin. Invest.* **84,** 656–664.

32. Chamberlain, J. S., Gibbs, R. A., Ranier, J. E., Nguyen, P. N., and Caskey, C. T. (1988) Deletion screening of the Duchenne muscular dystrophy locus via multiplex DNA amplification. *Nucleic Acids Res.* **16,** 11,141–11,156.

33. Whittall, R., Gudnason, V., Weavind, G., Day, L. B., Humphries, S., and Day, I. N. M. (1995) Utilities for high throughput use of the single strand conformational polymorphism method: screening of 791 patients with familial hypercholesterolaemia for mutations in exon 3 of the low density lipoprotein receptor gene. *J. Med. Genet.,* **32,** 509–515.

34. Day, I. N. M., Whittall, R., Gundason, V., and Humphries, S. E. (1995) Dried template DNA, and dried PCR oligonucleotides and mailing in 96-well plates: LDL receptor gene mutation screening. *BioTechniques* **18,** 981–984.

35. Day, I. N. M. and Humphries, S. E. (1994) Electrophoresis for genotyping: microtitre array diagonal gel electrophoresis (MADGE) on horizontal polyacrylamide (H-PAGE) gels, Hydrolink or agarose. *Anal. Biochem.* **222,** 389–395.

36. Sheffield, V. C., Beck, J. S., Kwitek, A. E., Sandstrom, D. W., and Stone, E. M. (1993) The sensitivity of single-strand conformation polymorphism analysis for the detection of single base substitutions. *Genomics* **16,** 325–332.

37. Wood, W. I., Gitschier, J., Lasky, L. A., and Lawn, R. M. (1985) Base composition independent hybridization in tetramethylammonium chloride: a method for oligonucleotide screening of highly complex gene libraries. *Proc. Natl. Acad. Sci. USA* **82,** 1585–1588.

38 Cariello, N. F. and Skopek, T. R. (1993) Mutational analysis using denaturing gradient gel electrophoresis and PCR. *Mutat. Res.* **288,** 103–112.

39. Leren, T. P., Solberg, K., Rodningen, O. K., Rosby, O., Tonstad, S., Ose, L., et al. (1993) Screening for point mutations in exon 10 of the low density lipoprotein receptor gene by analysis of single-strand conformation polymorphisms: detection of a nonsense mutation-FH469 → Stop. *Hum. Genet.* **92,** 6–10.

40. Sekiya, T. (1993). Detection of mutant sequences by single-strand conformation polymorphism analysis. *Mutat. Res.* **288,** 79–83.

41. Cai, Q.-Q. and Touitou, I. (1993) Excess PCR primers may dramatically affect SSCP efficiency. *Nucleic Acids Res.* **21,** 3909,3910.

42. Hongyo, T., Buzard, G. S., Calvert, R. J., and Weghorst, C. M. (1993) "Cold SSCP": a simple, rapid and non-radioactive method for optimized single-strand conformation polymorphism analyses. *Nucleic Acids Res.* **21,** 3637–3642.

43. Yap, E. P. H. and McGee, J. O. (1993) Nonisotopic discontinuous phase single strand conformation polymorphism (DP-SSCP): genetic profiling of D-loop of human mitochondrial (mt) DNA. *Genomes* **21,** 4155.

44. Spinardi, L., Mazars, R., and Theillet, C. (1991) Protocols for an improved detection of point mutations by SSCP. *Nucleic Acids Res.* **19,** 4009.

45. Savov, A., Angelicheva, D., Jordanova, A., Eigel, A., and Kalaydjieva, L. (1992) High percentage acrylamide gels improve resolution in SSCP analysis. *Nucleic Acids Res.* **20,** 6741,6742.

46. Baxter, S. M., Greizerstein, M. B., Kushlan, D. M., and Ashley, G. W. (1993) Conformational properties of DNA hairpins with TTT and TTTT loops. *Biochemistry* **32,** 8702–8711.

47. Mayer, P., Slater, G. W., and Drouin, G. (1993) Exact behaviour of single-stranded DNA electrophoretic mobilities in polyacrylamide gels. *Appl. Theoret. Electrophor.* **3,** 145–155.

48. Ainsworth, P. J., Surh, L. C., and Coulter-Mackie, M. B. (1991) Diagnostic single strand conformational polymorphism, (SSCP): a simplified non-radioisotopic method as applied to a Tay-Sachs B1 variant. *Nucleic Acids Res.* **19,** 405,406.

49. Mohabeer, A. J., Hiti, A. L., and Martin, W. J. (1991) Non-radioactive single strand conformation polymorphism (SSCP) using the Pharmacia "PhastSystem." *Nucleic Acids Res.* **19,** 3154.

50. Bassam, B. J., Caetano-Anollés, G., and Gresshoff, P. M. (1991) Fast and sensitive silver staining of DNA in polyacrylamide gels. *Anal. Biochem.* **196,** 80–83.

51. Beck, S. and Pohl, F. M. (1984) DNA sequencing with direct blotting electrophoresis. *EMBO. J.* **3,** 2905–2909.

52. Ellison, J., Dean, M., and Goldman, D. (1993) Efficacy of fluorescence-based PCR-SSCP for detection of point mutations. *BioTechniques* **15,** 684–691.

53. Yang, M. M. and Youvan, D. C. (1989) A prospectus for multispectral-multiplex DNA sequencing. *Biotechnology* **7,** 576–581.

20

Quality Assurance in Molecular Diagnosis

The UK Experience

Susan A. R. Stenhouse and Helen Middleton-Price

1. Introduction

Molecular genetic diagnosis is a relatively young discipline and also one of the fastest growing among clinical laboratory sciences. The majority of diagnostic laboratories in this field emerged from groups active in research into human genetic disease, and the development of a service-oriented structure from more loosely organized research laboratories was the first priority for the provision of an efficient diagnostic service. In April 1988, the Clinical Molecular Genetics Society (CMGS) was constituted as the professional body representing molecular geneticists working in a diagnostic capacity in the United Kingdom (UK). This organization quickly saw the need for a central system of external quality assurance (EQA), and a subcommittee was set up to establish such a scheme.

The first trial of EQA took place in 1991 and required simple genotyping of DNA samples for three disorders: Duchenne muscular dystrophy (DMD), cystic fibrosis (CF), and Huntington disease (HD). The majority of laboratories in the UK offering a service for these diseases participated in the scheme. In the second trial in 1993, CF, DMD, and fragile X syndrome (FRAXA) were covered. The scheme was expanded on this occasion to include interpretation of the results with risk calculations and recommendations for further analysis, which were submitted in the form of a full clinical report.

Encouraged by the success of these trials, the EQA subcommittee applied to the UK Department of Health for funding of a 2-yr pilot project with a view toward moving to a subscription-based scheme at the end of that period. This application was successful and the CMGS EQA subcommittee was reconsti-

From: *Methods in Molecular Medicine: Molecular Diagnosis of Genetic Diseases*
Edited by: R. Elles Humana Press Inc., Totowa, NJ

tuted as an independent body known as the steering committee for Molecular Genetics External Quality Assurance (MGEQA), since independence from the professional organization is required for formal recognition by the Department of Health. In 1994, the first pilot scheme was established for five disorders: DMD, CF, HD, FRAXA, and myotonic dystrophy (distroplia myotonica [DM]).

2. Structure of EQA Schemes in the United Kingdom

Most clinical laboratory disciplines are subject to EQA and participation in such a scheme is generally required for laboratory accreditation. EQA schemes in the UK are overseen at the highest level by the Joint Working Group, which is comprised of representatives from the professional organizations of all the pathology laboratory sciences and members of the Royal College of Pathologists. The Joint Working Group approves each EQA scheme and reports directly to the government via the Secretary of State for Health. Advisory panels for individual disciplines constitute the next level of management, and the Chairs of the Advisory Panels report directly to the Joint Working Group regarding the progress of individual schemes. Advisory panels are composed of experts in the field, and their primary function is to deal with poor performance and to advise the scheme organizers. The steering committee of the MGEQA plans the structure of the EQA scheme, devises the questions, and supplies the DNA samples. It is also responsible for the scoring of final reports.

The scheme organizer is responsible for the practical administration of the EQA and is the main direct contact with participating laboratories. A key function of the scheme organizer is to maintain the anonymity of the individual laboratories, which are otherwise identified by numerical code. He or she is responsible for sample distribution and receipt of final reports. Any queries or problems related to the EQA are directed through the scheme organizer. Figure 1 outlines the overall structure of clinical laboratory external EQA schemes in the UK.

3. Present Scheme

The UK scheme currently involves 37 participating laboratories, including recently 8 in the Netherlands and 1 in the Republic of Ireland. Laboratories may choose from eight diseases offered: DMD, CF, FRAXA, HD, DM, Prader-Willi/Angelman syndromes (PWS/AS), familial adenomatous polyposis coli (FAP), and spinal muscular atrophy (SMA). There are two sample distributions per year with four disorders covered in each distribution.

Samples and relevant clinical details are provided by members of the steering committee and distributed to all participating laboratories by the scheme organizer. The EQA samples are supplied with a clinical request as if referred by a clinician. Each will require either direct mutation testing or the analysis of linked markers, but the choice of the appropriate test is normally left to the individual laboratory. Four or five DNA samples are provided for each

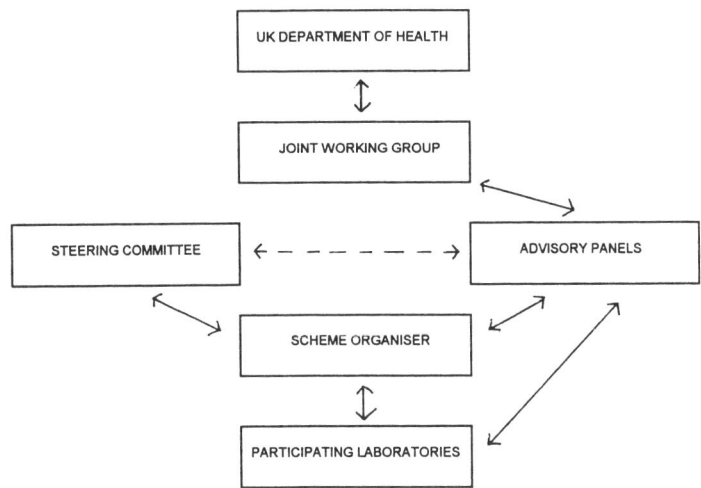

Fig. 1. Structure of clinical laboratory EQA schemes in the UK. —, Direct interaction; ---, interaction through observers.

disorder, and they may be a family group or single individuals. Results and reports must be returned to the scheme organizer within 6 wk and are identified by a number code. Only the scheme organizer knows the identity of the individual laboratories.

Performance is assessed on two levels, correct genotyping and appropriate interpretation. Clear criteria for the scoring of each disorder are agreed to by the steering committee. The individual who supplied the samples and posed the clinical request marks the returns first before passing them to a second committee member for independent scoring using the same agreed on criteria. Discrepancies in the scoring are discussed and resolved by the full committee. The scoring system is described in full in this chapter.

Feedback to the participating laboratories is provided annually after the second sample distribution. Each center will receive a general overview of the returns and an anonymous table of results, including the scoring criteria plus specific comments from assessors on the individual performance of their laboratory.

At every stage in the development of the EQA scheme, the choice of disorders has reflected those that are most commonly offered in diagnostic service, and EQA is now provided for all disorders which are tested for in more than eight laboratories in the UK. However, some disorders are so rare or specialized that only a few centers offer testing. It will not be possible to provide comprehensive EQA for such conditions, but the MGEQA steering committee intends to coordinate transfer of samples between the laboratories involved in order to give a measure of EQA.

4. Scoring

In contrast to many other pathology disciplines, reports from molecular genetics laboratories in the UK are expected to contain a full interpretation of the results in addition to raw genotyping data. Most referring clinicians require the addition of an explanatory paragraph or two interpreting the data in concise English. In order to reflect this, each report is scored for the accuracy of the genotype data and for the presence of a number of interpretative points, which are judged by the MGEQA steering committee to be elements of a good report.

The marking scheme is best illustrated by an example. In the 1994 EQA, DNA samples were provided from a family in which there was an isolated case of Becker muscular dystrophy (BMD) (Fig. 2). Sufficient DNA was provided for polymerase chain reaction (PCR)-based analysis, but not for Southern blots. Laboratories were asked to write reports for individuals BMD1 and BMD3, who wished to know their carrier status, and BMD4, who is affected.

DNA analysis should have shown a deletion of exons 45–47 of the dystrophin gene in BMD4. BMD1 was homozygous/hemizygous at the (CA)n marker locus STR45 from within the deleted region, whereas BMD3 was heterozygous at STR45. In addition, there had been a recombination 5' to the deletion between BMD1 and BMD3 or between BMD1 and BMD4. The most likely approach to the problem would be a multiplex deletion screen followed by analysis with markers from within and flanking the deletion.

The genotyping data were scored as follows:

Correct genotypes	2 Marks
Correct but incomplete genotypes	1 Mark
One or more incorrect genotypes	0 Marks

A report written following this analysis ideally should have contained the following five interpretative points:

1. BMD4 was deleted for exons 45–47 of the dystrophin gene.
2. BMD3 was heterozygous at STR45 from within the deleted region and was, therefore, at very low risk of being a carrier of BMD.
3. BMD1 was either homozygous or hemizygous at STR45 from within the deleted region, and her carrier status could not be resolved by this analysis alone.
4. A calculation of BMD1's carrier risk (90% on pedigree alone, which rises if an estimate of the likelihood of homozygosity at STR45 in BMD1 is included).
5. A suggestion of further analyses (e.g., pulsed-field gel electrophoreses [PFGE], fluorescent *in situ* hybridization [FISH], dosage densitometry), which would resolve the carrier status in BMD1.

A report that contained four to five of these points was awarded 2 marks, one containing two to three was awarded 1 mark, and a report with one or no points

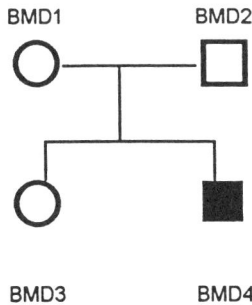

BMD1   BMD2

BMD3   BMD4

Fig. 2. DNA samples of BMD.

was awarded 0 marks. These interpretative points assumed that laboratories adopted the most likely approach to the analysis. The scheme must be adaptable, however, and should accommodate alternative ways of tackling any problem. In fact, one laboratory analyzed the BMD pedigree by PCR-based dosage densitometry using an automated fluorescent sequencer, which gave the correct answer for BMD3 and also allowed the carrier status of BMD1 to be resolved. Clearly, this report received full marks for the genotype data and interpretation.

The level of interpretation required will vary depending on the clinical question and type of analysis involved. In some cases, increased flexibility was introduced by using half marks. The criteria necessary for a full interpretation of each report are agreed to by the steering committee, and each report is marked independently by two committee members. The anonymity of laboratories is maintained throughout since the markers have access only to the laboratory number code.

Scores are reported back to the steering committee for validation before results are returned to the laboratories. In the future, the style and clarity of the final report will also be considered with a view toward establishing minimum criteria for reporting.

The object of using this sort of criteria-based marking scheme was to reduce the subjective nature of the process as far as possible and to allow average performance for each disease to be calculated. Circulation of the collected results for all laboratories and diseases is, of course, anonymous, and although it should not in any way be considered a league table, it does allow a laboratory to check that its standard of reporting is acceptable compared to the average. Publication of the criteria used in the scoring can provide guidance to laboratories for the future, as well as making the steering committee accountable to the participating laboratories to some extent.

EQA schemes in other countries seem to follow broadly similar approaches, although the College of American Pathologists EQA scheme puts more emphasis on interpretation and less on DNA analysis. In the American scheme samples are sent out as cell pellets for DNA extraction. In the EQA scheme for Australia and New Zealand, returns are scored on time taken to issue the report, accuracy of clerical information, accuracy of genotype, and appropriateness of comment of report. Anonymous scores are distributed in a similar way to the UK MGEQA (G. Suther, personal communication). The UK MGEQA is attempting to cover all aspects of laboratory work and reporting, although speed of reporting has not been addressed and is discussed in Section 8.

5. Performance

In general, the quality of results and reports submitted for EQA. EQA has been very good, with most laboratories achieving a high degree of accuracy in genotyping and appropriate interpretation. Where problems have arisen, the laboratory concerned has been approached informally by the scheme organizer offering advice and, where appropriate, practical help. The primary function of the advisory panel is to deal with persistent poor performance, a problem that has not yet been encountered. This would involve a more formal approach to the head of the laboratory concerned. In the future, satisfactory performance in an approved EQA scheme is likely to be a prerequisite for molecular genetic laboratory accreditation. In the UK National Health Service, the purchasing agencies for health care may also provide pressure on laboratories to maintain high standards, one measure of which is EQA performance scores.

6. Topic-Based Discussion Meetings

One of the most successful aspects of the MGEQA scheme has been the introduction of topic-based discussion meetings. These have been held either in response to demand from the participating laboratories or following new developments in the field.

Disease-based meetings allow current practice to be discussed and agreement to be reached on a common approach to service provision. Such meetings can be particularly helpful for laboratories wishing to expand their service to include the disease in question. Technique-based meetings can also be very useful for the evaluation of a new method or piece of equipment with advice available from scientists with experience of its use. Discussion meetings have been held on DMD, CF, DM, HD, SMA, FAP, FRAXA, hereditary non-polyposis colon cancer (HNPCC), internal quality control (QC), and fluorescent DNA analysis.

Following many of these meetings and in light of the discussion there, the steering committee has drawn up consensus guidelines for many aspects of service provision, including "best practice" for individual diseases and internal QA. These are distributed to all participating laboratories and have helped to ensure a high quality of diagnostic service throughout the UK.

7. Bench-Level QC

Participation in external QC schemes is intended to assist molecular genetics laboratories to monitor their performance by providing an independent assessment of results and reporting. Internal QC refers to the additional measures that should be in place in each laboratory to maintain the highest possible standard of service. The following guidelines were drawn up following a discussion meeting on internal QC.

7.1. Specimen Reception

Care should be taken to ensure that specimens are received and stored in such a way that the chance of errors and mix-ups is minimized. The laboratory should ideally have a designated reception area that is clear of other activities or apparatus. Logging in of specimens includes responsibility for checking that the condition of the specimen is suitable (i.e., whether the tube is intact, if the sample is clotted, whether the blood volume is sufficient for the proposed analysis, and so on) that the details on the form and specimen container (usually a blood tube) are complete, and that the referral is appropriate. Unlabeled or incompletely labeled specimens should not be accepted. The operator logging in specimens should also be responsible for drawing the attention of the referring clinician to the need for a further/different specimen if appropriate. At this stage, the specimen is usually given a sample reference number, which is then used throughout the subsequent analysis. Many laboratories find that the use of printed numbered labels helps to reduce transcription errors.

7.2. DNA Extraction

It could be argued that DNA extraction is the most critical stage of sample handling; an error here cannot be rectified at a later stage and may be difficult to detect. Consideration should therefore be given to the employment of rigorous checking procedures at this stage.

The greatest chance for error at DNA extraction is associated with the transfers that must necessarily occur during preparation. Some laboratories prefer to use a DNA extraction method that avoids phenol/chloroform extraction steps, improving the safety of the procedure, and cutting down on sample transfer. Other laboratories have opted for DNA extraction machines, which minimize operator handling. When appropriate, these techniques may be combined with an independent checking system where the checker observes each transfer, which is signed and witnessed as correct.

7.3. DNA Storage

DNA samples for storage should carry at least the unique identifier (laboratory number) as well as the name of the individual on the tube. Other appropriate information to add to the tube is the date of birth, date of preparation, or any additional data that would assist in tracing the sample through the laboratory. Efforts should be made to store duplicate samples or at least a blood spot at a separate location in order to protect this valuable resource in case of fire or other mishap. Special care should be taken to label samples fully when sending them to another laboratory.

7.4. Laboratory Handling of DNA Samples

In order to minimize errors during analysis, sample transfers should be reduced to a minimum, and systematic tube handling procedures employed. Some laboratories have extended the independent checker system to all sample handling procedures, including PCR setup, restriction enzyme digestion, and gel loading. This is not a substitute for careful work, which is still required, but it does provide evidence of the care taken.

7.5. Control Size Markers and Gel Orientation

Most molecular genetics diagnostic procedures involve running samples on agarose or polyacrylamide gel systems. Molecular-weight markers, negative controls, normal male and/or female samples, and specific mutation controls should always be used when appropriate. Since gels, particularly polyacrylamide gels, can be inverted, it is wise to incorporate a vacant track or some other method that will allow unambiguous orientation of the gel. The MGEQA steering committee has been active in obtaining standard-size markers, available to all laboratories for use as controls in specific diseases, such as DM and HD.

7.6. Checking of Results for Reporting

Results should always be read independently by two scientists who must agree on their suitability for reporting. It is recommended that results are graded according to their quality. A suggested scheme grades as follows: (1) a clear result; (2) a less good, but reportable result; and (3) a failure. Final reports should be independently checked when all data, including the referral sheet, experimental details, raw data, and risk calculations, should be scrutinized. Final reports should carry the signatures of the scientist who carried out the analysis and wrote the report, and also of the scientist who checked the report.

7.7. Paternity Testing

Where family relationships are different from those indicated by the pedigree, this is often uncovered by chance in the course of a family analysis. However, correct paternity should only be specifically tested for when it is vital for the inference of the genotype in an individual or fetus.

7.8. Maternal Contamination of Chorionic Villus Biopsy (CVB)

The contamination of fetal material with maternal cells could result in a genotyping error at prenatal diagnosis. This is only a consideration when the fetus shows an identical genotype to that in the mother. Such results should be checked by using highly polymorphic repeat markers to confirm the presence of one maternal and one paternal allele in the fetal material.

7.9. Audit Trail and Standard Protocols

Audit trail refers to the efficient storage of information on each individual sample so that information on its passage through the laboratory from reception to report can be easily retrieved. This issue will be highlighted as laboratories seek accreditation, at which time they will have to expose their systems for recording and tracing samples to inspection. In addition, laboratories will be expected to keep accessible, up-to-date standard protocols for each analysis, so that quality of service can be maintained regardless of the operator.

8. Future Issues

8.1. Reporting Times

In the present EQA system, 6 wk are allowed between sample distribution and submission of returns. This recognizes the fact that EQA testing must be fitted around the routine work of the laboratory and cannot take precedence over urgent diagnostic requests. However, reporting time is an important element of a service and should be measured. One way would be to establish a national average reporting time for each disorder as a guideline. Laboratories could then be asked to calculate the percentage of samples reported within this time. This is certainly an issue that will need to be addressed, since it is likely to be a requirement as evidence of the quality of service.

8.2. EQA for Rare Diseases

The question of rare diseases analyzed in a few specialized centers has already been mentioned briefly. One way to address this issue would be to exchange samples between the laboratories involved, which may be centrally coordinated by the MGEQA steering committee. Involvement of other countries in Europe would be helpful in this respect in order to give a broader population base and the potential to assess more diseases.

8.3. Size of the EQA Scheme

At present in the UK, only four participating laboratories test for all eight diseases offered in the EQA scheme, and so will receive the maximum number of samples; FRAXA is the most commonly tested disorder with 31 laboratories offering diagnosis, and FAP is the least common with only 10 participating laboratories. The eventual size of the scheme will be determined in part by the proportion of laboratory work load that can be devoted to EQA. Even for a large laboratory, the EQA for HD probably represents as much as 5–10% of the annual work load for this disease, and this would be accentuated for a smaller laboratory. This is very different from EQA in chemical pathology, for example, which represents a much smaller proportion of the annual work load. A balance must be found between adequate EQA and excessive interference with routine diagnostic work. As more diseases become amenable to molecular diagnosis, the EQA scheme will need to adapt, perhaps by not testing all diseases every year or by offering a more flexible time-scale for the analysis of a larger number of diseases. The availability and quality of DNA samples for EQA testing are already an issue as the scheme expands both in numbers of participating laboratories and the range of diseases covered. This may be addressed by establishing cell lines from suitable patient samples after informed consent. This will require additional resources and facilities for maintenance of cell lines, extraction of DNA from cells, and validation testing of the final samples. Such developments will also be more complex to administer efficiently, and will require full-time technical and clerical support for the EQA scheme.

8.4. Assessors

The work involved in administration and execution of the MGEQA has increased considerably over the years of its operation. The MGEQA steering committee has been solely responsible for all aspects of the scheme. In order to spread this responsibility more widely, it has been proposed that a panel of assessors be recruited from senior laboratory scientists from around the UK. These independent assessors would score the anonymous reports according to criteria agreed on by the steering committee, and their scores would finally be ratified by that committee.

8.5. Cost of EQA

In its first 2 yr, the financial cost of the QA was met entirely by the CMGS. The pilot scheme was funded by the UK Department of Health. At the end of the 2-yr pilot study, the scheme will become self-financing, and this will be achieved by setting a charge per disease with participating laboratories subscriptions being dependent on how many diseases they offer.

In setting the subscription rate, the cost of technical and clerical support will have to be taken into account to allow further development of the scheme as outlined in Section 8.3. EQA subscription costs will also have to be taken into account when laboratories are setting their annual budgets.

8.6. Adoption of Common Standards and Reporting Systems

It is clearly desirable that the minimum service offered by all molecular genetics laboratories should be consistent and standardized as far as possible. Although all laboratories offering testing for a disorder should provide the accepted minimum service, specialist laboratories will offer a more extensive service in their field of expertise and accept referrals from outside their own normal catchment population. To try to establish minimum service provision, the MGEQA steering committee has produced a guidelines booklet with details of the most useful markers for the various diseases, recombination frequencies where appropriate, and suggested best practice for the analysis of families. The guidelines also provide recommendations for sample labeling and internal QC. Much of the information in this booklet was gained during disease-based meetings with the participating laboratories and is regularly updated in light of new developments.

Recommendations for the basic elements of a good report are also included in the guidelines. MGEQA feedback to laboratories included critical appraisal of the report format with the emphasis on ensuring clear, concise, and unambiguous information, and the inclusion of pedigree structure where this is appropriate. Local preference and protocols from individual clinical teams will mean that true standardization will never be achieved, but information provided by MGEQA should encourage a convergence to best practice.

8.7. Expansion of the UK EQA Scheme in Europe

In 1995, eight molecular genetics laboratories from The Netherlands and one from the Republic of Ireland participated in the UK MGEQA. This was the first time that laboratories outside the UK had been involved in the scheme and resulted from the absence of any similar facility in continental Europe.

In 1994, the European Concerted Action on Cystic Fibrosis initiated a quality-control study for CF only, which was coordinated by Jean-Jaques Cassiman of Leuven. Sixty-nine laboratories throughout Europe were invited to take part, and 40 of these agreed, 22 of which were in the UK. Nine DNA samples were provided for CF mutation analysis with no additional information. Distribution of these samples within the UK was organized by the MGEQA steering committee. A summary of the results was published in the autumn of 1994 *(1)* and also sent out to the participating laboratories, but no comments were included. This was an exercise that provided some lessons for both the organizers and the laboratories and the results show that there is a need for some formal EQA throughout Europe *(2)*. The best way to organize a European EQA scheme is not clear, but some of the problems involved can be anticipated.

The use of a common language for written EQA reports would be inappropriate, but language differences would have to be overcome. For disorders like

CF in which the most common mutations are routinely sought, laboratories Europe-wide may screen for a very different spectrum of mutations according to the prevalence in their population. Within the UK, MGEQA provision of adequate DNA samples of uniform quality for all the participating laboratories has proven to be problematic, and this would be exacerbated if a single scheme attempted to cover the whole of Europe.

One approach would be for each country or group of small countries to run an internal scheme, perhaps drawing on the experiences of the UK schemes. Central coordination of all the approved schemes by a European MGEQA committee would ensure similar standards and facilitate communication between the separate countries. Such a system could prove extremely valuable in the sharing of resources, experience, and techniques.

Acknowledgments

The authors thank Walter Noll of the College of American Pathologists and Karen Snow of the Human Genetics Society of Australasia for helpful information on EQA schemes in other parts of the world.

References

1. Cassiman, J. J. (1994) *A Quality Control Study of CFTR Mutation Screening in 40 Different European Laboratories.* Newsletter of the European Community Concerted Action for Cystic Fibrosis, Autumn 1994 vol. 2, no. 4., pp. 7–10.
2. Cuppens, H. and Cassiman, J. J. (1995) A quality control study of CFTR mutation screening in 40 different European laboratories. *Eur. J. Hum. Genet.* **3,** 235–245.

Index

A

Accreditation in clinical molecular genetics, 13
Adult polycystic kidney disease, heterogeneity, 163, 164
Agarose,
blocks for PFGE, 274
gel electrophoresis, 286
ARMS,
CAH analysis, 125
fluorescent assay, 188, 195, 196
hemoglobin analysis, 171, 178–181
in analysis of fetal material from maternal blood, 238, 239
multiplex for CF diagnosis, 100, 104
Allele-specific oligonucleotides, 114–116
Amelogenin gene analysis in preimplantation diagnosis, 249, 253
Angelman syndrome/Prader Willi syndrome, 219–236
Audit in clinical molecular genetics, 11–13
Automated genotyping in diagnosis, 185–204

B

Bayesian calculation, 155–158
Becker Muscular Dystrophy, 283–298
diagnosis-external quality assessment, 344, 345

Blastomere preparation,
in PCR-based preimplantation diagnosis, 248, 250
in FISH-based preimplantation diagnosis, 263, 264

C

Carrier testing,
counseling for, 210, 211
in CF, 107–109
in DMD,
direct methods, 18–21
indirect methods, 21
within families, 3
within populations, 3
Chemical cleavage of mismatch, 66, 67, 69–74, 76, 77, 80–86, 90–92
Clonality in tumor cell lines, 143
Congenital adrenal hyperplasia, 121–140
Cycle sequencing, 300–302
Cystic fibrosis, 99–119
clinical presentation, 110, 111
cost of mutation detection service, 5
diagnosis-external quality assessment, 351, 352
fluorescent analysis, 197
mutations detected by sequencing, 310
preimplantation diagnosis, 245–247
risk analysis, 161–163
testing strategy, 102